1991

HOW BRAVE A NEW WORLD?

HOW BRAVE A NEW WORLD?

Dilemmas in Bioethics

Richard A. McCormick, S.J.

Georgetown University Press, Washington, D. C. 20057

Library of Congress Cataloging in Publication Data

McCormick, Richard A., 1922–
How brave a new world?

Includes index.
1. Bioethics.   2. Medical ethics.   I. Title.
QH332.M32   1985   174'.2   84-25840
ISBN: 0-87840-417-1

With various changes and adjustments, the chapters in this volume appeared in other earlier books and journals, to which acknowledgment is hereby made:

1. "The Judaeo-Christian Tradition and Bioethical Codes" in *Human Rights and Psychological Research*, ed. Eugene C. Kennedy (New York: Crowell, 1975), 23–36.
2. "The Teaching of Medical Ethics" in *The Teaching of Medical Ethics*, ed. Robert M. Veatch, Willard Gaylin, and Councilman Morgan (New York: Hastings Center, 1973), 103–14.
3. "Some Neglected Aspects of the Moral Responsibility for Health" in *Perspectives in Biology and Medicine*, 22 (1978), 31–43.
4. "Proxy Consent in the Experimentation Situation," *Perspectives in Biology and Medicine*, 18 (1974), 2–20.
5. "Public Policy and Fetal Research" in the *Hastings Center Report*, 5 (n. 3, 1975), 26–31.
6. "Sharing in Sociality: Children and Experimentation" in the *Hastings Center Report*, 6 (n. 6, 1976), 41–46.
7. "The Rights of the Voiceless" in *The Journal of Medicine and Philosophy*, 3 (n. 3, 1978), 211–21.
8. "The Abortion Dossier" in *Theological Studies*, 34 (1974), 312–59.
9. "Rules for Abortion Debate" in *America*, 139 (1978), 26–30.
10. "Public Policy on Abortion" in *Hospital Progress*, 60 (Feb. 1979), 36–44.
11. "The Encyclical *Humanae Vitae*" in *Theological Studies*, 29 (1968), 718–41.
12. "The Tenth Anniversary of *Humanae Vitae*" in *Theological Studies*, 40 (1979), 80–97.
13. "Sterilization and Theological Method" in *Theological Studies*, 37 (1976), 471–77.
14. "Sterilization as a Catholic Institutional Problem" (previously unpublished).
15. "Genetic Medicine: Notes on the Moral Literature" in *Theological Studies*, 33 (1972), 531–52.
16. "Ethics and Reproductive Interventions" is a synthesis of three studies from The Encyclopedia of Bioethics (1978), *America*, 139 (1978), 74–78, and *Theological Studies*, 40 (1979), 97–112.
17. "To Save or Let Die: The Dilemma of Modern Medicine" in *Journal of the American Medical Association*, 229 (1974), 172–76, and *America*, 130 (1974), 6–10.

18. "Saving Defective Infants: Options for Life or Death" with John J. Paris in *America*, 146 (1983), 313–317.
19. "The Moral Right to Privacy" in *Hospital Progress*, 57 (n. 8, 1976), 38–42.
20. "The Case of Joseph Saikewicz" with André E. Hellegers in *America*, 138 (1978), 257–60.
21. "Preservation of Life and Self-determination" with Robert M. Veatch in *Theological Studies*, 41 (1980).
22. "The Quality of Life, the Sanctity of Life" in *Hastings Center Report*, 8 (n. 1, 1978), 30–36.
23. "Legislation and the Living Will" with André E. Hellegers in *America*, 136 (1977), 210–13.
24. "Living-Will Legislation, Reconsidered" with John J. Paris in *America*, 144 (1981), 86–89.
Appendix: "The Principle of the Double Effect" in *Concilium*, 120 (1976) entitled *Discerner les valeurs pour fonder la morale*.

FOR

Edward and Mary Jane,
Carol and Bill,
Kathleen and Bob,
Mary Jo and Bob

WHO
HAVE TAUGHT ME SO MUCH
ABOUT WHAT IT IS TO BE
A FAMILY

Preface

Why another book in bioethics?

Aside from the transient exhilaration and youthful folly of see-ing one's own name on a book, I believe there is a place for an ap-proach to these problems by those who are thoroughly stamped by and unabashedly proud of a historic religious faith, and are con-vinced that it has something to do with our deliberations in the area of bioethics. I write as a Catholic moral theologian, proud of the richness of the tradition in which I have been privileged to share. That is not to say that this tradition is the sole proprietor of enlightening perspectives in bioethics, nor that it has not en-joyed its share of distorted perspectives. Nor is it to say that one is or ought to be a slave to papal formulations or conciliar docu-ments, whether ancient or contemporary—much as some Catho-lics of a classicist mentality view the matter in this way. Nor is it to say that one is or ought to be constantly constrained to appeal to explicitly theological warrants for everything one says. Still less is it to suggest that all Catholics will agree with the analyses at-tempted or the conclusions drawn. My own stumbling errors of the past are chastening reminders that such an expectation is un-warranted, and even arrogant.

To say that I write as a Catholic moral theologian means to suggest above all, though not exclusively, three things: (1) Reli-gious faith stamps one at a profound and not totally recoverable depth. (2) This stamping affects one's instincts, imagination, etc., and hence influences one's perspectives, analyses, and judgments. (3) Analyses and judgments of such a kind are vitally important in our communal deliberations about bioethics. Put simply, I am convinced that those who believe that theology and theologians are out of place in these discussions have got it all wrong, difficult as it may be to specify the exact contribution of theology, especially in a very concrete problem of bioethics. If God is present and self-communicative to us in His glorified Son—the exemplary human being—through His Spirit and if this presence is mediated to us by a historical religious community, then surely this faith in that presence as formed by this community will have a powerful influence on one who tries to sort out the complexities of modern scientific problems in light of it. That is one reason why a Catholic moral theologian might succumb to the temptations to expose his gropings to others.

But there are two more. The second is autobiographical-historical. I was trained in and for some years taught a moral theology with deep roots in what is now called a "classicist mentality." It is easy—and at some point terribly wrong and unfair—to caricature here. And no careful scholar will do so. Nonetheless, it remains true that the ecclesiological and moral theological perspectives introduced by Vatican II have led to a consciousness that is much more historically oriented. This has meant a new willingness to re-examine some traditional formulations that were authoritatively proposed to the Catholic community. The task of doing this is far from easy and, obviously, not always successful. Nonetheless, I believe there is a real value in our time in opening the shutters to allow others to see attempts at this re-examination. There are some who have resisted such a re-examination and have remained comfortable with a relatively traditional outlook and vocabulary. There are others who have felt no need to do so because they have never been thoroughly trained in the "traditional Catholic categories." The present author fits somewhere in between. Trained in the classicist mentality, he has become conscious of both its strengths and its weaknesses—and the need to correct or modify the latter.

My third reason for exposing my thought to a wider public is the eager anticipation of constructive criticism. I have already received such from friends and colleagues and I treasure it as an indispensable aid in growth toward understanding in a difficult and sometimes controversial area such as bioethics.

A small explanatory note is in place here. I have left the essays virtually the same as they originally appeared. Since some touch on the same subjects, even if in different ways (for example, "Genetic Medicine: Notes on the Moral Literature" and "Ethics and

Reproductive Interventions"), and since I have modified my own views over the years, there will be instances where a later essay takes a different view from an earlier one. This is the case, for instance, with regard to some of the arguments surrounding *in vitro* fertilization. I have made no attempt to alter this since there is no little value in seeing why one originally held a certain view and then why one modified it.

This volume could never have been compiled but for the friendly and generous assistance of Emilie Dolge, Mary Ellen Timbol, and Mary Baker. My thanks to them is profound and repeated, and will take the peculiar form of relying upon them even more in the future.

Richard A. McCormick, S.J.

Contents

HOW BRAVE A NEW WORLD?

SECTION I

GENERAL METHODOLOGICAL REFLECTIONS

1. The Judaeo-Christian Tradition and Bioethical Codes

It has been said that medicine is too important to be left to doctors alone. The same is usually true of theology. It is too important to be left to theologians alone. And I believe that psychology is too important to be left to psychologists alone. All disciplines are aware of their intersecting and interdisciplinary character in our time. Theologians have recently become aware of their deep reliance on disciplines other than their own. The title of this chapter indicates a confidence that there is perhaps something that psychology can wrest from theological reflection, and I think that confidence is justified.

The title of this chapter would be more accurate if it read: "how one individual in the Judaeo-Christian tradition sees the relevance of this tradition for the development of a code of ethics in professional psychology." There is an acknowledged pluralism of theologies and methods in contemporary moral reflection, and no one individual can speak with assurance for a whole fraternity. Furthermore, when speaking of the "Judaeo-Christian tradition" one must locate himself carefully. The continuity of the Old and New Testaments, and the broad coincidence of value judgments in both certainly justify the usage "Judaeo-Christian." My emphasis, however, will fall on the term "Christian," since I would not presume to speak for a contemporary dimension with which I am not personally familiar.

Let me begin by saying that to determine the insights of the Judaeo-Christian tradition on the development of an ethical code in psychology, we must treat two major themes. First, we must see what a code is and how it is developed. A code is, I take it, the conclusion of a process. We must lift up, therefore, those things that go into this process to see at what point a religious tradition might exert its influence. I hope to make it clear that the Judaeo-Christian tradition does indeed influence a code of ethics, but only at a certain point in the developmental process that issues in a code, and only in a carefully restricted way. Second, we must determine the meaning of the Judaeo-Christian tradition and how it influences morals in general. This will reveal, I hope, how it may be expected to influence the specific matter of a code for professional psychologists.

How a Code Is Developed

A code is the concretization in a certain sphere of more general moral convictions or postures. Hence to see how the Judaeo-Christian tradition influences the development of a code, we must first see how moral positions arise and are maintained. This is a huge and wearying undertaking and I can do no more here than suggest the barest outlines of one approach to this question.

The first thing to be said is that moral convictions do not originate from rational analyses or arguments. Let us take slavery as an example. We do not hold that slavery is humanly demeaning and immoral chiefly because we have argued to this rationally. Rather, first our sensitivities are sharpened to the meaning and value of human persons. We then *experience* the out-of-jointness, inequality, and injustice of slavery. We then *judge* it to be wrong. At this point we develop "arguments" to criticize, modify, and above all communicate this judgment. Reflective analysis is an attempt to reinforce rationally, communicably, and from other sources what we grasp at a different level. Discursive reflection does not discover the good but only *analyzes* it. The good that reason seems to discover is the good that was already hidden in the original intuition.[1]

This needs more explanation. How do we arrive at definite moral obligations, prescriptions, and proscriptions? How does the general thrust of our persons toward good and away from evil become concrete, even as concrete as a code of do's and don'ts and caveats? It happens somewhat as follows—and in this I am following closely the school of J. de Finance, G. de Broglie, G. Grisez,

[1] J. M. Finnis, "Natural Law and Unnatural Acts," *Heythrop Journal*, 11 (1970), 365–87.

John Finnis, and others. We proceed by asking: What are the goods or values man can seek, the values that define his human opportunity, his flourishing? We can answer this by examining man's basic tendencies, for it is impossible to act without having an interest in the object, and it is impossible to be attracted by, to have an interest in something without some inclination already present. What then are the basic inclinations?

With no pretense at being exhaustive, we could list some of the following as basic inclinations present prior to acculturation: the tendency to preserve life; the tendency to mate and raise children; the tendency to explore and question; the tendency to seek out other men and obtain their approval—friendship; the tendency to use intelligence in guiding action; the tendency to develop skills and exercise them in play and in the fine arts. In these inclinations our intelligence spontaneously and without reflection grasps the possibilities to which they point, and prescribes them. Thus we form naturally and without reflection the basic principles of practical or moral reasoning. Or as philosopher John Finnis renders it:

> What is spontaneously understood when one turns from contemplation to action is not a set of Kantian or neo-scholastic "moral principles" identifying this as right and that as wrong, but a set of values which can be expressed in the form of principles such as "life is a good-to-be-pursued-and-realized and what threatens it is to be avoided."[2]

We have not yet arrived at a determination of what concrete actions are morally right or wrong; but we have laid the basis. Since these basic values are equally basic and irreducibly attractive, the morality of our conduct is determined by the adequacy of our openness to these values, for each of these values has its self-evident appeal as a participation in the unconditioned Good we call God. The realization of these values in intersubjective life is the only adequate way to love and attain God.

Further reflection by practical reason tells us what it means to

[2] Ibid.

remain open and to pursue these basic human values. First, we must take them into account in our conduct. Simple disregard of one or other shows we have set our mind against this good. Second, when we can do so as easily as not, we should avoid acting in ways that inhibit these values, and prefer ways that realize them. Third, we must make an effort on their behalf when their realization in another is in extreme peril. If we fail to do so, we show that the value in question is not the object of our efficacious love and concern. Finally, we must never choose against a basic good. When one of the irreducible values falls immediately under our choice, to choose against it in favor of some other basic value is arbitrary, for all such values are equally basic and self-evidently attractive. What is to count as "turning against a basic good" is, of course, the crucial moral question in some concrete and controversial ethical discussions in which I find myself in disagreement with G. Grisez, John Finnis, and others. My only point here is that particular moral judgments are incarnations of these more basic normative positions, which have their roots in spontaneous, prereflective inclinations.

Even though these inclinations can be identified as prior to acculturation, still they exist as culturally conditioned. We tend toward values as perceived. And the culture in which we live shades our perception of values. Philip Rieff in *The Triumph of the Therapeutic* notes that a culture survives by the power of institutions to influence conduct with "reasons" that have sunk so deeply into the self that they are implicitly understood—"the unwitting part of it," as Harry Stack Sullivan puts it.[3] In other words, decisions are made, policies are set not chiefly by articulated norms, codes, regulations, and philosophies, but by "reasons" that lie below the surface. This is the dynamic aspect of a culture, and in this sense the moral problems of psychology and medicine are cultural. Our way of perceiving the basic human values and relating to them is shaped by our whole way of looking at the world. James Gustafson has made this very clear in a recent study.[4]

[3] P. Rieff, *The Triumph of the Therapeutic: Uses of Faith After Freud* (New York: Harper & Row, 1966).
[4] James Gustafson, "Theology Confronts Technology and the Life Sciences," *Commonweal*, 105 (1978), 386–92.

Let me take an example from an allied area of concern, that of bioethics. In relating to the basic human values, several images of man are possible, as Callahan has observed.[5] First, there is a power-plasticity model. In this model, nature is alien, independent of man, possessing no inherent value. It is capable of being used, dominated, and shaped by man. Man sees himself as possessing an unrestricted right to manipulate in the service of his goals. Death is something to be overcome, outwitted. Second, there is the sacral-symbiotic model. In its religious forms, nature is seen as God's creation, to be respected and heeded. Man is not the master; he is the steward and nature is a trust. In secular forms, man is seen as a part of nature. If man is to be respected, so is nature. We should live in harmony and balance with nature. Nature is a teacher, showing us how to live with it. Death is one of the rhythms of nature, to be gracefully accepted.

The model that seems to have "sunk deep" and shaped our moral imagination and feelings—shaped our perception of basic values—is the power-plasticity model. We are, corporately, *homo technologicus.* The best solution to the dilemmas created by technology is more technology. We tend to eliminate the maladapted condition (defectives, retardates, and so on) rather than adjust the environment to it. Even our language is sanitized and shades from view our relationship to basic human values. We speak of "surgical air strikes" and "terminating a pregnancy," ways of blunting the moral imagination from the shape of our conduct. My only point here is that certain cultural "reasons" qualify or shade our perception of and our grasp on the basic human values. Thus these reasons are the cultural soil of our moral convictions and have a good deal to say about where we come out when a code is concerned.

Once the basic values are identified along with their cultural tints and trappings, we attempt in a disciplined, rational way to develop "middle axioms" or mediating principles. These relate the basic values to concrete choice. The major problem any professional ethic faces is to reinterpret the concrete demands of the basic values in new circumstances without forfeiting its grasp on these values.

[5] Daniel Callahan, "Living with the New Biology," *Center Magazine,* 5 (1972), 4–12.

This is what I take to be the process whereby a code of professional ethics is generated.

Judaeo-Christian Influence on the Development of a Code of Ethics for Psychologists

There are undoubtedly those who grow nervous and apprehensive at the thought of a religious influence on professional codes. This is most likely traceable to a misunderstanding. At least very many psychologists might conjure up the picture of a theologian citing a text from Scripture as decisive for clinical practice. Or worse yet, some would see a Pope or a bishop—supposedly in possession of arcane wisdom that yields solutions to difficult human dilemmas—meddling into what is regarded as an essentially autonomous discipline and telling its practitioners what to do. Even though some theologians remain to a degree biblical fundamentalists, and even though not all hierarchical processes are as rehabilitated to modern times as we would like, these fears are essentially unfounded—precisely because it is almost universally accepted in theological circles that the authoritative sources of Christian tradition (Scripture, teaching authority) do not directly translate into independent, concrete moral prescriptions and proscriptions. This may come as a surprise to some. I hope it is not a disappointment. To understand why this is so, we must see the meaning of the term "Christian morality."

The term "Christian morality" suggests that there is a morality specific to Christians, one that is drawn from Christian sources and is in principle unavailable to the insights and reasoning of other persons, and inapplicable to them. Of course, this is true in one sense; but in another it is not. Here it is important to distinguish several levels and senses of the term "ethics." First there is *essential* ethics, those concrete demands thought to be valid of and to apply to all persons precisely as human persons. In this sense the individual is but an instance of what is equally true of others. Then there is what we might call *existential* ethics—that is, those moral claims that fall upon the individual precisely as an individual, with unique aspirations, capacities, circumstances, etc. Third, there is a level identifiable as *essential Christian* ethics. This refers to those moral demands that touch all Christians precisely as members of the Christian community (for example, to provide Christian education for their children, to worship together as a community, etc.). Finally, there is an *existential Christian* ethic, one having reference to those moral claims that visit a Christian precisely as an individual Christian (for example, the priestly or religious vocation).

I am concerned here with the first sense, *essential* ethics, and indeed at the concrete or behavioral level (in contrast to the general or formal level). At this level it has been a Catholic Christian conviction at least since the time of Thomas Aquinas that revelation and the faith experience originate no new concrete moral demands that are in principle unavailable to human insight and reasoning.

This means that there is a *material* identity between Christian moral demands and those perceivable by reason. Whatever is distinct about Christian morality is found essentially in the style of life, the manner of accomplishing the moral tasks common to all men, not in the tasks themselves. Christian morality is, in its concreteness and materiality, *human* morality. The theological study of morality accepts the human in all its fullness as its starting point. It is the *human* that is then illumined by the person, teaching, and achievement of Jesus Christ. The experience of Jesus is regarded as normative because he is believed to have experienced what it is to be *human* in the fullest way and at the deepest level.[6] Christian ethics does not and cannot add to human ethical self-understanding as such any material content that is, in principle, strange or foreign to man as he exists and experiences himself.

Therefore, the Judaeo-Christian tradition does not add to the human. Rather it is an outlook on the human, a community of privileged access to the *human,* if you will. The Judaeo-Christian tradition is anchored in faith in the meaning and decisive significance of God's covenant with men, especially as manifested finally in the saving incarnation of Jesus Christ and the revelation of his final coming, his eschatological kingdom that is here aborning but will finally only be given. Faith in these events, love of

[6] Enda McDonagh, "Towards a Christian Theology of Morality," *Irish Theological Quarterly,* 37 (1970), 187–98.

and loyalty to their central figure yield a decisive way of viewing and intending the world, of interpreting its meaning, of hierarchizing its values, of reacting to its apparent surds and conflicts. In this sense the Judaeo-Christian tradition only illumines human values, supports them, provides a context for their reading at given points in history. It aids us in staying human by underlining the truly human against all cultural attempts to distort the human. This is one of the meanings of the traditional Catholic assertion that concrete moral problems must be approached by "reason informed by faith." The phrase is "informed by" not "replaced by." And it is in this way, I believe, that the faith tradition exercises its major influence on professional codes—by steadying our gaze on the basic human values that are the parents of more concrete rules and ethical protocols. When we examine several of its key emphases, we will see how they support the human, and we will get some idea of how this tradition exerts its influence on the development of a code.

The Dignity of the Individual Person

The Judaeo-Christian tradition has always seen persons as "in relationship to God." This means that persons are the bearers of an "alien dignity," a dignity rooting in the value God puts in them. No one has stated this better than Helmut Thielicke:

> This "alien dignity" expresses the fact that it is not man's own worth—his value for producing "good works," his functional proficiency, his pragmatic utility—that gives him his dignity, but rather what God has "spent upon him," the sacrificial love which God has invested in him (Dt. 7:7 f). Therefore this alien dignity actualizes itself at the very point where man's own value has become questionable, the point where his functional value is no longer listed on society's stock market and he is perhaps declared to be "unfit to live."[7]

The greatest affirmation of this alien dignity is, of course, God's Word—become flesh. As Christ is of God, and Christ is *the* man,

[7] H. Thielicke, *The Ethics of Sex* (New York: Harper & Row, 1964).

so all persons are God's, his darlings, deriving their dignity from the value He is putting in them. This perspective stands as a profound critique of our tendency to assess persons functionally, to weaken our hold on the basic value that is human life. It leads to a particular care for the weakest, most voiceless, voteless, defenseless members of society: orphans, the poor, the aged, the mentally and physically sick, the unborn. All violations of the ethics of experimentation root in and reflect a slipped grasp of man's lovableness, at root an "alien" lovableness in Thielicke's sense.

It can be persuasively argued, I believe, that the peculiar temptation of a technologically advanced culture such as ours is to view and treat persons functionally. Our treatment of the aged is perhaps the sorriest symptom of this. The elderly are, it can be argued, probably the most alienated members of our society. "Not yet ready for the world of the dead, not deemed fit for the world of the living, they are shunted aside. More and more of them spend the extra years medicine has given them in 'homes for senior citizens,' in chronic hospitals, in nursing homes—waiting for the end. We have learned how to increase their years, but we have not learned how to help them enjoy their days."[8] Their protest is eloquent because it is helplessly muted and silent. It is a protest against a basically functional assessment of their persons. "Maladaptation" is a term used to describe *them,* rather than the environment. Hence we intervene against the maladapted individual rather than against the environment.

I do not know in detail or by experience the peculiar temptations of psychologists to reproduce in their policies a functional assessment of human beings. But I presume that psychologists are not unlike the rest of men and women, and therefore have their feet buried deep in a pragmatic culture, and do experience the temptation to use and manipulate generally in terms of that notorious nonpatient, the human race. The Judaeo-Christian tradition will not dictate to you what acts are justifiable, and what are not. It will not give you a code. That is your task and responsibility and risk. But it will insist that there is an ethic of means, because you deal with someone who is of more value than the sum of his —or her—parts, someone who is an end value in all human deci-

[8] Leon R. Kass, "The New Biology: What Price Relieving Man's Estate?" *Science,* 174 (1971), 784.

sions. That is the way the Judaeo-Christian tradition functions, I think, where the development of a professional code is concerned. It supports our grasp of the basic human values against cultural counterfeits. If you look for more, you will not find it. But if you acknowledge less, you are, I think, in trouble. For a sure grasp on the alien dignity of persons is, where a code of ethics is concerned, both very little and very much. It is a kind of compass to steer our deliberations, constrain our eugenic enthusiasms, and control our scientific aspirations. But a compass is not a rudder.

The Social Character of the Human Person

If the person's dignity is radically in his relationship to God, and if this is a relationship pursued and matured only through relationships to other persons, then this relationship to God is unavoidably social. God covenanted with the Jewish *people*, with a group. It was within a group and through a group that the individual was responsible and responsive to God. This is even clearer in the New Testament. "Being in Christ" is a shared existence. Man's new being, of which St. Paul speaks so frequently, is being in a community. Assumption into Christ means assumption into His Body, His People. We cannot exist as Christians except in a community, and we cannot define ourselves except as "of a Body." Hence it is Christianly axiomatic that the community of believers (the Church) is the extension of the Incarnation. It is similarly axiomatic that those actions wherein we initiate into, fortify, restore, and intensify the Christlife (the Christian sacraments) are at once Christ's actions and the actions of the community.

This sense of community, sunk deep into the spontaneous consciousness of Christians, has meant two things to them over the centuries. First, it has meant that my freedom to realize my potentialities as a person is conditioned by the authenticity of the other members of the community, and vice versa—that is, the community exists for the individual. It is not an independent superentity to which we are subordinate, and whose good absorbs our own. It does not serve an abstract ideal; rather that ideal is incarnate in each of its members.

Second, it means that if we cannot exist in isolation, neither can we know as Christians in isolation, and it would be un-Christian to think we do or hope that we could. Our shared knowledge is concerned with God's wonderful saving events and their moral implications. True moral insight, in St. Paul's understanding, is mediated to the individual through participation in the community. Just as the Christian's mode of being is a sharing, so the moral knowledge necessary to its continuation and development is the result of a communal experience, a communal discernment that prolongs knowledge into the twilight human areas where there are no sharp contours, no bright colors.[9] The Christian is one who spontaneously seeks correction for his own biases within a community of shared loyalty, but of more diverse experience and perspectives.

These two perspectives have enormous implications for moral conduct, and for the protocols of a professional code. I see especially two of major importance. They can be sketched only briefly here. First of all, there is the relation of the individual to the community. Sometimes the individual and the community are conceived as two separable and competing values. The Judaeo-Christian tradition resists this and sees them as coimplicating and interpenetrating each other as inseparable complementarities. It is not a question of the individual versus the community as if they were atomized. Rather the individual and the community are related like only partially overlapping circles. At points there is identification of concerns and goods, at other points there is distinction. Thus, while the individual is an integral part of the community and must take it into account in defining his or her own prerogatives and rights, still the individual does not exist for the community in a way that *totally* subordinates him or her to it. The balance is delicate, and probably in constant flux and tension. Individuals ought to—indeed, can—be rightfully forced to make certain sacrifices for the common good (for example, conscription, proportionate taxation).

Yet where positively harming individuals in medical practice for the sake of others is concerned, there must be the strongest possible presumption against such a practice. Put simply, we do not harm one for the sake of the other. Harming individuals in a choice or policy is justifiable only to the extent that this individ-

[9] For this emphasis, see, for example, the many writings of noted exegete Jerome Murphy-O'Connor, O.P.

ual would himself be exposed to more harm over the long term if
such a policy did not exist. Therefore, for instance, if you conclude in a code that it is sometimes legitimate to deceive an individual or expose that individual to harm, it is only because you
have shown clearly that this is the best policy in terms of this individual in the long run. The Judaeo-Christian tradition does not
tell us this, but human reason informed by this tradition moves in
this direction.

Second, moral knowledge as a community possession and
achievement says a good deal about the manner in which a code
ought to be developed. Codes developed within a single profession, without the benefit of other competences, are very likely to
be inadequate. We are learning in the Catholic community that
the moral teaching authority of the Church should not be viewed
as an isolated club—the hierarchy—in prior possession of the
truth. Rather wisdom is resident in the entire community and all
must share in the teaching-learning process if we are to escape the
isolation of our own reflections and if moral stands are to be cred-
ible and persuasive. I believe that the Judaeo-Christian tradition
suggests something similar for psychologists. Your policies should
be the result of a discernment process collaborative in character,
involving laypersons from a variety of disciplines as partners in the
conversation. Thus the tradition functions as a constant corrective
against our tendencies toward fragmentation and isolation in the
development of moral policies.

Love as the Crowning Human Relationship

When a person is no longer related to other persons, he is
quite literally dead. Suicide is the ultimate way of shutting out all
other people from one's life. At a time when it is possible to keep
lungs breathing and hearts pumping by machines, our attention is
refocused on what it means to be human. The answer most frequently given is that to be human means to have a capacity, actually or potentially, for significant human relationships. It is, I
believe, not a Christian discovery, but a typically Christian insistence that the crowning achievement of human relationships
is love. For St. Paul, love is the epitome of the entire law, the root
of other virtues, the bond of perfection, more elevated than all

charisms. It is the dominant characteristic of the new mode of being that Paul calls "belonging to Christ," "being in Christ." In the Pauline literature the "old man" is contrasted with the new. The "old man" is characterized by isolation and selfish withdrawal. His traits—all dominantly antisocial—are anger, wrath, malice, slander, dissension, envy, and so on. The "new man's" characteristics are all other-centered: compassion, kindness, lowliness, meekness, patience.

These things are familiar to all of us; but their implications may be easily overlooked. The tradition referred to insists that man's response to God occurs only through relating to others *lovingly*. This is definitive of our growth and maturity as human beings, of the ultimate significance of our lives whatever else they might be. Our actions are right to the extent that they are in their external shape and effects, describable as *actually* beneficent—that is, loving. To derogate from this capacity to love, to bypass it, to stultify it is to dehumanize both ourselves and others.

It is this insight that stands behind and illumines the consent canon where experimentation is concerned. Christian ethicians maintain that an individual can become (in carefully delimited circumstances) more fully a person by donation of an organ to another; for by communicating to another of his or her very being, the person has more fully integrated himself into the mysterious unity between person and person. Something analogous can be said of experimentation undertaken for the good of others. It can be an affirmation of one's solidarity and Christian concern for others (through the advancement of medicine). Becoming an experimental subject can involve any or all of three things: some degree of risk (at least of complications), pain, and associated inconvenience (for example, prolonging hospital stay, delaying recovery, and so on). To accept these for the good of others could be an act of charitable concern, of genuine love.

While admitting this, we have always excluded those incapable of consent from such procedures. Why? Because, I believe, these undertakings become human goods for the donor or subject precisely because and therefore only when they are voluntary; for the personal good under discussion is the good of expressed charity. This demands freedom by its very definition.

The Christian tradition's heavy emphasis on affective and effec-

tive love as the most radical human mandate, reductively the only
mandate, necessarily fortifies our grasp on freedom as the highest
of instrumental values. All things that attack or subvert man's
freedom are violative of the *humanum*. Laws are inherently defensible only because in constricting freedom they actually protect
and expand it. There is, it is correctly said, no liberty without law.
Codes are nothing more than attempts to set up rules that will
guarantee the maximum amount of freedom. All violations of professional ethics are equivalently and reductively encroachments on
human freedom.

For instance, misuse of confidential information not only hurts
an individual in clinically detectable ways, but also, in so doing, it
ultimately restricts that individual's freedom. Similarly, an exorbi-
tant fee scale in professional work is unethical because it renders
the profession less available, thus restricting freedom of access to a
needed service. Deception in patient care is an obvious example of
diminished freedom.

These are but three recurring emphases in the Judaeo-Christian
tradition. There are many more—for example, the sinfulness of
man and therefore frequently of his plans and aspirations. Or
again, the eschatological view of life and of human ethical action
whereby we are led to admit that the final validation and trans-
formation of human effort is given by God with the ultimate coming of His kingdom. These emphases do not yield a code. But
they affect it. The stories and symbols that relate the origin of
Christianity and nourish the faith of the individual, affect one's
perspectives. They sharpen and intensify our focus on the human
goods definitive of our flourishing. It is persons so informed, persons with such "reasons" sunk deep in their being, who face new
situations, new dilemmas, and reason together as to what is the
best policy, the best protocol for the service of all the values. They
do not find concrete answers in their tradition, but they bring a
world view that informs their reasoning—especially by allowing
the basic human goods to retain their attractiveness and not be
tainted by cultural distortions. This world view is a continuing
check on and challenge to our tendency to make choices in light
of cultural enthusiasms that sink into and take possession of our
unwitting, pre-ethical selves. Such enthusiasms can reduce the
good life to mere adjustment in a triumph of the therapeutic; col-

lapse an individual into his functionability; exalt his uniqueness into a lonely individualism or crush it in a suffocating collectivism. In this sense I believe it is true to say that the Judaeo-Christian tradition is much more a value-raiser than an answer-giver. And it affects our values at the spontaneous, prethematic level. One of the values inherent in its incarnational ethos is an affirmation of the goodness of persons and all about them—including their reasoning and thought processes. The Judaeo-Christian tradition refuses to bypass or supplant human deliberation and hard work in developing ethical protocols within a profession. For that would be blasphemous of the Word of God become human. On the contrary, it asserts their need, but constantly reminds people that what God did and intends for us is an affirmation of the human and therefore must remain the measure of what persons may reasonably decide to do to and for themselves.

2. The Teaching of Medical Ethics

In this chapter I should like to propose a way of conceiving a medical ethics program. This is distinct from a group of cases or even a "how to" description for illuminating bioethical problems, though these certainly have their place and key importance. I am rather concerned to establish a kind of general framework for organizing and thinking about these problems. I suggest the notion of issue areas as a useful beginning. It is possible, of course, to conceive of several possible frameworks for a medical ethics program. For instance, one such framework would be departmental in orientation, organizing problems as they apply above all to the various departments in medicine: pediatrics, obstetrics-gynecology, psychiatry, legal medicine, and so on. Another would organize problems according to the personnel most nearly responsible for the decision: thus, duties of doctors, patients, chaplains, hospitals, nurses, etc. Former medical-moral textbooks represent a combination of these. But ultimately such frameworks represent divisions of convenience. Serviceable as they are, they do not really point out how issues are generated; rather they presuppose the existence of already generated issue areas and simply proceed to sort them out. I shall take a different path.

How one identifies issue areas for a medical ethics program will depend on two general judgments: (1) what one judges to be the concrete purpose or goal of a medical ethics program and (2) how one assesses the contemporary medical situation—its problems, possibilities, and dangers. These judgments in turn involve a whole series of previous assumptions or presuppositions that must be made explicit. They are the following: (1) a certain idea about what a doctor ought to be; (2) what medical ethics is all about; (3) how medical policies and decisions ought to be made; (4) the structure of a health-care system in a certain culture; (5) the level of ethical sensitivity in a certain culture; and (6) the assessment of the strengths and weaknesses of contemporary medical students, and therefore their present and future needs. The form our issue areas take and the emphases they reveal will depend on what judgments we make with regard to these assumptions. Let me say a brief word about each of these assumptions to indicate how they have led me to structure issue areas as I have.

What a doctor ought to be. I am supposing that a doctor is not and ought not to be a mere technician, disposing of medicines and machines toward the palliation or removal of disease. He is one who ought to relate to the whole patient-person. Furthermore, as a member of a community, a physician is, as physician, one with social-medical responsibilities.

What medical ethics is all about. Some will conceive of medical ethics as a form of indoctrination, the appropriation of set-piece answers (or directions) to case problems. A technologically sophisticated and pragmatic people is likely to have an overly codal and mechanical idea of what ethics in medicine means. Contrary to this perspective, I would urge two points. First of all, medical ethics, like any ethics, is much more search and tentative discovery than indoctrination. This search involves several steps: a descriptive analysis of the hard facts, a determination of the values at stake, a normative statement about the values, and finally the "why" or vindication of this judgment. Second, beyond this rational reflection on individual problem cases, a program must attempt, insofar as possible, to develop in the physician a sensitivity to human values against which rational reflection alone may aspire to steer a human course. Here, clearly, the relation of faith commitments is of enormous relevance. One's whole outlook on the meaning of life, death, suffering, and eternity is brought into play. I do not see how an adequate medical ethics can be nontheological, at least in this sense.

How medical decisions ought to be made. I assume that we are and ought to be moving away from an "individualistic" orientation where medicomoral policies and decisions are involved. It is true that medicomoral decisions are always highly personal decisions—decisions about persons. However, in our time it is clearer than ever that there are many dimensions to personal good—dimensions that range beyond the special expertise and perspectives of physician and moral theologian. Increasingly medicomoral policies can be established only when the perspectives of psychiatry, sociology, law, etc., are involved in the dialogue. This means that the direction of such policies is increasingly a community concern, perhaps even quasipublic in character. This gradual *aggiornamento* of ethical reflection in health care is ultimately, I believe, in the best interests of both patient and physician. Nader is, after all, just around the corner.

The structure of a health-care delivery system. I assume that in our time a health-care delivery system must and will take shape around the conviction that adequate health care is an individual right, not simply a privilege of those who can pay. This means unavoidable government partnership in the delivery system, and probably therewith an increasing depersonalization and bureaucratization in health care.

The level of ethical sensitivity in our culture. I assume that the level of ethical sensitivity to life and personal integrity is likely to be somewhat blunted in a culture whose dominant values are efficiency, immediacy, comfort, affluence, technological progress, and eugenic ambitions. These tend to put a merely functional valuation on human beings (compare Pappworth's *Human Guinea Pigs*). Therefore, a truly adequate medical ethics program will call for certain countercultural correctives. Furthermore, I assume that moral judgments are likely to be given a highly individualistic interpretation in our culture. Concretely the physician's attitude toward medical decisions is likely to be structured on "freedom of conscience" in such a way that this freedom is liable to pass for the content of the decision and to be seen as legitimating it.

Strengths and weaknesses of medical students. Issue areas depend also on a realistic assessment of those to partake in the program. I cannot give an accurate composite of today's medical student with any assurance, but I assume the general directional validity of the following traits: a disinclination to rational and logical discourse; a strong reliance on "gut" reactions; antagonism to authority and imposed decisions, rules, and principles; a strong, if unstructured, sense of idealism and social concern; and a pragmatism of outlook and thought process.

These are the suppositions or "atmospheric" assumptions I would make in determining how the issue areas for a contemporary program in medical ethics ought to be organized. In combination they lead me to the following three conclusions: (1) The issue areas should be stated in terms of the basic values at stake in medical practice. (2) These values should be approached through the concrete problems which challenge us to clarify and perhaps modify our understanding of them. (3) The method to be used is so important that it is itself an issue area. It must be an ongoing dialogical process that includes: *communal* discussion of a *rational* kind that attempts to reinterpret the meaning of these values in a new set of medical and cultural circumstances. The task, therefore, of a medical ethics program is not to apply old and presumably invariable injunctions to new facts, but rather to discover in changing times the very meaning of our value commitments. We simply do not have the answers to many questions surrounding our adherence to these basic values. The organization of a program in terms of issue areas must reflect this.

The issue areas, then, as I see them, are constituted by a basic human value that has encountered a new set of circumstances—a set of circumstances that calls for a re-evaluation of the meaning of the value itself. For instance, the existence of effective contraception and the ability to fertilize *in vitro* force us to ask ourselves anew about the meaning of our sexuality, about the family. This is the structure that I see generating ethical problems, and usefully organizing a program for their systematic study. In what follows, I shall list several such values as examples, list the problems that seem to relate to them, identify the contemporary circumstances that call for re-examination of the meaning of the value, and pose some questions that seem inseparable from this reinterpretation.

1. *The sanctity of life.* The most basic value in the practice of medicine is obviously the sanctity of life itself. Every decision, every policy, every rule must both reflect and promote this value if medicine is to remain humane. However, contemporary advances in life-sustaining and resuscitative devices have thrown this value into a new light. It is no longer mere physical life that is at stake, but the quality of life. There are times when preserving life would go against our deepest convictions about its meaning and sanctity; there are other times when making a decision about the quality of life would seem to be an attack on the sanctity of life itself, an

assumption of power we tremble to accept. In other words, contemporary medicine has propelled to center stage the sanctity of life in a new guise: the quality of life. It asks us to view life *also* in terms of its quality, to admit that there comes a time when living is no longer *human* life—and to take the consequences of this admission.

The sanctity of life as embracing also its quality is at the heart of the following problems: keeping alive, allowing to die, hastening death, abortion, radical surgery, definition of death, allocation of scarce medical resources, treatment of retardation, drug use and abuse, alcoholism, and care of the elderly.

Let me propose but a single example here, one concerning the decision to allow to die or not to allow to die. It is the instance of spina bifida with a meningomyelocele. This is a birth defect involving an opening along the spinal column with protrusion of the spinal sac. It is often associated with paralysis from the site of the lesion down, with hydrocephalus, mental retardation, permanent incontinence, etc. Prior to the mid 1950s, few babies born with this defect survived for very long. Hence the moral problem was not seen as terribly urgent. Now, however, advances in medical knowledge and technology make it possible through surgery to prevent further contamination of the spinal fluid and lethal infection. If surgery is not performed, the infant will probably contract meningitis due to bacterial invasion of the open sac of spinal fluid and die. However, the surgical prognosis is highly variable. Sometimes it is quite poor. At other times, it is good, but even with a fairly good prognosis, these children can end up severely impaired and in a constantly deteriorating condition that represents a tremendous burden on the child and the family.

For instance, in many of these cases nerve function is impaired from the lesion downward, so that the child cannot walk without the aid of crutches and braces. Even to walk with crutches requires extensive physical therapy that continues throughout the life of the child. In 90 per cent of these cases hydrocephalus develops. With immediate treatment by surgical insertion of a shunt (a tube that drains off the cerebrospinal fluid), the child still has a fifty-fifty chance of being mentally retarded—and the shunt may need revision several times. Without such a shunt the infant will definitely be retarded and could quite possibly die as a result of intracranial pressure. Even if hydrocephalus does not develop, there is no guarantee that the child will not suffer some degree of mental retardation. Furthermore, this condition is not infrequently associated with lifetime loss of bladder and bowel control. The instance is complicated by the fact that the decision must be made within hours of birth if optimum results are to be had; but even at this optimal time it is difficult to predict its ultimate outcome.

Should the operation be performed, or should it be omitted with only supportive care provided? It must be noted that we are not dealing with the irreversible process of dying, but with a process that can be reversed, a life that can be saved at least in a notable number of instances. But should this life be saved? If one says "no," the decision seems clearly to be based on the quality of life available to the child. To operate may save the child—but for a crippled, painful, retarded existence. It seems, therefore, that if we judge that the surgery should not be performed in an individual case, we are implicitly saying that the quality of the infant's life is not worth it.

This type of judgment may be morally appropriate, or it may not be. At any rate, it raises a whole series of difficult questions: (a) Do we have the right to say what quality of life is tolerable and what is not? (b) If such decisions are unavoidable at some point (as I think they probably are), in light of what criteria are they to be made? (c) If in individual cases one may allow such infants to die, why cannot the process be hastened by active intervention? This list of questions expands to an even larger list of more general questions: What is the moral difference between active euthanasia and foregoing extraordinary means? Is the "sanctity of life" crucially dependent on a concept of God as Creator and ultimate destiny of life? Is there a right to die? What is the value of terminal suffering?

This case and similar ones force us to ask ourselves: How much dominion over life can be exercised compatibly with the claims others have on us in terms of respect for the integrity, the sanctity of life? Where is the line to be drawn, by whom, and with what checks, safeguards, and warrants? Each era must face these questions anew, with a vivid consciousness of its own biases and insensitivities. In other words, each era must redefine in changing cir-

cumstances the meaning of the values to which it ought to
adhere.

2. *The meaning of sexuality and the family.* Another very basic
value at stake in the practice of medicine is that of human sexuality. The meaning we give to our sexuality can have a good deal to
say about the quality of our lives. This value has been challenged
by two contemporary biological achievements: the separation of
sexual expression and procreation through effective contraception,
and the achievement of procreation apart from sexual expression.
These possibilities force us to ask ourselves: What is the meaning
of sexuality? What is the meaning of the family? Several medical
problems bring this value under direct scrutiny: sterilization, contraception, donor and husband insemination, genetic counseling,
in vitro fertilization, and eventually the exotic matter of cloning.

Take, for instance, the case of a sixteen-year-old girl who is notably retarded. She has the mental competence of a six- or seven-
year-old child, and an IQ ranging between 40 and 60. She does
not understand her menses, seems incapable of understanding or
sustaining a mothering relationship—yet is quite affectionate and
sexually aggressive. She is presently living in an institution that
gives excellent care, but the responsible authorities are quite
worried about her sexual activity. To control it with any degree of
security would involve inhumane isolation incompatible with the
basic affective needs of the girl—a kind of "institutional sterilization." Both the parents and the guardians begin to think of surgical sterilization—always, they insist, for the good of the girl, to
protect her against her own vulnerabilities. But they wonder and
hesitate, basically because they do not know what is in the best interests of the child in the long run.

One's whole approach to sterilization here will open on larger
questions such as these: Should the responsible guardians of a severely retarded person encourage, tolerate, or try to prevent sexual
encounters of the retardate? Would these encounters be good or
be destructive for the retardate? The discussion of this type of
question takes one back to one's basic view of sexuality. What is
the meaning and value of sexual relations? Are they the language
of permanency, exclusiveness, and fidelity? Would we trivialize
sexuality by expanding the relationships of which it is thought to
be an appropriate expression? In what circumstances should the

sexual experience of intimacy occur if sexual language is to retain its viability as truly *human* language? By his or her decision and policies the doctor will answer these questions in one way or another.

In the past, sexual expression was viewed as the language of relationship. It derived its fullest human meaning from the relationship it expressed and fostered. And the relationship that provides us with our best opportunity to integrate and humanize the fickle, fleeting, and frustrative character of sex and eros is the covenant relationship of marriage, for it is friendship (*philia*) that generates constancy, loyalty, and fidelity. And these are the qualities that allow sex to speak a truly human language. If sex is to have any chance at all to help us bridge the separateness of our lives and to escape the loneliness and isolation of our individuality, it cannot be lived merely in the present. It must celebrate the past and guarantee the future. It is as affirmation and promise that sexual exchange achieves quality. It has been a Judaeo-Christian conviction that it is a relationship lived in the promise of permanency that prevents the collapse of sexual expression into a divisive, alienating, and destructive trivialization. This is not a terribly popular idea these days; but we must face squarely the fact that this could be all the more reason why its strong countercultural statement is more necessary than ever now. Our narrow American pragmatism can easily lead us to overlook the depth of the problems we face, to identify the disappearance of a problem with its fully human solution. Contemporary perspectives generate isolated tactical decisions rather than over-all human strategy.

Another problem is that of *in vitro* fertilization with subsequent uterine implantation. Should we do it? Or is it a step we should resist? We know that there are any number of things that we can do but should not. Is this one of them? There are those who argue, as we shall see below, that moving procreation into the laboratory can possibly undermine the justification and support that biological parenthood gives to monogamous marriage. In other words, the family as we know it is basically (though not eminently or exclusively) a biological unit. Would weakening the biological link untie the family at its root and therefore undermine it? Would this be ultimately dehumanizing?

The procedure in question may seem minuscule. A child is, after all, a child regardless of how he came to be. If the parents desire their own child and this is the only way, what is objectionable? Ethically, however, the matter is not that easy. There are several problems inseparable from procedures such as these, and one of them is the family as we know it. The family, one might argue, embodies the ordinary conditions wherein we learn to become persons. In the stable, permanent man-woman relationship we possess the chance to bring libido and eros to the maturity of *philia* (friendship). Through monogamous marriage we experience the basic (but not the only) form of human love and caring—and learn thereby to take gradual possession of our own capacity to relate in love. Marriage is the ordinary societal condition of our coming to learn about responsibility, tenderness, fidelity, patience, the meaning of our sexuality, etc. Without its nourishing presence in our midst, do we not gamble with our best hope for growth and dignity, our chances of learning what it means to love and be loved? Would undermining the family in any way, especially at its biological rootage, compromise the ordinary conditions of our own growth as persons?

Obviously, marriages (and families) fail. And just as obviously, the surrogate arrangements that pick up the pieces of our weakness, failure, and irresponsibility can and do succeed. Furthermore, it seems undeniable that the contemporary shape of family life cries out for restructuring if monogamous marriage is to survive, grow, and realize its true potential. But do these facts negate the basic necessity of the monogamously structured family? They only say that it is worth criticizing vigorously because it is worth saving. Is *in vitro* fertilization a subtle but real attack on the family as we know it? These concerns seem to have been at the root of the fears of Pius XII, as we shall see below.

Medical problems involving sterilization, abortion, contraception, and procreation necessarily bring us back to basic questions of this kind. Medical ethics cannot solve these problems alone. But if it fails even to recognize their existence, it is playing the ostrich, and actually solving them without benefit of reflection and at considerable risk to all of us who have a stake in the good of our neighbor.

3. *The value of the personal physician-patient relationship.* For centuries this relationship has rightly been treasured by both phy-

sicians and patients. It is one of dependence and trust. The doctor treats not only a disease or a wound, but also a person with human hopes, desires, fears, failings, and worries. The physician knows that often the two are not unrelated and that to heal the body he must often heal the person in much less tangible ways. The challenge is enormous, even frightening. And it explains why the personal relationship of doctor-patient is so basic a value in medical practice, even if it is ultimately an instrumental value, and why doctors are so rightly jealous of the human and legal supports that protect this relationship. The quality of this relationship is inextricably bound up with the following problem areas: the patient's right to be informed, confidentiality, the physician as counselor, the canon of informed consent, the "closing-ranks syndrome" where protection of the physician is concerned, malpractice problems, and medical treatment of minors and dependents.

Let me focus for a moment on a single aspect of this relationship: confidentiality. There are many atmospheric conditions that tend to erode the value of confidentiality in contemporary medicine. First, there is the team approach to medicine with the taped or observed interview, the staff meeting, group practice, and so on. Second, there is the mechanization and depersonalization of health care. Increasingly machines do for people what people used to do. Efficient? Yes. But the removal of the patient from people contains a built-in tendency to depersonalize people—by depersonalizing the process that treats them. This tends to undermine confidentiality, for confidentiality is between persons. Third, there is the increasing role of paramedical and nonmedical personnel in medical care (for example, government). This means a multiplication of records and of those who see them. These and other factors indicate a tendency to deprivatize the physician-patient relationship, or at least to desensitize the physician to the value of confidentiality. The cynic says: "The professional secret is one that one professional person whispers to another."

The questions about confidentiality were relatively clear-cut in the past, because they occurred in an atmosphere where medicine was indeed "private practice." But now a shift is going on. Contemporary conditions raise this issue: What kind of doctor-patient relationship should we attempt to establish and insist on preserving? In our time, for instance, confidentiality does not raise so much the question of the airline pilot with heart disease (though that remains a classic case in its own right), but the problem of the availability of medical care within an atmosphere of privacy. One of the most frequent examples of this is the problem of minors and adolescents. Parents often feel that they have obligations and rights where the health of their children is concerned. "Generation gap" minors, on the other hand, will frequently not seek medical help if the parents must be informed. This is the problem of the fourteen-year-old drug addict or VD case, or the instance of desired abortion or the botched abortion. Even the laws are inconsistent in some of these cases. In Hawaii and Nebraska a doctor can treat an unemancipated minor for VD on his own consent, but then the doctor must inform the parents. In Illinois a minor with a baby can give consent for medical treatment for her child, but not for herself. In California, a girl can consent to an abortion at any age, but youngsters under fifteen cannot obtain the means of contraception. Here is the area of contemporary concern for the doctor-patient relationship. We have very few answers, only an extremely interesting issue—interesting because it touches on the very heart of the doctor-patient relationship and its quality.

4. *Individual and social justice in health-care delivery.* There are two distinct values that comprise this general category: the individual's right to health care, and the physician's right to autonomy. A proper understanding of these two values is at the heart of the problems associated with the following: group practice, volunteer medical work for the poor, fee structures, racial discrimination in physician training and hospital care, hospital fees, national health plans, conscience rights of physicians, and so on. We have been accustomed to think of "medicomoral" problems in terms of decisions about procedures touching the health and life of individual patients. In this sense medical ethics has suffered from the individualism that has infected ethics in general. It has equivalently excluded a whole crucial domain from the area of ethical concern, or at least it has not given proportionate attention to this area.

Here a single example will suffice: the physician's right to autonomy in medical practice. Until the relatively recent past, health care was viewed as a privilege of those who could afford it.

Now, however, contemporary consciousness views it much more as a right, ancillary to the right to life. If all individuals have a right to health care, at least in the sense of a decent minimum (as an outgrowth of their right to life and health), then obviously the duty to provide this care falls heavily on those who have the competence: physicians and paramedical personnel. This does not mean that any individual has a claim on a specific doctor's services. It does mean that the profession as a whole, since it is service-oriented in support of a fundamental right, must organize its delivery system in such a way that it brings the exercise of this right within the reach of as many as is humanly possible. In our country, however, because of the complexity and sophistication of medical care, it has become clear that an open, fee-for-service delivery system without any governmental partnership does not provide for this good adequately.

But a growing governmental partnership in health delivery appears to many as a threat to the physician's autonomy. Many physicians feel that a national health plan may be a form of, for example, economic coercion, forcing the physician to come under its aegis in a way that violates his right to dispose freely of his services. He may also be unable to collect remuneration commensurate with his training. Coercion, then, suggests a possible double loss of autonomy: in the determination and disposal of services, and in remuneration.

It is understandable that the right of the physician to his autonomy has received a very high valuation. Loss of full autonomy tends to introduce a third party into the doctor-patient relationship with all the dangers associated with such an intrusion. Second, there is the time-consuming multiplication of paperwork. Third, autonomy promotes specialization, with the consequent advance of medicine (not least because specialists can charge commensurately for their services). Fourth, government involvement could lead to a growing apathy and loss of initiative on the part of health providers, and to eventual carelessness and routine in medical practice. And so on. In view of such considerations the medical profession has tended to defend its autonomy as a near absolute right, to be infringed upon by no need or system.

The contemporary conscience is challenging this—especially in view of the right of individuals to adequate health care. In other words, the medical profession is being asked to redefine the meaning of its autonomy in light of a changed situation. I judge this issue area with all its social ramifications to be the most crucial, perhaps, at the present time. Autonomy is a definite value. But it can be underestimated or overestimated. By underestimating autonomy we could get trapped in a stifling collectivism that would eventually undermine the provision of sound health care. By overestimating it, the medical profession could be its own worst enemy by failing to face the nation's health problems in a creative, service-minded way. Such a failure would all but constitute a mandate to the government to intervene in bungling and inefficient ways, since the intervention would not enjoy the co-operation and consultation of the medical profession. If government partnership is to be supportive of the rights of all—physician as well as patient—the medical profession must be a partner in the planning. And if it is wise, it will bring to this planning an attitude toward its rights that interprets them within a service-minded structure. This requires a good deal of rethinking.

These are but four of the issue areas I believe should be included in a medical ethics program. Another might be *the meaning of individuality and sociality.* Man is both an individual and a social being. What is the proper balance that respects both aspects of his being? This basic value is at stake in questions touching experimentation (as I shall point out below), transplants, eugenic planning, and consent requirements. Or again, there is the whole issue area of *human freedom,* its value and limits. The population problem in some countries has raised this issue in a very pressing way. How much freedom is compatible with the success of population policies? How much coercion is compatible with human dignity where determination of family size is involved? I am sure that there are other such issue areas, but those I have mentioned cannot be avoided.

What I am basically proposing, therefore, is a notion of issue areas that will insist on organizing a medical ethics program in terms of the basic values that contemporary medical-moral casuistry involves. The results of such a program will not always be tidy, certain, or reassuring, especially in transitional and pluralistic times. Such a program will appear to many to be "speculative" and "unrealistic." But if medicomoral problems are approached in any other way, I fear that they will be solved in isolation by tradition, power, fiat, prestige, economics—a whole host of influences that reflect and support the interests of the moment, but less clearly the interests of the patient, and therefore ultimately of the medical profession.

3. Some Neglected Aspects of the Moral Responsibility for Health

The public is increasingly becoming a partner in discussions of health and health-care delivery. That is as it should be. But too often these discussions confine themselves to the neon problems of abortion, euthanasia, suicide, genetic screening and manipulation, allocation of scarce resources, etc., as if an answer to these very difficult problems exhausted the notion of moral responsibility for health. We are not likely to neglect or to forget such problems.

Furthermore, there are other general aspects of the question of responsibility for health that we are not likely to neglect. One can list them quickly and easily, as one rises with the late Mayor Richard Daley and his beloved Chicago to "higher and higher platitudes." Yes, there is an obligation to promote health. Yes, there is an obligation to keep it. No, there is not—at least in Catholic Christian tradition—a right to suicide, since every right is concerned with a good, whether instrumental or consummatory. Yes, revelation does have something to say about the moral responsibility for health. And so on. These are things we are *not* likely to neglect because very little effort was expended in learning them and because what was learned was minimal, even if important. They are so general in character that we know them down our pulses as human beings—even though they contain the seeds of some serious moral disputes, as, for example, in the case of euthanasia in some instances.

In what follows I should like to outline some neglected aspects of responsibility for health. Because my purpose is provocative and suggestive, I shall paint with a broad brush. In doing so I shall spare the reader the extensive footnote documentation that could be adduced to support the claims made or extend the probes initiated.

I

In thinking about responsibility for health, one of the first things we are likely to forget is that "health" is both too broad and too narrow a term to convey our over-all responsibilities. Health is a notion defined by its relation to disease. But the term "disease" has had an interesting evolutionary history and therefore so has health.[1] "Disease" first meant an identifiable degenerative or inflammatory process which, if unchecked, would lead to serious organic illness and sometimes eventually to death. The next stage of development was statistical—at least some diseases being identified by deviation from a supposed statistical norm. Thus we referred to *hyper*thyroidism or *hypo*thyroidism, *hyper*cholesterolemia, *hypo*glycemia, etc. One was said to be unhealthy, to have a disease if he or she were *hypo* or *hyper* anything, not in the sense of an existing, tangible degenerative process, but in the sense that the individual was more than others likely to suffer some untoward event, what my colleague Dr. André Hellegers is fond of calling "hyperuntowardeventitis."

The third notion of disease is inability to function in society. For instance, there is a good deal of surgery being performed to enlarge breasts, to shrink buttocks, to remove wrinkles—in brief, to conform to someone's notion of the attractive and eventually of the tolerable. We live in a society that cannot tolerate aging. At some point, then, this question arises: Who is the patient here, who is sick—the individual, or society? I mean, of course, that this broad understanding of "health" can too easily reflect a sickness of society, in its judgments about the meaning of the person. In our time and in some societies, people are hospitalized because of nonconformity. That suggests that the notion of "health" is becoming increasingly nonsomatized and getting out of control.

The final stage of development is the definition of health popularized by the World Health Organization. Health is a "state of

[1] These reflections I owe to Dr. André Hellegers (Charles Sumner Bacon Lecture).

complete physical, mental, and social well-being, not simply the absence of illness and disease." This description of health was adopted in the *Doe* v. *Bolton* abortion decision of the U. S. Supreme Court. The Court stated that the "medical judgment may be exercised in the light of all factors—physical, emotional, psychological, familial, and the woman's age—relevant to the well-being of the patient."[2] Following this notion of health, the quite preposterous situation could arise where a person's sense of well-being is threatened by the size of his or her car. The appropriate medical judgment would be a prescription for a Chrysler Imperial to replace one's Dodge Dart.

Through the expansion of the notions of health and disease, contemporary medicine is increasingly treating the desires of people in a move toward a discomfortless society. Desires, of course, are notoriously the product of many suspect sources. What we can easily forget, then, is that under this burgeoning notion of health and disease, "moral responsibility for health" can too easily lead to an endorsement of a notion of the person that is highly distorted and at some point radically un-Christian.

On the other hand, the term "health" is far too narrow. If we define and delimit our moral responsibilities under such narrowing, we very easily forget that our responsibilities extend to the living even in their dying. A narrow notion of health as delimiting responsibility can lead us to forget that one of our most urgent moral tasks is care and comfort of the dying. Particular temptations of a highly technological health-care system are to abandon the dying, to approach our responsibilities by narrowing the options to pulling the plug or not pulling the plug. "Orders not to resuscitate" are too often carried out as if they were orders to do nothing—not even care.

II

The second thing we can easily forget is that health problems are traceable to and root in cultural priorities and the structures that embody these priorities. It is popular now, perhaps even faddish to speak of "sinful structures" in society. What is meant

[2] *Doe* v. *Bolton*, 410 U.S. 179, 192 (1973).

here, in a general way, is that enslavement of persons occurs through structures.

To understand this, we must distinguish two types of structures. The first I refer to as "operational structures." These are zoning laws, welfare systems, tax systems, health-delivery systems, international monetary systems, etc.—the concrete organizational patterns that make up our environment. Since our environment profoundly shapes our lives, these structures can be either liberating or enslaving. They are very often enslaving—and that brings me to the second type of structure, "ideological structures." An ideological structure is nothing more nor less than a corporately adopted priority. An ideological structure becomes enslaving when it makes some value other than individual persons the organizing and dominating value. I say "organizing"—that is, this value produces reciprocal expectations, patterns of action, decisions, policies. I say "dominating"—that is, individuals are subordinated to this value.

For example, one could argue that American business or economic life is structured around, dominated by, a single value: Make money. The GNP is the index of economic health. The Cadillac is the sign of social status. Boards of trustees are often composed of men of money. Banks have replaced cathedrals as our largest buildings. Our American culture rewards this value in many subtle and nonsubtle ways. This means that other values will be pursued only within this over-all priority. Thus justice in education, housing, medical services, and job opportunity is promoted within the dominance of the financial criterion—"if we can afford it." That means, of course, "if we can achieve it without changing our life-style." In summary, then, when large numbers of people are suffering or are denied their rights and opportunities, look for a value that subordinates them and one that has been made a structure by becoming the organizing force of policies and decisions.

What we are likely to forget, where responsibility for health is concerned, is that health is deeply affected by the life-style of a culture or nation, a life-style that is the embodiment of certain value priorities. In the United States, our dominant instrumental values are technology, efficiency, and comfort, for these support the "good life" of consumerism that is ours. Many of our health problems are directly or at least heavily traceable to this so-called good life. It would be typically American to face these problems with more technology and more pain relief, more uppers and downers, better filters on the cigarette. Actually, if we get our heads on straight—that is, if we are truly responsible—what is needed is a change in structures, above all the ideological structures or value priorities involved. For instance, I believe there would be far less smoking and excessive drinking in a society organized differently than ours. Changing value priorities is not easy, for it means changing hearts and minds and outlooks on life. We are likely to forget this when we think of "moral responsibility for health."

III

Another aspect of moral responsibility for health that must concern us is that which gathers around the notion of public morality. By that term I do not mean public participation in the directions and priorities of medical practice, getting representatives of the public on committees and decision-making bodies. Nor do I mean simply the law. Since one acid test of law is feasibility, reducing public morality to the law could all too easily collapse it into the utterly pragmatic considerations that so often decide what is feasible.

Public morality is something quite different. I would outline the notion by highlighting the fact that health-care delivery is increasingly mediated very heavily by institutions. We have group practice, insurance coverage, medication controlled by the FDA, Medicare, Medicaid, etc., hospitals built by government, and research supported and controlled by its agencies. Groups, it must be noticed (whether hospitals, companies, or governments), have interests and concerns other than the immediate good of the patient. For instance, the federal government has a legitimate interest in population control; reducing the welfare rolls; control of illegitimate parenthood; advance of diagnostic, therapeutic, and preventive medicine; protection of life.

All of this suggests that whenever other values are the legitimate concern of the mediators of health care, the good of the patient can easily become one of several values, in competition for attention and priority. This means that the individual is in danger of being subordinated to these values. Public morality is precisely the pursuit of these other values without violating individual rights. Or stated differently, it is harmonizing public concerns with individual needs and rights—the pursuit of these other public values while keeping the good of the individual primary.

When the biomedical enterprise is mediated by groups with other legitimate concerns, the danger of mistreatment of the individual is real. The ones who are likely to suffer most are the poor, the dependent (the elderly, retarded, prisoners), and the "ordinary" patient who is neglected in favor of exquisite technological virtuosities that consume disproportionate energies, time, and funds. We are likely to forget that moral responsibility for health means keeping a sharp eye on the harmonization of public concerns with the needs of individuals, on public morality—so that the "little people" are not short-suited.

IV

The fourth dimension of responsibility for health care that is easy to forget is directly attributable to the technological and impersonal aspect of health care, especially in its hugeness. When sickness calls for hospitalization, one is often ushered into a vast system. Certain symptomatic conditions call for certain responses. Certain turns of events dictate still other responses. Medical and paramedical personnel are trained to respond swiftly, efficiently, and in standard or orthodox ways to certain phenomena. Gradually, if imperceptibly, the impression grows that "*we* (the medical system) are responsible for *them*," that the medical system makes the decisions about treatment—and eventually that it is necessary to subtract ourselves from systematic or institutional treatment decisions by legislating living wills.

I realize that it is possible to caricature here. But I am trying to paint a picture of health-care delivery in our society that has tended to create and reinforce the impression that it is the attending physician who makes the decision to treat or not to treat. The Karen Ann Quinlan case is a dramatic and symbolic example of this mislocation of the onus of decision-making. In that case, the Quinlan family sought to subtract their daughter from the jurisdiction of her physicians. The way events developed in that case, the presumptions seem to be that physicians have a right to treat a patient unasked—indeed, opposed. This premise is wrong in itself and dangerous in its implications—and responsibility for health demands that we be clear on these points.

It is wrong in itself because the individual, having the prime obligation for his own health care, has also thereby the right to the necessary means for such basic health care—specifically, the right of self-determination in the acceptance or rejection of treatment. When an individual puts himself into a doctor's hands, he engages the doctor's services; he does not abdicate his right to decide his own fate. Patients retain the right to refuse a physician's advice, however ill advised the patients might be in doing so.

Furthermore, this subtle shift in the doctor-patient relationship is threatening in its value implications, for in lessening the patients' rights, it will tend to blunt those perspectives that are intended to inform the exercise of those rights. The Judaeo-Christian tradition maintains that there are values more important than life in the living of it. So it also holds that there are values more important than life in the dying of it. For this reason the accumulation of minutes of life is not the moral guideline by which dying must be done. For instance, the justification for administration of pain-killing drugs, even if they should shorten life, recognizes that there is a value in being free, which permits the pursuit of other values, such as prayer.

What I fear is that a system that increasingly reinforces the notion of physician mastery over patients will at the same time undermine those altogether balanced perspectives within which patient choice ought to occur, for the very notion that a dying patient has a moral choice as to how he will live while dying is an outgrowth of these basic perspectives. A system that undermines that choice attacks, however subtly, the perspectives that generated it. To forget this is to fail in moral responsibility for health care.

V

Another aspect of responsibility for health that we are likely to forget is the possible implication of quality-of-life judgments.

Much of contemporary health care and very many decisions about treatment are concerned with not just the preservation of life and avoidance of disease, but also with a certain quality of life. This is absolutely as it should be. Thus we are concerned not just with keeping a patient alive by surgery or medication, but with a certain level of being alive, a certain acceptable mix of freedom, painlessness, and ability to function. Problems like this are particularly acute and anguishing where resuscitation is in question. Sissela Bok, composing a possible living will in the *New England Journal of Medicine*, has put into words what most of us feel about the technological potential of modern medicine:

> I wish to live a full and long life, but not at all costs. If my death is near and cannot be avoided, and if I have lost the ability to interrelate with others and have no reasonable chance of regaining this ability, or if my suffering is intense and irreversible, I do not want to have my life prolonged. I would then ask not to be subjected to surgery or resuscitation. Nor would I then wish to have life support from mechanical ventilators, intensive-care services, or other life-prolonging procedures, including the administration of antibiotics and blood products. I would wish, rather, to have care which gives comfort and support, which facilitates my interaction with others to the extent that this is possible, and which brings peace.[3]

I believe that most of us would agree with that and hope that we are treated in line with the value mix expressed so well by Bok.

However, what we are likely to forget is that the extension of such a mix backward to the incompetent child or baby is not quite as easy. We are likely to forget in making such quality-of-life judgments about the newborn that we can be discriminatory and be exercising a racism of the adult world. Extrapolation backward to babies of the criteria we might use for Karen Ann Quinlan— and use reasonably, in my judgment—has these characteristics. First, it is extremely difficult for an adult to draw the line at the right place, because in attempting to do so, that adult would una-

---

[3] Sissela Bok, "Personal Directions for Care at the End of Life," *New England Journal of Medicine*, 295 (1976), 369.

voidably be saying what he or she would want to be (what kind of life), not what kind of life they could come to live with God's grace and sufficient supports were they terribly deprived. Second, the tiny infant has no background, no history, no biography of aspirations and perspectives against which we can make a judgment. And third, therefore, the kind of judgment we make about defective newborns is in principle applicable to all babies. It is generalizable. That means that all babies are at risk in our quality-of-life judgments about instigation or withdrawal of treatment at this time.

On the other hand, I am in agreement with Dr. Judson G. Randolph (surgeon in chief, Children's Hospital National Medical Center, Washington, D.C.) when he states, "I think it is well within the guidelines of right and wrong to make certain qualitative judgments about human life. . . ." Dr. Randolph continues: "If a severely handicapped child were suddenly given one moment of omniscience and total awareness of his or her outlook for the future, would that child necessarily opt for life? No one has yet been able to demonstrate that the answer would always be 'yes.' "[4] In my judgment, the perspectives of the Christian tradition on life and its meaning would suggest that in some instances the answer would be "no." Our main task as reasonable persons is to discover where the line is to be drawn and why. Our temptation as adults in a highly function-oriented and comfort-biased world is to draw it in terms of adult perspectives on comfort and functionability. What we are likely to forget—and therefore what is eminently part of our responsibility for health—is that these decisions are terribly anguishing, terribly risky, and utterly final. Moral responsibility demands sensitivity to this and a corresponding humility.

VI

In reflecting on "man's moral responsibility for health," we may easily forget any number of things about the notion of morality. The first thing we are tempted to forget is the distinction between "moralism" and "morality." Moralism is that attitude or mind-set

[4] J. G. Randolph, "Ethical Considerations in Surgery of the Newborn," *Contemporary Surgery*, 7 (1975), 17.

that approaches human problems with a dominating, perhaps even exclusive concern, for the prescriptive and proscriptive, for the permissible and the nonpermissible, the do's and the don'ts. This is particularly the temptation of the Anglo-Saxon mind, which thinks of law as being the answer to all problems, the only answer, and a fully adequate answer. When this attitude enters the realm of moral discourse and reflection, it becomes preoccupied with norms and rules.

Now, there is nothing objectionable about norms and rules— indeed, they are utterly essential. But they are basically generalizations on the significance of human conduct. If that is the case, our first task is always to understand the significance of our conduct. It is only then that we are positioned to formulate and apply norms. Preoccupation with norms is moralism, and the problem with moralism is that it bypasses and therefore effectively subverts the processes leading to understanding. Without adequate understanding—as fully informed as possible by all the disciplines that can enlighten the human—we fall into education by edict, which is no education at all. And we fall into practice by conformity, which neglects important human aspects of conduct. This happens all too often in the area of sexual morality, where our preoccupation with the rights and wrongs hurries us over the very understanding that alone yields the true rights and wrongs.

In the area of health care, there is, I submit, an enormous amount of moralizing going on—a phenomenon that can block the development of a genuine morality, thus subverting our moral responsibility for health care. For instance, the morality of care for the dying is often popularly framed in terms of "pulling the plug" or "not pulling the plug." We discuss whether there should be a law controlling DNA recombinant research. We wonder whether a patient may elect to forego hemodialysis. We ask whether the incompetent retarded person may be protectively sterilized. We conduct long discussions about the moral propriety of *in vitro* fertilization. And so on. These are all important issues, of course. But their resolution must occur within a much broader context if we are to avoid moralism, the context of profound deliberation about human and Christian being and end, about who we are.

It is conversation about who we are that is so often bypassed in

contemporary discussions about health care. But it is precisely
who we are that will inform us about the shape of our health-care
responsibilities. (For a fuller treatment of those issues see Chapters
6 and 7.) For the moment, however, let me take but a single example. It is axiomatic that we are social beings, that we move and literally have our being not as atomized individuals, but as interrelated beings. We exist in relationships and are dead without
them. This is not surprising to those who believe that man is
created in the image and likeness of God, for the more we know
of God, the more we know that He is relation, that His very being
is "being in and for another." As man comes to know more about
himself through psychiatry and clinical psychology, it should not
be surprising that his Godlikeness becomes more obvious, that he
sees that he is made for relational life, and that everything in his
makeup (including instincts and emotions) conspires to relational
possibility or, as undeveloped, hinders it.

The ultimate meaning of this relational constitution of the
human person is love. In Christian perspective, we could put it as
follows: The great commandment, in a sense the only commandment, is the love of God and of neighbor for God's sake. All other
Christian duties are simply specifications of this command. But
not only is this a command; God's commands are also affirmations
about ourselves. In telling us that the great commandment is love
of God and neighbor, Christ was actually telling us what is good
for us and what we are. He was saying that our own completion
and fulfillment are to be found here, hence that ultimately our
eternal happiness depends on love and is love. If one is to find
life, one must lose it—in the divestment of self that is love.

Now, what is interesting here is that just as my ability to love
God is His gift to me, so our ability to love each other is our gift
to each other. The greatest human need is to be loved; for
unloved, I remain unloving, withdrawn, self-encased. But when I
am loved in a full human way, selfhood, personal dignity, a feeling of security, a sense of worth and dignity are conferred upon
me—the very things that enable me to respond to others as persons, to love them. Thus it is clear that because my greatest
fulfillment is the other-centeredness of love, my greatest human
need is for that which creates this possibility—that is, love from
others, their acceptance of me as a person. Similarly, my greatest

gift to them is my self-donation to them, because this is also their greatest need. Modern psychology, in uncovering the growth process that leads to the ability of self-donation in interpersonal relationships, has not only described a capacity, it also has at once described a need. And in doing this it has painted in bold colors the ultimate meaning of any concrete act of charity, justice, fairness toward men.

What has all this to do with responsibility for health care? The following, I would suggest: Unless prevention, cure, and care are experienced as extensions of genuine human caring and love, they are less than they could be. They do not touch the whole person; rather, they minister to a body. They may heal a body, but we long for and need a deeper healing from each other as the body is healed, or even at times if it is to be healed. That is one good reason why persons of deep faith and religious consecration should be in health care, for in our time, it is far too easy for health care to be reduced to only bodily care, in a very impersonal way. That is why there is a profound difference between physicians, paramedical personnel, and a hospital with a self-image of vocation, on the one hand, and those with a self-image of only "being in business" on the other. This difference manifests itself in subtle but very important ways. Unless we are aware of this, we drift toward moralism, the extension into the moral sphere of a merely technological assessment of man.

What I am driving at is that moralism, and excessive preoccupation with "problems" and the rights and wrongs of omissions and commissions, too readily leads us to overlook the human quality of care and cure—that which we need no matter what our condition. I believe we are likely to forget this in discussing moral responsibility for health. The New York *Times* recently reported the remarks of a surgeon whose kidney-transplant recipient was undergoing anxiety and depression after his transplant: "Well, I gave him a good kidney; I can't help what's wrong with his brain."[5]

[5] New York *Times* (May 11, 1977).

VII

The next aspect of moral responsibility for health we are likely
to forget is the affective component in moral conviction. Judgments of the moral "ought," what I as a Christian should do or
avoid, and action upon such conclusions, originate not simply in
rational analysis, book learning, or exposure to sociological fact.
They have deep roots in our sensitivities and emotions. This has
particular relevance where the health needs of the elderly and dependent (fetuses, infants, retarded, the poor) are concerned.

What I mean to suggest here is the difficulty we experience in a
media culture in remaining sensitive to human hurt, deprivation,
and injustice. The efficiency of the media means that human
suffering and loneliness are dished up to us both frequently and
mediately. By "mediately" I mean that we learn of the sickness,
suffering, starving, death, and isolation of others several levels removed from the happening—often enough in a cozy chair with a
glass of standard swank Beefeaters ready to soften any overly severe blows and to soothe our quivering ganglia. Thus the body
counts in Vietnam night after night had inevitably the effect of
chipping away at our moral horror at what was happening. Being
surrounded by sickness, pain, and death, we get hardened to it.
The phenomenon has been noted in nurses frequently. I speak as
an American when I say that in far too many areas it is true to say
that "the feeling has gone out of it." "Oh just another rape" is a
phrase that, God forbid, can become as common as a comment
on the weather.

I will pursue this for a moment, because it is utterly essential.
What is so often lacking in contemporary life is passion. For example, couples talk of affection and tenderness and read manuals
of marital gymnastics to find them. The more they desire feeling
and passion, the more it escapes them. We are the clinicians of
quality where quality escapes the mere clinician. We talk about
the poor, their terrible situation; yet we eat well, drink well. We
get mad (passionate) at injustice only when it hits us or our family. Those who get mad when it hits others (the neighbor as the
self, so to speak) are often viewed as marginal characters.

Passion is the beginning of any true moral responsibility and therefore of responsibility for health. It is the inner identification with the suffering and the downtrodden. It is that personal start-up that gets us off-center a bit—self-center—and propels us to examine our consciences, comforts, and priorities. To develop genuine passion and concern, I believe we have to be exposed to those who suffer. There is a qualitative difference in the approach of those who have seen, touched, and hugged a hydrocephalic child and those who have not. There is a qualitative difference in the concern of those who have companied with the dying and those who only write statistics and articles about the experience. Those who have seen some retirement homes know in a dimensionally different way the health problems of the elderly; those who have seen know, for example, how our society has failed to come to grips with this problem.

Moral responsibility for health means, far more than we have admitted in our lives and policies, firsthand exposure to the problems of health; for without such experience, we are likely to remain without passion—and therefore without one of the basic ingredients of moral responsibility.

VIII

The next point to advert to in unpacking the notion of "moral responsibility" is the cultural shaping of our grasp of basic human values. In the first chapter I adverted to the fact that we are corporately *homo technologicus* in our attitudes. This prethematic shaping tends to affect profoundly our moral judgments.

Something of a highwater mark in this technological bias is reached in the writings of Joseph Fletcher, as I note in Chapter 15. For instance, Fletcher writes: "Man is a maker and a selector and a designer and the more rationally contrived and deliberate anything is, the more *human* it is." On this basis he continues: "Laboratory reproduction is radically human compared to conception by ordinary heterosexual intercourse. It is willed, chosen, purposed, and controlled, and surely these are among the traits that distinguish *Homo sapiens* from others in the animal genus. . . .

Coital reproduction is, therefore, less human than laboratory reproduction."[6]

My only point here—but it is a very serious point and one we are likely to overlook—is that responsibility for health demands that we attend to and lift out those cultural leanings and biases that may distort our grasp on the basic values and hence prejudice our notion of what moral responsibility means and requires.

IX

My final point in dealing with health and care for health is that our responsibility must be "holistic." Otherwise it begins to suffer erosion and is simply incredible as a form of witness to others. By holistic I mean that responsibility must be conceived and spoken of as covering all of those things that affect life and health. It must be part and parcel of an attitude toward persons that defends their rights, is strongly prophetic about warfare, about poverty, about quality of life in all aspects and at all ages. Why is this important? Because without such a reach and universality, our own sense of responsibility begins to erode by being selective. One cannot responsibly care for the person—the self of others—by caring for only a single aspect of the person.

We know this notionally, but it is terribly hard to make it part of ourselves, to know it evaluatively. I recall a panel I was on at Georgetown University on the problem of abortion. Three of us participated: a pro-abortionist, a prolifer, and I. The students were, by and large, strongly opposed to abortion, but the language used by the prolife lawyer involved all but "turned them off." At one point I noted that we must also be concerned with what happens to children once they are born. We must be concerned about whether they are starving, are beaten, are abandoned in gutters and on front steps. "Otherwise," I argued, "our abortion stand is selective and one-eyed." To my consternation, the lawyer responded: "That has nothing to do with the problem of abortion." I submit that it has everything to do with it, with our own sense of responsibility and with our credibility. This same tunnel vision can overtake us as we reflect on our responsibilities for health.

[6] Joseph Fletcher, "Ethical Aspects of Genetic Controls," *New England Journal of Medicine*, 285 (1971), 776.

These are but some of the things we are likely to forget when discussing "man's moral responsibility for health." I am sure there are many more. But if one details too many things we are likely to forget, one becomes a self-fulfilling prophet and all but guarantees our memory failure.

SECTION II

EXPERIMENTATION AND THE INCOMPETENT

4. Proxy Consent in the Experimentation Situation

It is widely admitted within the research community that if there is to be continuing and proportionate progress in pediatric medicine, experimentation is utterly essential. This conviction rests on two closely interrelated facts. First, as Alexander Capron has pointed out,[1] "Children cannot be regarded simply as 'little people' pharmacologically. Their metabolism, enzymatic and excretory systems, skeletal development and so forth differ so markedly from adults' that drug tests for the latter provide inadequate information about dosage, efficacy, toxicity, side effects, and contraindications for children." Second, and consequently, there is a limit to the usefulness of prior experimentation with animals and adults. At some point or other, experimentation with children becomes necessary.

At this point, however, a severe problem arises. The legal and moral legitimacy of experimentation (understood here as procedures involving no direct benefit to the person participating in the experiment) are founded above all on the informed consent of the subject. But in many instances, the young subject is either legally or factually incapable of consent. Furthermore, it is argued, the parents are neither legally nor morally capable of supplying this consent for the child. As Dr. Donald T. Chalkley of the National Institutes of Health puts it: "A parent has no legal right to give consent for the involvement of his child in an activity not for the benefit of that child. No legal guardian, no person standing *in loco parentis*, has that right."[2] It would seem to follow that infants and some minors are simply out of bounds where clinical research is concerned. Indeed, this conclusion has been explicitly

---

[1] Alexander Capron, "Legal Considerations Affecting Clinical Pharmacological Studies in Children," *Clinical Research*, 21 (1973), 141.

[2] *Medical World News* (June 8, 1973), p. 41.

drawn by well-known ethician Paul Ramsey. He notes: "If children are incapable of truly consenting to experiments having unknown hazards for the sake of good to come, and if no one else should consent for them in cases unrelated to their own treatment, then medical research and society in general must choose a perhaps more difficult course of action to gain the benefits we seek from medical investigations."[3]

Does the consent requirement taken seriously exclude all experiments on children? If it does, then children themselves will be the ultimate sufferers. If it does not, what is the moral justification for the experimental procedures? The problem is serious, for, as Ramsey notes, an investigation involving children as subjects is "a prismatic case in which to tell whether we mean to take seriously the consent requirement."

Before concluding with Shirkey that those incompetent of consent are "therapeutic orphans,"[4] I should like to explore the notion and validity of proxy consent. More specifically, the interest here is in this question: Can and may parents consent, and to what extent, to experiments on their children where the procedures are nonbeneficial for the children involved? Before approaching this question, it is necessary to point out the genuine if restricted input of the ethician in such matters. Ramsey has rightly pointed up the difference between the ethics of consent and ethics in the consent situation. This latter refers to the meaning and practical applications of the requirement of an informed consent. It is the work of prudence and pertains to the competence and responsibility of physicians and investigators. The former, on the other hand, refers to the principle requiring an informed consent, the ethics of consent itself. Such moral principles are elaborated out of competences broader than those associated with the medical community.

A brief review of the literature will reveal that the question raised above remains in something of a legal and moral limbo. The Nuremberg Code states that "the voluntary consent of the human subject is absolutely essential. This means that the person

3 Paul Ramsey, *The Patient as Person* (New Haven, Conn.: Yale University Press, 1979).

4 H. Shirkey, Editorial Comment: "Therapeutic Orphans," *Journal of Pediatrics*, 72 (1968), 119.

involved should have legal capacity to give consent."[5] Nothing specific is said about infants or those who are mentally incompetent. Dr. Leon Alexander, who aided in drafting the first version of the Nuremberg Code, explained subsequently that his provision for valid consent from next of kin where mentally ill patients are concerned was dropped by the Nuremberg judges "probably because they did not apply in the specific cases under trial."[6] Be that as it may, it has been pointed out by Beecher[7] that a strict observance of Nuremberg's Rule 1 would effectively cripple study of mental disease and would simply prohibit all experimentation on children.[8]

The International Code of Medical Ethics (General Assembly of the World Medical Association, 1949) states simply: "Under no circumstances is a doctor permitted to do anything that would weaken the physical or mental resistance of a human being except from strictly therapeutic or prophylactic indications imposed in the interest of his patient."[9] This statement is categorical and if taken literally means that "young children and the mentally incompetent are categorically excluded from all investigations except those that directly may benefit the subjects."[10] However, in 1954 the General Assembly of the World Medical Association (in *Principles for Those in Research and Experimentation*) stated: "It should be required that each person who submits to experimentation be informed of the nature, the reason for, and the risk of the proposed experiment. If the patient is irresponsible, consent should be obtained from the individual who is legally responsible for the individual."[11] In the context it is somewhat ambiguous whether this statement is meant to apply beyond experimental procedures that are performed for the patient's good.

The Declaration of Helsinki (1964) is much clearer on the point. After distinguishing "clinical research combined with pro-

---

[5] H. K. Beecher, *Research and the Individual* (Boston: Little, Brown, 1970).

[6] Ramsey, *Patient as Person*, 26, 6.

[7] Beecher, *Research and the Individual*, 231.

[8] Most of the codal documents subsequently cited can be found in Beecher, *Research and the Individual*.

[9] Beecher, *Research and the Individual*, 236.

[10] Franz J. Ingelfinger, "Ethics of Experiments on Children," *New England Journal of Medicine*, 288 (1973), 791.

[11] Beecher, *Research and the Individual*, 240.

fessional care" and "nontherapeutic clinical research," it states of
this latter: "Clinical research on a human being cannot be undertaken without his free consent, after he has been fully informed; if
he is legally incompetent the consent of the legal guardian should
be procured."[12] In 1966 the American Medical Association, in its
Principles of Medical Ethics, endorsed the Helsinki statement.
The AMA statement distinguished clinical investigation "primarily for treatment" and clinical investigation "primarily for the accumulation of scientific knowledge." With regard to this latter, it
noted that "consent, in writing, should be obtained from the subject, or from his legally authorized representative if the subject
lacks the capacity to consent." More specifically, with regard to minors or mentally incompetent persons, the AMA statement reads:
"Consent, in writing, is given by a legally authorized representative of the subject under circumstances in which an informed
and prudent adult would reasonably be expected to volunteer
himself or his child as a subject."[13]

In 1963, the Medical Research Council of Great Britain issued
its *Responsibility in Investigations on Human Subjects.*[14] Under
title of "Procedures Not of Direct Benefit to the Individual" the
Council stated: "The situation in respect of minors and mentally
subnormal or mentally disordered persons is of particular
difficulty. In the strict view of the law parents and guardians of
minors cannot give consent on their behalf to any procedures
which are of no particular benefit to them and which may carry
some risk of harm." Then, after discussing consent as involving a
full understanding of "the implications to himself of the procedures to which he was consenting," the Council concluded:
"When true consent in this sense cannot be obtained, procedures
which are of no direct benefit and which might carry a risk of
harm to the subject should not be undertaken." If it is granted
that every experiment involves some risk, then the MRC statement would exclude any experiment on children. Curran and
Beecher have pointed out[15] that this strict reading of English law

[12] Ibid., 278.
[13] Ibid., 223.
[14] Ibid., 262 ff.
[15] William J. Curran and H. K. Beecher, "Experimentation in Children,"
Journal of the American Medical Association, 210 (1969), 77.

is based on the advice of Sir Harvey Druitt, though there is no statute or case law to support it. Nevertheless, it has gone relatively unchallenged.

Statements of the validity of proxy consent similar to those of the Declaration of Helsinki and the American Medical Association have been issued by the American Psychological Association[16] and the Food and Drug Administration.[17] A recent formulation touching on proxy consent is that of the Department of Health, Education, and Welfare in its *Protection of Human Subjects, Policies, and Procedures.*[18] In situations where the subject cannot himself give consent, the document refers to "supplementary judgment." It states: "For the purposes of this document, supplementary judgment will refer to judgments made by local committees in addition to the subject's consent (when possible) and that of the parents or legal guardian (where applicable), as to whether or not a subject may participate in clinical research." The DHEW-proposed guidelines admit that the law on parental consent is not clear in all respects. Proxy consent is valid with regard to established and generally accepted therapeutic procedures; it is, in practice, valid for therapeutic research. However, the guidelines state: "When research might expose a subject to risk without defined therapeutic benefit or other positive effect on that subject's well-being, parental or guardian consent appears to be insufficient." These statements about validity concern law in the sense (I would judge) of what would happen should a case determination be provoked on the basis of existing precedent.

After this review of the legal validity of proxy consent and its limitations, the DHEW guidelines go on to draw two ethical conclusions. First, "When the risk of a proposed study is generally considered not significant, and the potential benefit is explicit, the ethical issues need not preclude the participation of children in biomedical research." Presumably, this means that where there is risk, ethical issues do preclude the use of children. However, the DHEW document did not draw this conclusion. Rather, its second ethical conclusion states: "An investigator proposing research

---

[16] Beecher, *Research and the Individual*, 256 ff.
[17] Ibid., 299 ff.
[18] Department of Health, Education, and Welfare, *Federal Register*, 38 (1973), 31,738.

activities which expose children to risk must document, as part of the application for support, that the information to be gained can be obtained in no other way. The investigator must also stipulate either that the risk to the subjects will be insignificant or that, although some risk exists, the potential benefit is significant and far outweighs that risk. In no case will research activities be approved which entail substantial risk except in the cases of clearly therapeutic procedures." These proposed guidelines admit, therefore, three levels of risk within the ethical calculus: insignificant risk, some risk, and substantial risk. Proxy consent is, by inference, ethically acceptable for the first two levels but not for the third.

The documents cited move almost imperceptibly back and forth between legal and moral considerations, so that it is often difficult to know whether the major concern is one or the other, or even how the relationship of the legal and the ethical is conceived. Nevertheless, it can be said that there has been a gradual move away from the absolutism represented in the Nuremberg Code to the acceptance of proxy consent, possibly because the Nuremberg Code is viewed as containing, to some extent, elements of a reaction to the Nazi experiments.

Medical literature of the noncodal variety has revealed this same pattern or ambiguity. For instance, writing in the *Lancet*, Dr. R. E. W. Fisher reacted to the reports of the use of children in research procedures as follows: "No medical procedure involving the slightest risk or accompanied by the slightest physical or mental pain may be inflicted on a child for experimental purposes unless there is a reasonable chance, or at least a hope, that the child may benefit thereby."[19] On the other hand, Franz J. Ingelfinger, editor of the *New England Journal of Medicine*, contends that the World Medical Association's statement ("Under no circumstances . . ." [above]) is an extremist position that must be modified.[20] His suggested modification reads: "Only when the risks are small and justifiable is a doctor permitted. . . ." It is difficult to know from Ingelfinger's wording whether he means small and therefore justifiable or whether "justifiable" refers to the hoped-for benefit. Responses to this editorial were contradictory. N. Baumslag and R. E. Yodaiken state: "In our opinion

---

19 R. E. W. Fisher, in Letters to the Editor, *Lancet* (Nov. 1953), 993.
20 Ingelfinger, "Ethics of Experiments on Children," 791.

there are no conditions under which any children may be used for experimentation not primarily designed for their benefit."[21] Ian Shine, John Howieson, and Ward Griffen, Jr., came to the opposite conclusion: "We strongly support his [Ingelfinger's] proposals provided that one criterion of 'small justifiable risks' is the willingness of the experimentor to be an experimentee, or to offer a spouse or child when appropriate."[22]

Curran and Beecher had earlier disagreed strongly with the rigid interpretation given the statement of the Medical Research Council through Druitt's influence. Their own conclusion was that "children under fourteen may participate in clinical investigation which is not for their benefit where the studies are sound, promise important new knowledge for mankind, and there is no discernible risk."[23] The editors of Archives of Disease in Childhood recently endorsed this same conclusion, adding only "the necessity of informed parental consent."[24] Discussing relatively minor procedures such as weighing a baby, skin pricks, venipunctures, etc., they contend that "whether or not these procedures are acceptable must depend, it seems to us, on whether the potential gain to others is commensurate with the discomfort to the individual." They see the Medical Research Council's statement as an understandable but exaggerated reaction to the shocking disclosures of the Nazi era. A new value judgment is required in our time, one based on the low risk/benefit ratio.

This same attitude is proposed by Alan M. W. Porter.[25] He argues that there are grounds "for believing that it may be permissible and reasonable to undertake minor procedures on children for experimental purposes with the permission of the parents." The low risk/benefit ratio is the ultimate justification. Interestingly, Porter reports the reactions of colleagues and the public to a research protocol he had drawn up. He desired to study the siblings of children who had succumbed to "cot death." The research

21 N. Baumslag and R. E. Yodaiken, in Letters to the Editor, New England Journal of Medicine, 288 (1973), 1,247.
22 I. Shine, J. Howieson, and W. Griffen, Jr., in Letters to the Editor, New England Journal of Medicine, 288 (1973), 1,248.
23 Beecher, Research and the Individual, 81.
24 Editorial in Archives of the Diseases of Childhood, 48 (1973), 751.
25 A. W. Franklin, A. M. Porter, and D. N. Raine, "New Horizons in Medical Ethics," British Medical Journal, 2 (1973), 402.

involved puncturing a vein (venipuncture). A pediatric authority told Porter that venipuncture was inadmissible under the Medical Research Council code. Astonished, Porter showed the protocol to the first ten colleagues he met. The instinctive reaction of nine out of ten was: "Of course you may." Similarly, a professional market researcher asked (for Porter) ten laymen about the procedure, and all responded that he could proceed. In other words, Porter argues that public opinion (and therefore, presumably, moral common sense) stands behind the low risk/benefit ratio approach to experimentation on children.

This sampling is sufficient indication of the variety of reactions likely to be encountered when research on children is discussed.

The professional ethicians who have written on this subject have also drawn rather different conclusions. John Fletcher argues that a middle path between autonomy (of the physician) and heteronomy (external control) must be discovered.[26] The Nuremberg rule "does not take account of exceptions which can be controlled and makes no allowance whatsoever for the exercise of professional judgment." It is clear that Fletcher would accept proxy consent in some instances, though he has not fully specified what these would be.

Thomas J. O'Donnell, S.J., notes that, besides informed consent, we also speak of three other modalities of consent.[27] First, there is presumed consent. Life-saving measures that are done on an unconscious patient in an emergency room are done with presumed consent. Second, there is implied consent. The various tests done on a person who undergoes a general checkup are done with implied consent, the consent being contained and implied in the very fact of his coming for a checkup. Finally, there is vicarious consent. This is the case of the parent who consents for therapy on an infant. O'Donnell wonders whether these modalities of consent, already accepted in the therapeutic context, can be extended to the context of clinical investigation (and by this he means research not to the direct benefit of the child). It is his conclusion that vicarious consent can be ethically operative "pro-

26 John Fletcher, "Human Experimentation: Ethics in the Consent Situation," *Law and Contemporary Problems*, 32 (1967), 620.

27 Thomas J. O'Donnell, "Informed Consent," *Journal of the American Medical Association*, 227 (1974), 73.

vided it is contained within the strict limits of a presumed consent (on the part of the subject) proper to clinical research and much narrower than the presumptions that might be valid in a therapeutic context." Practically, this means that O'Donnell would accept the validity of vicarious consent only where "danger is so remote and discomfort so minimal that a normal and informed individual would be presupposed to give ready consent." O'Donnell discusses neither the criteria nor the analysis that would set the "strict limits of a presumed consent."

Princeton's Paul Ramsey is the ethician who has discussed this problem at greatest length.[28] He is in clear disagreement with the positions of Fletcher and O'Donnell. Ramsey denies the validity of proxy consent in nonbeneficial (to the child) experiments simply and without qualification. Why? We may not, he argues, submit a child either to procedures that involve any measure of risk of harm or to procedures that involve no harm but simply "offensive touching." "A subject can be wronged without being harmed," he writes. This occurs whenever he is used as an object, or as a means only rather than also as an end in himself. Parents cannot consent to this type of thing, regardless of the significance of the experiment. Ramsey sees the morality of experimentation on children to be exactly what Paul Freund has described as the law on the matter: "The law here is that parents may consent for the child if the invasion of the child's body is for the child's welfare or benefit."[29]

In pursuit of his point, Ramsey argues as follows: "To attempt to consent for a child to be made an experimental subject is to treat a child as not a child. It is to treat him as if he were an adult person who has consented to become a joint adventurer in the common cause of medical research. If the grounds for this are alleged to be the presumptive or implied consent of the child, that must simply be characterized as a violent and false presumption." Thus he concludes simply that "no parent is morally competent to consent that his child shall be submitted to hazardous *or other*

[28] Ramsey, *Patient as Person*. Ramsey has also continued his discussion of this matter in *Biological Revolution: Theological Impact*, 51. This title contains the proceedings of a conference held April 6, 1973 (see footnote 31).
[29] Paul Freund, "Ethical Problems in Human Experimentation," *New England Journal of Medicine*, 273 (1965), 691.

experiments having no diagnostic or therapeutic significance for the child himself" (emphasis added). Though he does not say so, Ramsey would certainly conclude that a law that tolerates proxy consent to any purely experimental procedure is one without moral warrants—indeed, is immoral because it legitimates (or tries to) treating a human being as a means only.

A careful study, then, of the legal, medical, and ethical literature on proxy consent for nontherapeutic research on children reveals profoundly diverging views. Generally, the pros and cons are spelled out in terms of two important values: individual integrity, and societal good through medical benefits. Furthermore, in attempting to balance these two values, this literature by and large either affirms or denies the moral legitimacy of a risk/benefit ratio, what ethicians refer to as a teleological calculus. It seems to me that in doing this, current literature has not faced this tremendously important and paradigmatic issue at its most fundamental level. For instance, Ramsey bases his prohibitive position on the contention that nonbeneficial experimental procedures make an "object" of an individual. Consent is the heart of the matter. If the parents could legitimately consent for the child, then presumably experimental procedures would not make an object of the infant and would be permissible. Therefore, the basic question seems to be: Why cannot the parents provide consent for the child? Why is their consent considered null here while it is accepted when procedures are therapeutic? To say that the child would be treated as an object does not answer this question; it seems that it presupposes the answer and announces it under this formulation.

There is in traditional moral theology a handle that may allow us to take hold of this problem at a deeper root and arrive at a principled and consistent position, one that takes account of all the values without arbitrarily softening or suppressing any of them. That handle is the notion of parental consent, particularly the theoretical implications underlying it. If this can be unpacked a bit, perhaps a more satisfying analysis will emerge. Parental consent is required and sufficient for therapy directed at the child's own good. We refer to this as vicarious consent. It is closely related to presumed consent—that is, it is morally valid precisely insofar as it is a reasonable presumption of the child's wishes, a construction of what the child would wish could he consent for himself. But here the notion of "what the child would wish" must be pushed farther if we are to avoid a simple imposition of the adult world on the child. Why *would* the child so wish? The answer seems to be that he would choose this if he were capable of choice because he *ought* to do so. This statement roots in a traditional natural-law understanding of human moral obligations such as I have outlined in Chapter 1 (pp. 3).

In summary, then, the natural-law tradition argues that there are certain identifiable values that we *ought* to support, attempt to realize, and never directly suppress because they are definitive of our flourishing and well-being. It further argues that knowledge of these values and of the prescriptions and proscriptions associated with them are, in principle, available to human reason— that is, they require for their discovery no divine revelation.

What does all this have to do with the moral legitimacy of proxy consent? It was noted that parental (proxy, vicarious) consent is required and sufficient for therapy directed to the child's own good. It was further noted that it is morally valid precisely insofar as it is a reasonable presumption of the child's wishes, a construction of what the child would wish could he do so. Finally, it was suggested that the child *would* wish this therapy because he *ought* to do so. In other words, a construction of what the child *would* wish (presumed consent) is not an exercise in adult capriciousness and arbitrariness, subject to an equally capricious denial or challenge when the child comes of age. It is based, rather, on two assertions: (1) that there are certain values (in this case, life itself) definitive of our good and flourishing, hence values that we *ought* to choose and support if we want to become and stay human, and that therefore these are good also for the child; and (2) that these "ought" judgments, at least in their more general formulations, are a common patronage available to all men, and hence form the basis on which policies can be built.

Specifically, then, I would argue that parental consent is morally legitimate where therapy on the child is involved, precisely because we know that life and health are goods for the child, that he *would* choose them because he *ought* to choose the good of life, his own self-preservation as long as this life remains, all things considered, a human good. To see whether and to what extent this type of moral analysis applies to experimentation, we must ask: Are there other things that the child *ought*, as a human being, to choose precisely because and insofar as they are goods definitive of his growth and flourishing? Concretely, *ought* he to choose his own involvement in nontherapeutic experimentation, and to what extent? Certainly there are goods or benefits, at least potential, involved. But are they goods that the child *ought* to choose? Or again, if we can argue that a certain level of involvement in nontherapeutic experimentation is good for the child and therefore that he *ought* to choose it, then there are grounds for saying that parental consent for this is morally legitimate and should be recognized as such.

Perhaps a beginning can be made as follows. To pursue the good that is human life means not only to choose and support this value in one's own case, but also in the case of others when the opportunity arises. In other words, the individual *ought* also to take into account, realize, and make efforts in behalf of the lives of others also, for we are social beings, and the goods that define our growth and invite to it are goods that reside also in others. It can be good for one to pursue and support this good in others. Therefore, when it factually is good, we may say that one *ought* to do so (as opposed to not doing so). If this is true of all of us up to a point and within limits, it is no less true of the infant. He would choose to do so because he *ought* to do so. Now, to support and realize the value that is life means to support and realize health, the cure of disease, and so on. Therefore, up to a point, this support and this realization are good for all of us individually. To share in the general effort and burden of health maintenance and disease control is part of our flourishing and growth as humans. To the extent that it is good for all of us to share this burden, we all *ought* to do so. And to the extent that we *ought* to do so, it is a reasonable construction or presumption of our wishes to say that we would do so. The reasonableness of this presumption validates vicarious consent.

It was just noted that sharing in the common burden of progress in medicine constitutes an individual good for all of us *up to a point*. That qualification is crucially important. It suggests that there are limits beyond which sharing is not or might not be a good. What might be the limits of this sharing? When might it no longer be a good for all individuals and therefore something that all need not choose to do? I would develop the matter as follows.

Let me repeat here what I noted earlier. Adults may donate (*inter vivos*) an organ precisely because their personal good is not to be conceived individualistically but socially—that is, there is a natural order to other human persons that is in the very notion of the human personality itself. The personal being and good of an individual do have a relationship to the being and good of others, difficult as it may be to keep this in a balanced perspective. For this reason, an individual can become (in carefully delimited circumstances) more fully a person by donation of an organ, for by communicating to another of his very being he has more fully integrated himself into the mysterious unity between person and person.

Something similar can be said of participation in nontherapeutic experimentation. It can be an affirmation of one's solidarity and Christian concern for others (through advancement of medicine). Becoming an experimental subject can involve any or all of three things: some degree of risk (at least of complications), pain, and associated inconvenience (for example, prolonging hospital stay, delaying recovery, etc.). To accept these for the good of others could be an act of charitable concern.

There are two qualifications to these general statements that must immediately be made, and these qualifications explain the phrase "up to a point." First, whether it is personally good for an individual to donate an organ or participate in experimentation is a very circumstantial and therefore highly individual affair. For some individuals, these undertakings could be or prove to be humanly destructive. Much depends on their personalities, past family life, maturity, future position in life, etc. The second and more important qualification is that these procedures become human goods for the donor or subject precisely because and therefore only when they are voluntary, for the personal good under discussion is the good of expressed charity. For these two reasons I would conclude that no one else can make such decisions for an individual—that is, reasonably presume his consent. He has a right to make them for himself. In other words, whether a person *ought* to do such things is a highly individual affair and cannot be generalized in the way the good of self-preservation can be. And if we cannot say of an individual that he *ought* to do these things, proxy consent has no reasonable presumptive basis.

But are there situations where such considerations are not involved and where the presumption of consent is reasonable, because we may continue to say of all individuals that (other things being equal) they *ought* to be willing? I believe so. For instance, where organ donation is involved, if the only way a young child could be saved were by a blood transfusion from another child, I suspect that few would find such blood donation an unreasonable presumption on the child's wishes. The reason for the presumption is, I believe, that a great good is provided for another at almost no cost to the child. As the scholastics put it, *parum pro nihilo reputatur* (very little counts for nothing). For this reason we may say, lacking countervailing individual evidence, that the individual *ought* to do this.

Could the same reasoning apply to experimentation? Concretely, when a particular experiment would involve no discernible risks, no notable pain, no notable inconvenience, and yet hold promise of considerable benefit, should not the child be constructed to wish this in the same way we presume he chooses his own life, because he *ought* to? I believe so. He *ought* to want this not because it is in any way for his own medical good, but because it is not in any realistic way to his harm, and represents a potentially great benefit for others. He *ought* to want these benefits for others.

If this is a defensible account of the meaning and limits of presumed consent where those incompetent to consent are concerned, it means that proxy consent can be morally legitimate in some experimentations. Which? Those that are scientifically well designed (and therefore offer hope of genuine benefit), that cannot succeed unless children are used (because there are dangers involved in interpreting terms such as "discernible" and "negligible," the child should not unnecessarily be exposed to these even minimal risks), that contain no discernible risk or undue discomfort for the child. Here it must be granted that the notions of "discernible risk" and "undue discomfort" are themselves slippery and difficult, and probably somewhat relative. They certainly involve a value judgment and one that is the heavy responsibility of the medical profession (not the moral theologian) to make. For example, perhaps it can be debated whether venipuncture involves "discernible risks" or "undue discomfort" or not. But if it can be concluded that, in human terms, the risk involved or the discomfort is negligible or insignificant, then I believe there are sound reasons in moral analysis for saying that parental consent to this type of invasion can be justified.

Practically, then, I think there are good moral warrants for adopting the position espoused by Curran, Beecher, Ingelfinger, the Helsinki Declaration, the *Archives of Disease in Childhood*, and others. Some who have adopted this position have argued it in terms of a low risk/benefit ratio. This is acceptable if properly understood—that is, if "low risk" means for all practical purposes and in human judgment "no realistic risk." If it is interpreted in any other way, it opens the door wide to a utilitarian subordination of the individual to the collectivity. It goes beyond what individuals would want because they *ought* to. For instance, in light of the above analysis, I find totally unacceptable the DHEW statement that "the investigator must also stipulate either that the risk to the subjects will be insignificant, or that *although some risk exists, the potential benefit is significant and far outweighs that risk*" (emphasis added). This goes beyond what all of us, as members of the community, necessarily *ought* to do. Therefore, it is an invalid basis for proxy consent. For analogous reasons, in light of the foregoing analysis I would conclude that parental consent for a kidney transplant from one noncompetent three-year-old to another is without moral justification.

In arguing a position that would not allow even that amount of experimentation on children proposed here, Ramsey has stated that this presumptive consent "must simply be characterized as a violent and a false presumption."[30] In developing this thought, he states that "a well child, or a child not suffering from an unrelated disease not being investigated, is not to be compared to an unconscious patient needing specific treatment. To imply the latter's 'constructive' consent is not a violent presumption, it is a life-saving presumption, though it is in some degree 'false.'" A careful analysis of this argument will reveal that for Ramsey the presump-

[30] Ramsey, *Patient as Person*, 14.

tion is nonviolent precisely because it is life-saving for the individual. Furthermore, he would in logic have to argue that whatever invasion is not life-saving for the individual concerned is violent if the individual does not consent thereto. I have attempted to show that this is too narrow. Rather, I would suggest that the presumption of consent to this life-saving therapy is nonviolent, not precisely and exclusively because it is life-saving but because, being such, it is something the individual would want because he *ought* to want it. I would further propose that there are good warrants for saying that there are other things an individual, as a social being, *ought* to want, and, to the extent that we may say this of him, then presumption of his consent is nonviolent—that is, reasonable.

This point is at the heart of the discussion and calls for a rewording. Ramsey does not believe we may "construct" or presume an infant's consent in nonbeneficial experimentation because submission to such experimentation pertains to the realm of charity; and one may not construe that an individual is consenting to works of charity.[31]

His argument moves in two steps. First, there is, he notes, "a difference between justice and charity. Charity, of course, is of highest excellence. But the thing one must imply about a child is not that he's charitable. In other words, let's not confuse the realms of nature and grace. You don't imply he's charitable. That comes by grace. That's his moral maturity. Later he can be charitable. Charity is itself not something one can extrapolate and presume to be the good of this child."

Second, to buttress this point, Ramsey attempts to see where such constructive consent would take us if once we allow it for any nonbeneficial experimentation. "Just think of the kind of constructive consents we could imply for children. You can imply, you can construe, that out of all charity this fetus doesn't want to be born because it's the seventeenth. If he's got any sense he doesn't want to fatally increase the poverty of his home. . . . I do not see where one could rationally stop in construing all sorts of works of mercy and self-sacrifice on the part of persons, not them-

31 Ramsey, in "Proceedings of the Institute for Theological Encounter with Science and Technology (ITEST)," 27 (Apr. 1973).

selves capable by nature or grace yet of being the subjects of charity."

This is a very strong argument and deserves to be taken with utmost seriousness. However, I believe some qualification is called for. Does all nonbeneficial experimentation on this infant pertain to what Ramsey calls "charitable works"? By this term, Ramsey obviously refers to works of supererogation, works that not all men just by being members of the human race are held to or *ought* to do. This is the key. It can be argued, and I think successfully, that there are some things that all of us, simply as members of the human community, *ought* to do for others. These are not works of supererogation, nor works of "charity" in this sense. Here the problem of semantics intrudes. If any involvement in nontherapeutic experimentation must be said to be "charitable" (in the strict sense—that is, beyond what is required of all of us and supererogatory), then Ramsey is correct. But some of these choices seem to pertain to the area of social justice, one's personal bearing of his share of the burden that all may flourish and prosper. Therefore, they are choices that all *ought* to make. In other words, these choices do not pertain to charity, or not at least to charity in Ramsey's sense, a sense where ordinary, nonheroic responses get collapsed into and identified with heroic and extraordinary responses.

The distinction I am suggesting, therefore, is that between those works that not all of us can be expected to make and those that all of us can be expected to make. To the former category belong choices involving notable risk, discomfort, inconvenience. Whether it is good for one to make these choices, whether therefore he *ought* to make them, is a highly circumstantial affair and cannot be said of all of us in general. These are the works to which, theologically, the particular invitations of the Spirit inspire. They are the works of individual generosity and charity. No presumptive consent is in place here.

But we can establish a baseline and discover other works that involve no notable disadvantages to individuals yet offer genuine hope for general benefit. It is good for all of us to share in these (unless we are by particular and accidental circumstances so weakened that even trivial procedures would constitute a threat to us), and hence we all *ought* to want these benefits for others. And if that is true, a presumption of consent is reasonable, and vicarious consent becomes legitimate. In summary, there are some experiments in children that do not pertain to charity in Ramsey's sense —charity as supererogation—and hence do not demand individualization before they can be said to be goods the individual would choose.

Now to Ramsey's second buttressing argument—the slippery slope. "I do not see where one could rationally stop in construing all sorts of works of mercy and self-sacrifice, etc." One stops and should stop precisely at the point where "constructed" consent does indeed involve self-sacrifice or works of mercy, the point beyond which not all of us are called but only individuals inspired by the Spirit to do "the more," the sacrificial thing. This dividing line is reached when experiments involve discernible risk, undue discomfort, or inconvenience.

Ramsey's reluctance or inability to make this distinction is traceable to the fact that he has not analyzed more deeply the validity of proxy consent in therapeutic situations. He states: "An 'implied' or 'constructive' consent—proxy consent—clearly is in order in the case of investigational therapeutic trials (beneficial research) when the patient/subject is incapable for any reason of giving actual consent." True. But why true? If one answers, as Ramsey does, that it is true because where therapeutic research is involved the patient/subject *would* give consent, he has not gone far enough. The patient *would* give consent because therapeutic research is (or can be) something for his own good and to which, therefore, he *ought* to consent. Reasonable presumption or construction of consent is rooted in this. And it suggests immediately the possibility that there may be other procedures that are not necessarily to the individual's therapeutic good but that still represent a good to others, a good to which he, like all of us, *ought* also to consent. Once, therefore, the validity of proxy consent is traced to its deepest roots, we will see both its further legitimate extensions and its limitations.

These considerations do not mean that all noncompetents (where consent is concerned) may be treated in the same way, that the same presumptions are morally legitimate in all cases. For if the circumstances of the infant or child differ markedly, then it is possible that there are appropriate modifications in our construction of what he *ought* to choose. For instance, I believe that institutionalized infants demand special consideration. They are in a situation of peculiar danger for several reasons. First, they are often in a disadvantaged condition physically or mentally, so that there is a temptation to regard them as "lesser human beings." Medical history shows our vulnerability to this type of judgment. Second, as institutionalized, they are a controlled group, making them particularly tempting as research subjects. Third, experimentation in such infants is less exposed to public scrutiny. These and other considerations suggest that there is a real danger of overstepping the line between what we all ought to want and what only the individual might want out of heroic, self-sacrificial charity. If such a real danger exists, then what the infant is construed as wanting because he *ought* must be modified. He need not *ought to want* if this involves him in real dangers of going beyond this point.

One test of an analysis is its appeal to common sense. Indispensable as this test certainly is, common sense can occasionally trip us up and turn out to be an appealing but deceptive cover for our own distorted perspectives and enthusiasms. Therefore, the validity of the analysis of proxy consent proposed here needs to be further tested by sampling its connections and consistency with other related matters. Transplantation of organs between infants has already been mentioned. Relatively trivial invasions (blood transfusions?) that are life-saving for the recipient would seem to be a sound basis for proxy consent if the benefit envisaged is otherwise unobtainable. It is suggested that the same is not true where more substantial deprivation is concerned. Case precedent has so far failed either to confirm or to deny this analysis, since, in allowing a kidney transplant from a noncompetent, it has based the decision on the donor's good—the psychological harm he would suffer if the transplant were not done now.

Another instance is that of parental decision over supporting an infant's life or allowing the child to die. It would be generally accepted among both moral theologians and physicians that not every infant need be saved by use of all available means. This is but an application to infants of a rather standard and settled moral teaching about the use of ordinary and extraordinary means to sustain life. Some means are extraordinary (or "heroic," as physicians often say), and generally speaking (per se or as a general rule, as theologians say) no one is morally bound to preserve his own life by use of such means, though he is free to do so if he wishes. The same reasoning surely should apply to infants. There are contemporary instances, of course, where application of the distinction between ordinary and extraordinary measures becomes extremely difficult and the source of a good deal of controversy. This is especially true of infants in cases involving crippling deformity and/or severe retardation. That need not concern us here. What is important is the general validity of the distinction.

Once it is accepted that one need not per se use extraordinary measures to preserve life and that this is true also of infants, it remains only to ask who is to make this decision for the child. It is generally granted that this is a parental responsibility. In other words, just as parental consent is required and sufficient for therapeutic measures in this child, so it is the parents who must decide when this consent to therapy is to be withheld. However, just as parental consent to therapy is not arbitrary and capricious but represents a reasonable presumption of the infant's wishes because he *ought* to want to preserve his life, so denial of consent must be traced to what the child would not want because it is beyond what he *ought* to want. This is a more difficult construction, of course, because though one need not employ extraordinary measures, he is free to do so. And it is difficult to construct the consent of a child in those areas where anyone is free to accept or reject certain measures. Nevertheless, it seems to be true that the only basis on which to found the moral meaningfulness and validity of parental denial of consent is that the infant is in a situation where we need no longer say that he *ought* to choose to preserve his life. It is because of this that proxy denial of consent makes sense and avoids being simply an exercise of parental utilitarianism. To base this denial of consent on what the child *would* do without further specification hinges the decision to considerations that are both too individualistic and too adult to form the basis of an intelligible generalization.

This is confirmed, it would seem, by occasional court overrule of parental denial of consent. Whether this or that overrule was in fact correct is, of course, debatable. But the very fact that we grant that a court can overrule parental denial of consent is instructive. The very possibility of court overrule implies two things. First, it implies that parental consent or denial thereof cannot be unrelated to the good of the child, but is sometimes judged to be so unrelated. Second, it implies that the court recognizes this unrelatedness, knows what is for the good of the child, and has criteria for its determination. Otherwise its overrule would be as arbitrary as the decision overruled. But the court cannot know better than the parents (or any of us) what is for the good of the child, and therefore what the child *would* choose unless this *would* roots in what the infant would do because he *ought*. In summary, if we cannot say of the child that life is a good to him and a good he *ought* to choose to preserve, then court overrule of parental denial of treatment seems arbitrary—indeed, an exercise of medical vitalism.

The editor of the *Journal of the American Medical Association,* Robert H. Moser, in the course of an editorial touching on, among other things, the problem of experimentation, asks whether we are ever justified in the use of children. His answer: "It is an insoluble dilemma. All one can ask is that each situation be studied with consummate circumspection and be approached rationally and compassionately."[32] If circumspection in each situation is to be truly consummate, and if the approach is to be rational and compassionate, then the situation alone cannot be the decisional guide. If the situation alone is the guide, if everything else is a "dilemma," then the qualities Moser seeks in the situation are in jeopardy, and along with them human rights. One can indeed, to paraphrase Moser, ask more than that each situation be studied. He can ask that a genuine ethics of consent be brought to the situation so that ethics in the consent situation will have some chance of surviving human enthusiasms. And an ethics of consent finds its roots in a solid natural-law tradition that maintains that there are basic values that define our potential as human beings; that we ought (within limits and with qualifications) to choose, support, and never directly suppress these values in our conduct; that we can know, therefore, what others would choose (up to a point) because they ought; and that this knowledge is the basis for a soundly grounded and rather precisely limited proxy consent.

[32] R. H. Moser, in an editorial entitled "An Anti-Intellectual Movement in Medicine?" *Journal of the American Medical Association,* 227 (1974), 432.

5. Public Policy and Fetal Research

[The National Research Act (July 1974) created the National Commission for the Protection of Human Subjects of Biomedical and Behavioral Research. The Act also mandated an investigation of fetal research and asked for a recommendation about the circumstances, if any, under which DHEW ought to conduct or support such research. The following study resulted from a mandate by the National Commission to suggest what public policy on this matter ought to be.]

Before sound public-policy proposals can be developed, for the regulation of fetal research as for any other public issue, the relationship between public policy and morality must be clarified.

Morality concerns itself with the rightness or wrongness of our conduct. Law or public policy, on the other hand, is concerned with the common good. Clearly, then, morality and public policy are both related and distinct. They are related because law or public policy has an inherently moral character due to its rootage in existential human ends (goods). The common good of all persons cannot be unrelated to what is judged to be promotive or destructive to the individual—in other words, judged to be moral or immoral. Morality and public policy are distinct because it is only when individual acts have ascertainable public consequences on the maintenance and stability of society that they are the proper concerns of society, fit subjects for public policy.

Once this point has been made, several additional clarifications are in order. First, what actions ought to be controlled by policy is determined not merely by the immorality of the action, but beyond this by a single criterion: feasibility. Feasibility is "that quality whereby a proposed course of action is not merely possible but practicable, adaptable, depending on the circumstances, cultural ways, attitudes, traditions of a people. . . ."[1] Feasibility, therefore, looks to questions such as: Will the policy be obeyed? Is it enforceable? Is it prudent to undertake this or that ban in view of possibly harmful effects in other sectors of social life? Can control be achieved short of coercive measures? The answer to the feasibility test depends on the temperature of a society at any given moment in its history.

I make this point in discussing fetal experimentation because the feasibility test is particularly difficult in our society and will profoundly affect the Commission's policy proposals. Ultimately public policy must find a basis in the deepest moral perceptions of the majority or, if not, at least in principles the majority is reluctant to modify.[2] This means that it is especially difficult to apply the feasibility test where fetal experiments are concerned, for the good itself whose legal possibility is under discussion is an object of doubt and controversy—that is, the moral assessment of fetal life and value differs.

A second point to be made is that policy will not infrequently go beyond morality. Concretely, while one might morally justify this or that experimental procedure on the fetus, the danger of abuse or miscalculation might be so considerable as to call for a policy ban, or safe-side regulatory cautions. It is one thing, for instance, to justify morally a single sterilization on a mentally retarded girl in her own best interests. However, when one sees five years later that one's moral reasoning has been used to sterilize a hundred thousand indigent blacks, then an exceptionless policy may be called for, or at least safe-side regulations to prevent such abuse.

By the term "experimentation" as used here, I understand all procedures not directly beneficial to the subject involved. (There is little moral problem and should be little policy problem where procedures are experimental but represent the most hopeful therapy for an individual.) By the term "nonviable fetus" I understand a fetus incapable of extra-uterine survival. (Attention in this study will be restricted to the nonviable fetus because I shall sup-

[1] Paul J. Micallef, "Abortion and the Principles of Legislation," *Laval théologique et philosophique*, 28 (1972), 294.

[2] Roger L. Shinn, "Personal Decisions and Social Policies in a Pluralist Society," *Perkins Journal*, 27 (1973), 58–63.

pose that in all decisively relevant moral and policy respects touching experimentation, the viable fetus should be treated as a child.) The nonviable fetus, as an experimental subject, could be further subdivided as follows:

in utero	*ex utero*
no abortion planned	spontaneous abortion
abortion planned	living
dead	
during abortion	induced abortion
	living
	dead

The literature on morality and fetal experimentation (to be reported below) is very sparse.[3] What does exist has drawn attention to the analogies with experiments on children. However, at least two things must be noted about this analogy. First, whether the question of fetal experimentation approximates, and indeed is, in most crucial respects identical with experimentation on children depends on one's assessment of fetal life. If one regards the fetus as "disposable maternal tissue" or as "potential human life" only, then the questions are sharply different and will yield a different moral conclusion, and ultimately a different public policy. If, however, the nonviable fetus is viewed as "protectable humanity" or a "person" with rights, then the problems are quite similar. Second, the nonviable fetus (whether abortion is contemplated or not) is in a dependency relationship, its health and growth being linked more or less to maternal health. This relationship can be read in a variety of ways in terms of its ethical yield. But one thing all would agree on is that whatever fetal experimentation is judged to be warranted, it must take account of maternal health.

Thus while there are possible differences in these two problems (experiments on children and fetuses), there are important continuities. If one judges all experimentation on living children (even if they are dying) to be an abuse and immoral, and at the same time regards the nonviable fetus as a person in its own right

[3] See especially Paul Ramsey, *The Ethics of Fetal Research* (New Haven: Yale University Press, 1975); LeRoy Walters, "Ethical Issues in Experimentation on the Human Fetus," *Journal of Religious Ethics*, 2 (1974), 33–75.

(even though within a dependency symbiosis), it is safe to say that one will condemn (morally) all experimentation on living fetuses in whatsoever condition they be. Contrarily, if one morally justifies some experimentation on children, it is quite possible, though not inevitable, that one could and would extend this justification to fetuses.

There are two identifiable schools of (moral) thought where experimentation on children is concerned. The first is associated with Paul Ramsey[4] and is supported by William E. May.[5] The second is the position of Curran,[6] O'Donnell,[7] and myself.[8] Ramsey argues that we may not submit a child to procedures that involve any risk of harm or to procedures that involve no harm but simply "offensive touching. . . ."

Thomas O'Donnell accepts the moral validity of vicarious consent where the "danger is so remote and discomfort so minimal that a normal and informed individual would be presupposed to give ready consent."[9] Charles Curran has drawn a similar conclusion. . . .[10]

I have attempted to argue for a position that would allow experimentation on children where there is no discernible risk or undue discomfort.[11] The position departs from Ramsey practically only if he disallows any give and play with the term "discernible risk." More importantly, it is at one with Ramsey's analysis in rejecting any utilitarian evaluation of children's lives that would submit their integrity to a quantity-of-benefits calculus far beyond any legitimately constructed consent. The heart of my argument is this: If we analyze proxy consent where it is accepted as legitimate—in the *therapeutic* situation—we will see that parental consent is morally legitimate because, life and health being goods for the

[4] Paul Ramsey, *The Patient as Person* (New Haven: Yale University Press, 1970), 27–40.
[5] William E. May, "Experimentation on Human Subjects," *Linacre Quarterly*, 41 (1974), 238–52.
[6] Charles E. Curran, "Human Life," *Chicago Studies*, 13 (1974), 293.
[7] Thomas J. O'Donnell, "Informed Consent," *Journal of the American Medical Association*, 227 (1974), 73.
[8] Richard A. McCormick, S.J., "Proxy Consent in the Experimentation Situation," *Perspectives in Biology and Medicine*, 18 (Autumn 1974), 2–20.
[9] O'Donnell, "Informed Consent," 73.
[10] Curran, "Human Life," 293.
[11] McCormick, "Proxy Consent," 2–20.

child, he would choose them because he *ought* to choose the good of life. In other words, proxy consent is morally valid precisely insofar as it is a reasonable presumption of the child's wishes, a construction of what the child would wish could he do so. The child would so choose because he *ought* to do so, life and health being goods definitive of his flourishing.

Once proxy consent in the therapeutic situation is analyzed in this way, this question occurs: Are there other things that the child *ought*, as a human being, to choose precisely because and insofar as they are goods definitive of his well-being? As an answer to this question I have suggested that there are things we *ought* to do for others simply because we are members of the human community. These are not precisely works of charity or supererogation (beyond what is required of all of us) but our personal bearing of our share that all may prosper. They involve no discernible risk, discomfort, or inconvenience, yet promise genuine hope for general benefit. In summary, if it can be argued that it is good for all of us to share in these experiments, and hence that we *ought* to do so (social justice), then a presumption of consent where children are involved is reasonable, and proxy consent becomes legitimate.

The moral reasoning outlined above yields a conclusion that is shared, at a practical level, by Curran, Beecher,[12] Ingelfinger,[13] the Helsinki Declaration,[14] the *Archives of Disease in Childhood*,[15] and others. Yet it has built into it rational limits and controls not always present in merely practical statements.

With this as a background we now turn to fetal experimentation itself. What one judges to be morally appropriate and acceptable where fetal experiments are concerned depends above all on his evaluation of the fetus. Here there are two general schools of thought. The first would regard the fetus as a nonperson or as "potential human life." These terms are used in the moral sense, not in the legal sense, though it is clear that one who

[12] H. K. Beecher, *Research and the Individual* (Boston: Little, Brown, 1970); see also W. J. Curran and H. K. Beecher, "Experimentation in Children," *Journal of the American Medical Association*, 210 (1969), 77.

[13] Franz J. Ingelfinger, "Ethics of Experiments on Children," *New England Journal of Medicine*, 288 (1973), 791.

[14] Beecher, *Research and the Individual*. Cf. Chapter 4.

[15] Editorial in *Archives of the Diseases of Childhood*, 48 (1973), 751.

is not a person morally should not be considered such legally. At any rate, one who is not a *moral* person, who is morally a nonperson—and therefore not the subject of rights and claims—seems to present little problem where experimentation is concerned. One who holds this position ought to conclude, if his moral reasoning is consistent, that experimentation on the fetus is legitimate and desirable, or if there are to be restrictions, they are rooted in values other than the fetus itself in its present state.

The second general school of thought is that the fetus is, indeed, protectable, a protectable humanity, and an appropriate subject of rights. Within this school of thought, three distinct tendencies or subdivisions are identifiable.

1. The fetus is protectable humanity but to be valued less than a viable fetus or a born infant. This school would probably tolerate experiments if the benefits are great, but no literature has made this conclusion explicit.

2. The fetus is a fellow human being and must be treated, where experimentation is concerned, exactly as one treats the child. Just as the child may not be exposed not only to harm and risk, but also to "offensive touching," so the fetus may not be exposed to any risk or even to "offensive touching." This would seem to be the position of Ramsey.[16] Concretely at one point the nonviable fetus is to be likened to an unconscious patient; at another point the nonviable living fetus (after instances of spontaneous or induced abortion) is to be likened to a dying patient; prior to an induced abortion the fetus is to be likened to the condemned. Since it is immoral to experiment on the unconscious, and without their consent, on the condemned or dying, it is immoral to experiment on the fetus—and this would apply even to "offensive touching." In logic Ramsey ought to conclude that *no* experimentation on living fetuses is morally warranted.

3. The fetus is a fellow human being and ought to be treated, where experimentation is concerned, exactly as one treats the child. However, experiments on children, where no discernible risk or discomfort is involved, are morally legitimate if appropriate consent is obtained and if the experiments are genuinely necessary (trials on animals being insufficient) for medical knowledge calcu-

[16] Ramsey, *The Ethics of Fetal Research.* Cf. note 3.

lated to be of notable benefit to fetuses or children in general. This is an extension to the fetus of the moderate position on children outlined above. It is, I believe, a defensible moral position— but the way the position is defended is utterly crucial (I shall return to this below) if sufficient protection of human subjects is to be assured.

The position just outlined is the one I would attempt to defend and the one I proposed to the Commission as the basis for its policy proposals. But since the fetus can be in a variety of postures or situations, this general approach must be carefully applied to this variety of postures. I emphasize here that I am discussing for the present a *moral* position (not immediately what public policy ought to be) and one that reflects *my own views*.

For purposes of clarity and precision, let me now return to the definition of those terms with which I began this section.

A. *The Fetus* in Utero

1. *No abortion planned.* Theoretically, if there is no discernible risk or discomfort to the fetus and to the mother, and appropriate proxy consent is obtained, such experimentation could be defended as morally legitimate—on the same grounds that identical experiments on children could be defended. Practically, however, one must question the necessity of experimentation here (a factual matter). If fetal material is otherwise available, experimentation here would be inappropriate precisely as unnecessary.

2. *Abortion planned.* Here a preliminary general reflection is in order. It applies to the fetus prior to abortion, during abortion, and after abortion (whether the fetus be living or dead). It is the issue of cooperation. If one objects to most abortions being performed in our society as immoral, is it morally proper to derive experimental profit from the products of such an abortion system? Is the progress achieved through such experimentation not likely to blunt the sensitivities of Americans to the immorality (injustice) of the procedure that made such advance possible, and thereby entrench attitudes injurious and unjust to nascent life? This is, in my judgment, a serious moral objection to experimentation on the products of most induced abortions (whether the fetus be living or dead, prior to abortion or postabortional). It is especially relevant in a society where abortion is widely done and legally protected.

However, I have no confidence that a society that does not share the underlying judgment on most abortions and is so highly pragmatic as to be insensitive to the issue of cooperation will be impressed by this moral consideration—factors that must be taken into account where public policy (feasibility) is concerned; that is, public policy must root in the deepest moral perceptions of the majority, or at least in principles the majority is reluctant to modify. Since there is such profound division on the moral propriety of abortion, the moral notion of cooperation in an abortion system will not function at the level of policy.

a. *Prior to abortion.* One cannot approach the position of the fetus without a further distinction. *If the planned abortion is morally legitimate* (for example, when without abortion both mother and fetus would die), we might say that the fetus is in the situation of the tragically but justly condemned individual. In this instance, if the proposed experimentation will involve no discernible risk to the fetus, I believe that proxy consent (of the mother) would be a defensible construction of fetal wishes. If, however, the proposed experimentation will involve discernible risks to the fetus, then proxy consent is an invalid construction. *If the planned abortion is not morally legitimate,* we might say that the fetus is in the situation of an unjustly condemned individual. In my judgment, this is the case with most abortions now being planned and performed. In this instance, the full moral weight of the cooperation issue strikes home—but once again, not at the policy level, as stated above. Second, there is the issue of consent and its validity. The consent requirement is premised on the fact that the parents are the ones who have the best interests of the child (here the fetus) at heart. But does such a premise obtain when an abortion (presumably immoral) is being planned? Does a mother planning an abortion in the circumstances described have the best interests of the fetus at heart? I think not. Third, there is the possible change of mind of the mother. Allowing experimentation prior to abortion—that is, experimentation that is potentially risky or harmful to the fetus—prejudices the freedom of the woman to change her mind about the abortion, and thus constitutes an infringement on fetal rights for this reason alone, if for no other. To those who do not share my evaluation of fetal life, these considerations will, of course, seem marginally relevant at best.

b. *During abortion.* Once again, a distinction. *If the abortion is morally legitimate,* then granted appropriate proxy consent, experimentation could be legitimate if it left the fetus in no worse position during its dying than it is in as a result of the abortion. If, however, the experimentation leaves the fetus in a worse position —for example, in pain—then it is equivalent to illegitimate experimentation on the dying. *If the abortion is not morally legitimate,* then experimentation on the fetus raises two of the points mentioned above (in subsection a.): cooperation and invalidity of consent. The question of "discernible risk" seems meaningless morally, since it seems meaningless to speak of exposing to risk one who has already been inserted into a lethal situation.

B. *The Fetus* ex Utero

1. *Spontaneous abortion.* The fetus may be either living or dead. If it is dead, there should be no moral objection to experimentation. If the fetus is living, the same conclusion obtains, providing experimentation imposes no pain; for the fetus may be legitimately constructed to consent to experiments involving no discernible risk, and he is in a situation (lethal) where the distinction between no discernible risk and discernible risk is meaningless.

2. *Induced abortion.* The fetus may be either living or dead. If the fetus is still living and the abortion was morally legitimate, then experimentation seems morally legitimate if it induces no pain or discomfort; for if the fetus may be constructed to consent to experiments where no discernible harm is involved, and if he is in a situation (lethal) where the difference between discernible harm or risk is meaningless, then he may be legitimately constructed to consent—given appropriate proxy consent. If the fetus is still living and the abortion was morally illegitimate, then the above issues (cooperation, consent) could intrude to prevent any morally legitimate proxy consent.

C. *Summary*

Within the parameters of *my* evaluation of fetal life, fetal experimentation would be clearly justified, with appropriate safeguards, distinctions, and consent, where the abortion is spontaneous or has been justifiably (morally) induced. Where it has been induced without moral justification, I believe there are moral objections of various sorts against experimentation. However, since these objections are premised on the moral character of the abortion, and since this is a difficult (at times) determination in itself, and since the ultimate judgment will hardly be shared by a majority, these objections will be extremely difficult—indeed, impossible—to formulate in policy proposals on fetal experiments. Moreover, one can question whether restriction on fetal experiments rooted in such considerations is the best way to highlight the moral illegitimacy of the abortion.

Where experimentation is morally justified, it is so because of the legitimacy and sharp limitations of proxy consent, extrapolated from the legitimacy of proxy consent where children are concerned. I wish to emphasize this point here. If proxy consent (with the clear limitations on the validity of this consent) is not the basis for the moral legitimacy of experimentation on fetuses, then the integrity of the individual will be "protected" not by soundly reasoned constructions of what the fetus—or any human being—would consent to because it *ought*, but by a very unpredictable and highly utilitarian assessment of its value and worth as over against great (alleged) scientific and medical benefits for others. Such an assessment does not provide but erodes—in a highly technological, pragmatic society—individual protection. Thus the DHEW's original but tentative version of *Protection of Human Subjects, Policies, and Procedures*[17] stated: "The investigator must also stipulate either that the risk to the subjects [children] will be insignificant, or *that although some risk exists, the potential benefit is significant and far outweighs that risk*" (emphasis added). In such thought and language is the germ—and even more—of the subordination of the individual to the collectivity. That germ is in the conclusion, to be sure; but it is far more insidiously present and threatening in the very way of thinking, in the form of moral reasoning undergirding it. We call it utilitarianism. And whatever the policy proposals this Commission recommends, it will have only gotten mired in the cultural

[17] Department of Health, Education, and Welfare, *Federal Register*, 38 (1973), 31,738.

status quo if its conclusions root in a utilitarian assessment of the value and integrity of man, fetal or otherwise.

Avoidance of this trap will not be easy; for if notable medical benefits do not justify *all* experimentation, they are the only things that justify *any* experimentation. And once that is said, the tendency will be to give medical benefits the preference. Furthermore, if fetal individuality and dignity do not prohibit *all* experiments, they certainly prohibit *some*. It is the first task of this Commission to discover the forms and structures of moral reasoning on which alone the proper protective balance can be based and spelled out in policy proposals. Those forms and structures center around proxy consent, its legitimation and limitations.

I raise this issue prior to an explicit consideration of policy proposals because I presume that in matters of law or policy, consistency is, at least to some extent, a desideratum. From a *moral* point of view fetal experimentation and abortion are in some respects separable issues—that is, even though a particular abortion is judged to be morally justifiable, one could maintain that experimentation on the living abortus is illegitimate experimentation on the dying. And that is a different question from the morality of the abortion itself. There are those who would convert such separability as follows: Even though the abortion was illegitimate, it does not follow that experimentation on the abortus is also illegitimate. (I do not believe the matter is that simple, as noted above.)

However, there is a point at which these issues converge, particularly in the popular mind. This convergence is best seen at the *policy* level. Under existing abortion law (*Doe* v. *Bolton*) fetal life enjoys no protection during the first two trimesters of pregnancy, and even in the third the compelling interest of the state in protecting fetal life is qualified by considerations of maternal health so broadly defined that it would be difficult to convict anyone of an illegal interruption of pregnancy anytime during pregnancy. The rationale for this policy is the predominance of maternal interests, especially privacy, over "potential human life." Now clearly, if fetal life is so totally unprotected *with regard to its very existence and survival*, and on the grounds that it is only "potential human life," then any policy restrictive of fetal experimentation must find other grounds (other than present fetal humanity and rights) for its restrictiveness—at least if legal consistency is to be preserved; for it is patently ridiculous to stipulate that fetal life may be *taken* freely because it is only "potential human life," and yet to prohibit experimentation on this same "potential human life," especially when great medical benefits may be expected from such experimentation, for such a prohibition would imply that the privacy or other interests of one woman are of more value than the survival and health of perhaps thousands of fetuses and infants.

I see no way out of this impasse where the Commission for the Protection of Human Subjects is concerned—except to say that perhaps even legal inconsistency has its values. But the only value perceptible to this commentator in such inconsistency is that it may be a first step toward reassessment of the Court's "potential human life." That may be a salutary step, but it reflects what appear to be the only two options open to this Commission: to reaffirm, by implication, the Court's philosophy in *Roe* v. *Wade*, or to establish proposals (restrictive in character) that are at some point inconsistent with this philosophy. This latter alternative is, in my judgment, the way to go.

In attempting to develop sound (feasible) policies on fetal experimentation, I suggest that the Commission must keep two points in mind: moral pluralism and cultural pragmatism. A word about each.

A. *Moral Pluralism*

Fetal life is variously evaluated, as the abortion decision shows. Even though abortion and experimentation are separable, they are closely related, as I have pointed out. Therefore the Commission is in a very delicate position and is faced potentially with another *Roe* v. *Wade* decision. In a sense the Commission cannot win in its conclusions. If it allows fetal experimentation without sufficient grounding and controls, it will alienate and galvanize those identified with right-to-life positions. If it disallows fetal experiments without sound and consistent reasoning, it will alienate and galvanize the "liberal" and research communities. If it tries to walk a middle path with a utilitarian sliding scale of costs and benefits, most ethicists in the country will be up in arms.

The only way out of this bind (and one that avoids utilitarian cost-benefits theory) is tied to the notion of proxy consent. In other words, that measure of proxy consent regarded as valid for children should be the measure of acceptable fetal experimentation. Where children are concerned, proxy consent is legitimate when the experimentation involves no discernible risks, discomforts, or inconvenience—in human judgment. Beyond that, the individual must be free to consent for himself. Analogously with the fetus. If the experimentation involves no discernible risk —or in cases where the nonviable fetus is dying and in no pain— proxy consent may be regarded as legitimate. (There is a moral problem, of course, with the legitimacy of proxy consent where the fetus is about to be aborted or has been aborted. However, since the moral legitimacy of the abortion itself is a highly disputed point in our society, the legitimacy of proxy consent in these cases cannot be decisive at the level of policy; to wit, it is not presently feasible.)

This practical policy structure (centering on permissibility and controls grounded in proxy consent) has the advantage of speaking to all segments of a divided community. To those convinced of fetal humanity and protectability, it says: Nothing more or less is allowed on the fetus than on the child. To the "liberal" and research community, it states the legitimacy and need of fetal experimentation. To the ethical community it states that the legitimacy and control of fetal experimentation is neither capricious nor utilitarian in character, but soundly and rationally based in and controlled by an intelligible principle.

B. *Cultural Pragmatism*

Our culture is one where: (1) technology, even medical, is highly esteemed; (2) moral judgments tend to collapse into pragmatic cost-benefit calculations; (3) youth, health, pleasure, and comfort are highly valued and tend to be sought and preserved at disproportionate cost; (4) maladaptations, such as senility, retardation, age, or defectiveness, are treated destructively rather than by adapting the environment to their needs. These factors suggest that the general cultural mentality is one that identifies the quickest, most effective way as the good way. Morality often translates into efficiency. This mentality constitutes the atmosphere in which the Commission's policies must be shaped. They are, I believe, calculated to be threatening and inimical to a careful implementation of proxy consent at the fetal-research level. Therefore, I believe that the Commission will best serve the community if it bends toward more protection of individuals, rather than toward more freedom for experimental research. The culture will bend this latter way, and the proposals ought to be conceived as a balancing influence, not simply as a reinforcing one.

If the above reflections are accurate, the task of the Commission (once it has accepted the proxy-consent rationale for experimentation on fetuses) is twofold: first, to spell out insofar as is possible what degree of risk may be regarded, in broad human terms, as equivalent to "no discernible risk"; and second, to detail the procedural demands that will best assure that this determination is realized in individual protocols.

C. Proposals

The following points are suggested as an attempt to bring this twofold task to the level of concrete proposals:

1. *The experiment must be necessary.* Use of animals and dead fetal tissue is not sufficient; the experiment is not repetitive (of work being done elsewhere); proportionate benefits are reasonably anticipated.

The onus of showing necessity is on the experimental researcher.

2. *There must be no discernible risk for the fetus or mother* or, if the fetus is dying, there must be no added pain or discomfort. (This would prohibit all experiments that are aimed at determining what harm might come to the fetus, and all experiments that prolong the dying process of the fetus.)

The onus of showing no discernible risk is on the experimental researcher.

3. *The above demands must be secured by prior approval and adequate review* of all fetal experiments. The reviewing group ought to include at least some members outside of the research community. (There is a tendency, as the literature shows, for researchers to minimize risk not only in terms of prospective benefits, but also in terms of the ability to "handle complications" that may arise.)

If these policies appear to some to be too restrictive, it must be recalled that we shall only know whether they are unduly restrictive if they are tried. It is always possible to liberalize; it is much more difficult to retrench—and retrenchment occurs only after rights have been exposed or violated. Where the rights of others are even and only *possibly* at stake, the part of wisdom and humanity is to try the less obvious, perhaps the more arduous, but more conservative (of rights) way.

6. Sharing in Sociality: Children and Experimentation

The use of children (incompetent to consent) in nontherapeutic research is an extremely delicate and difficult ethical problem. Here I wish to respond to Paul Ramsey's quite interesting commentary on some earlier writings of mine on this subject.[1] But first a public apology is due. In the course of his extended remarks, my colleague and friend confides to us that he had to "stifle his amazement" on at least two occasions. I publicly apologize for being the *agent provocateur* of such unaccustomed asceticism. However, when all is said and done, in his *Report* response to me, Ramsey's attempts at amazement stifling simply collapsed and bubbled-up—as they so often do—by implying that his summary of my argument only skims the surface of its faults. But even so, his attempts must have been painful; so an apology is due.

Now to the issues. First we ought to be clear on Ramsey's position, or better, positions, both of which he describes as "superior to McCormick's." The first regards *any* attempt to consent to experimentation for the child "as a false and violent presumption," for it is to treat a child as not a child. Thus Ramsey's first position

[1] Hereafter all citations of Ramsey are from "The Enforcement of Morals: Nontherapeutic Research on Children," *Hastings Center Report*, 6 (Aug. 1976), 21–30. Ramsey's citations are to my "Proxy Consent in the Experimentation Situation," *Perspectives in Biology and Medicine*, 18 (Autumn 1974), 2–20; these ideas are also expressed in my "Fetal Research, Morality, and Public Policy," *Hastings Center Report*, 5 (June 1975), 26–31, and *Federal Register*, 40 (1975), 335–38. Ramsey relates these two studies to the deliberations of the National Commission for the Protection of Human Subjects and says: "On whose deliberations his writings had considerable influence, as also did those of his colleague LeRoy Walters. . . ." Walters and I would be happy to think that is the case, but the matter of influence remains speculative.

rejects in principle any experimental procedures that involve *any* degree of risk of harm, however minimal. Further, he goes beyond even minimal risk and rejects procedures that involve no risk but simply "offensive touching." "A subject can be wronged without being harmed," he writes. That is certainly true in general; now, whether it is true of nonbeneficial experimentation on infants remains to be seen.

So in Ramsey's view those incapable of consent are simply, without qualification and in principle, out of bounds for nonbeneficial research. Any other view, he argues, involves using the child as a means only and not also as an end.

Whether it was an incipient and intuitive discomfort with the absoluteness of this position or not that led Ramsey to develop another position, I do not know. Nevertheless, he did so. To recapitulate, the position is as follows: "It is better to leave the research imperative in incorrigible conflict with the principle that protects the individual human person from being used for research purposes without either his expressed or correctly construed consent. Some sorts of human experimentation should, in this alternative, be acknowledged to be 'borderline situations' in which moral agents are under the necessity of doing wrong for the sake of the public good. Either way they are wrong. It is immoral not to do the research. It is also immoral to use children who cannot themselves consent and who ought not to be presumed to consent to research unrelated to their treatment." In other words, there are times when we must "sin bravely" in a broken and fallen world.

Ramsey admits that this second "solution" is peculiarly Protestant and he indulges it only as a thought experiment. His heart is with his first position. Yet it is important to ask why Ramsey ever yielded to the idea of departing even that much from his original and purist position. Is it that his own instincts counseled him that something is amiss with a deductive position that makes infants "therapeutic orphans"? I will not speculate further on this matter except to point out that the "sin bravely" and "don't deny the moral force of the imperative he violates" (that is, *must* violate) approach Ramsey suggests may be Protestant; but it is scarcely vintage Ramsey. For instance, he does not see the incidental killing of innocents when a nation repels the enemy's war machine as "sinning bravely" (against the imperative not to kill). He simply changes the rule that what is forbidden is all *direct* killing of innocents. Similarly, when he justifies contraception by appeal to the communicative good in marriage (and how it could harm the procreative good itself), he does not say, "Don't deny the moral force of the imperative you violate." He alters the imperative so that contraception is justified. As I said, his second solution is not vintage Ramsey.

One more introductory note is in order. Ramsey characterizes the position I proposed as "moralistic," and for two reasons. First he says that I want a smooth solution to "this conflict situation." Actually I would have thought that the force of my analysis would be to deny the conflict, a point that will become clearer below. Ramsey can only assert a conflict if he assumes that the position he expresses is the correct one. His second reason for viewing the position as "moralistic" (a pejorative term in most circles) is that it centers around what the child "ought" to do. Once again, such an "ought" is moralistic only if it can be shown to be a false or at least unsupportable construction. But this brings us to the heart of the issues separating us.

As I read Ramsey, he has two major objections against my analysis of the validity of proxy consent for nontherapeutic experimentation on children. First, it treats the child as a small adult by attributing obligations to him or her. Second, the controls on the criteria of the legitimacy of proxy consent appear to him to resemble an accordion—expandable and contractable according to the need for results. I will address each of these concerns and the issues that adhere to them.

In approaching this question I had argued that parental consent in therapy directed at the child's own good is, under analysis, morally valid precisely insofar as it is a reasonable presumption of the child's wishes. I further argued that behind this "*would* wish" (where therapy is concerned) is the conviction that the child *ought* to do so. Once this is stated—it is obvious that we are in the realm of construction—I suggested that there are other things that the child *ought*, simply as a human being, to choose. And I then suggested that minimal involvement in experimental procedures would be among these other things, not because they are of benefit to himself, but because at little or no cost to himself he could contribute to benefits for others. I argued this on the basis that "if this is true of all of us . . . it is no less true of the infant."

Ramsey's objection to this is that it "treats the child as a small adult," that "if McCormick does not treat the child *as* a moral agent, he nevertheless treats it *as if* it were a moral agent." Briefly, it analyzes the child as if he or she had moral obligations. In contrast, Ramsey argues that all that is necessary is a construction of what the child *would* want and consent to (in the therapeutic situation) if he could—a *would* inferred from the child's needs alone. To go beyond that *would* to a *should* is to co-opt the child into the adult world where it is the subject of moral obligation. Therefore, any analysis of the nontherapeutic in terms of an *ought* is similarly erroneous.

In response to that I would argue that by using the language of *ought* of the infant or incompetent child, one is not implying or imputing moral obligation and moral agency and thus introducing the infant to the adult world. Clearly, the infant has no obligations until he or she is the subject of moral claims and duties. But the language of *ought* need not imply actual obligations. It is simply a device, a construction (as is also the language of what the infant *would* choose) to get at the reasonableness of our expectations and interventions.

Let us put it another way. If we can say of adults (who can and do have obligations) that it is reasonable to expect that they will want certain goods for others and contribute to these goods if there is no discernible risk, discomfort, or inconvenience, it is not precisely because they are adults that we conclude this, but *because they are social human beings*. Being adults we assume that they will understand, acknowledge, and respond to the claims rooted in their sociality, their social nature. And we call the *experience* of such claims an *ought*. But the claims themselves are rooted in the sociality of our being. They are not primarily rooted in the adult's capacity or willingness to respond to them as an adult (freely, as a subject *experiencing claims*, a moral agent), but in the social nature of human beings.

Now, this sociality is shared quite as much by infants as by adults. *Ought* language is but an attempt to highlight this—that is, in using such language the focus is sociality, not age. The good of infants is inseparably interlocked and interrelated to the good of others, for infants are human beings. Clearly, they cannot experience this or respond to its implications as claims. But we may for them—to the extent that it is reasonable to do so, a reasonableness founded on their common share in our human nature. *On this basis* we conclude to the reasonableness of certain interventions and try to convey and limit this reasonableness (rooted in the continuity of our share in the sociality of human nature) by the language of *ought*.

In other words, in using the language of *ought* we concentrate on sociality, not age. And in doing so, I submit that we introduce the infant not to the world of adults, but to the world of *social* human beings, to the human world, not the adult world. In this sense *ought* language is two-layered: It refers to the social basis of what it is reasonable to expect of or do to others and to the *experience* of this reasonableness. Clearly when used of infants the language can mean only the former.

At the root of our disagreement, then, may be what I would suggest is Ramsey's narrowly individualistic notion of human nature. He treats the child as an unrelated entity, and thus refuses him entry not only into the adult world (rightly) but also into the human race (wrongly). This is clear from the argument he makes. He states of my argument: "His argument would *impose* a minimal *positive* sociability not only upon children but upon—indeed everyone else as well." And since Ramsey is rarely content to state once what can be repeated frequently, he adds: "McCormick's argument . . . is quite enough to justify the regimentation of any and all other human subjects into medical research, provided only that they are *needed* and that the risks are *minimal*."

That is exactly where my argument leads—indeed, exactly where it started—and it is exactly where I took it in an editorial in the *Journal of the American Medical Association* (an essay apparently unfamiliar to Ramsey at the time of his writing). Commenting on the recommendations of the National Commission for the Protection of Human Subjects on fetal research, I tried to expose the logical implications for all of us of treating the fetus as the recommendations did—namely, allowing minimal or no-risk experimental procedures. I wish to cite the substance of my conclusion.

At some point, then, our willingness to experiment on
children (and fetuses) when risk, discomfort, and pain
are minimal or nonexistent points to a duty that we all
have to be willing to bear our fair share that all may
prosper. If we as adults are unwilling to admit such a
duty and fulfill it, we should re-examine our attitudes toward children and fetuses. Otherwise, we are practicing
a racism of the adult world.

I am not speaking of heroic sacrifices or supererogatory
works, which call on and promote individual generosity.
I am speaking of the minimal duties that might fall into
the more basic category of social justice. If we really expect to, want to, and demand to enjoy the fruits of medical progress, we should be willing to bear our share in
the development of this progress. For too long we have
been transferring this task to the powerless—the retarded, the poor, the incarcerated. The associated inhu-
manities are all too clear.

Even though it can be argued that we all have duties
in this area, duties of readiness and willingness, it is understandable, even desirable, that informed consent ac-
company the fulfillment of these duties. For consensual
community is something to be promoted wherever possible. If, however, not enough volunteers are available for
minimal-risk experimentation and the research seems of
overriding importance to the public health, it would not
be unjust of the government to recruit experimental subjects, for example, by lottery, just as it is not unjust for
government to draft soldiers for national self-defense.
But just as a volunteer army is preferable, if adequate, to
a drafted one, so are volunteer experimental subjects.
Could they speak to the point, this is what children and
fetuses would probably be telling us.[2]

Thus I do not see Ramsey's fears about where my analysis
would take us as an objection at all. Indeed, I see his "objection"
as pointing up our social nature as human beings in a way Ramsey

[2] Richard A. McCormick, S.J., "Experimental Subjects—Who Should They
Be?" *Journal of the American Medical Association*, 235 (1976), 2,197.

is incapable of doing. He understands our needs and claims as persons in a very asocial and individualistic way and then extrapolates backward to the infant and fetus.

This personal isolationism reveals itself in two ways. The first is his treatment of rights. When I objected that Ramsey's position would not allow *any* nontherapeutic experimentation whatsoever, Ramsey replied:

> It shows, I think, that he began by granting a certain dominance to the *research imperative.* At least, he began with the assumption that the research imperative and the rights of unwilling experimental subjects *must* be harmonizable. Moreover, in doing so, he began with the assumption that a positive imperative to attain consequential goods may and must to a certain extent be weighted in the same balance with the rights of human subjects.

Not so at all. I began, as one ought to begin, with the idea that human rights ought not to be defined before the individual is viewed as a social being, before insertion into the web of human relationships that define our very being. Equivalently, Ramsey defines certain rights of an individual with no relation to the needs and claims of others, then sees these needs and claims as *opposed to individual rights.* I call that individualism: Ramsey must try to harmonize the rights of individuals with the "research imperative" (his phrase) because he has established those rights in total independence of other persons. There can be a conflict, of course; but the question is where it might occur. Ramsey sees it as occurring with *any* nontherapeutic experimentation (even "offensive touching") because he has first defined individual rights in such a way that they make any "touching" of a noncompetent "offensive." Not only is that juridical individualism, it also begs the entire question; for in saying that *any* nontherapeutic experimentation on an infant is violative of the infant's right, Ramsey must suppose that there is an established right precluding this—the very point to be proved. And it can be proved, I submit, only by a very one-sidedly individualistic notion of rights and claims. That is why Edouard Boné, S.J., is correct in pointing up the excessively individualistic dimension in a perspective otherwise rigorously Christian.[3]

Ramsey's second riposte, again revealing his individualism, is appeal to the Kantian maxim prohibiting use of an individual as a means *only* and not as an end *also*. To my original statement that Ramsey's position would allow no nontherapeutic experimentation, he responds: "McCormick will have to do better than that in moral argument if he ever succeeds in overturning Immanuel Kant and Paul Ramsey." Of course, I accept the Kantian axiom. But that is really not the issue. The issue is: What is to count as "treating an individual as a means *only*"? Ramsey would determine that issue prior to a consideration of any social relationships, then use this determination to exclude any procedures that might have their justificatory root in our nature as social human beings. This once again begs the question. And in doing so, it reveals the root of our difference: Ramsey's individualism in the delineation of human rights. If the individual's good transcends individuality and separateness from others, then to treat him or her with this in mind need not involve treating as a means *only*. This is not the key question; it is to establish the limits of the implications of our sociality once insertion into sociality has been done. On his rendering, for example, it is difficult to see how a nation could conscript an unwilling person (I speak not of a conscientious objector) for national self-defense; for such conscription would not only be without the consent of the individual, but more positively *against* it. In Ramsey's terms, is this not "to treat the individual as a means"? And in Ramsey's terms, is it not therefore a violation of right? If it is not, then it is only because we socialize a person before we say what is in violation of his right, before we say what procedures use him as a means *only*. If we do not, we beg the question and get mired in an individualism of rights.

Therefore, when Ramsey accuses me of seeking *"another ground for 'legitimate' proxy consent—from which, then, 'being made an object' takes its meaning"* (emphasis added) he is absolutely correct. But his point is barely an accusation, for that "other ground" is the social dimension of our being. Limits must

---

[3] Edouard Boné, S.J., "Quelques Thémes Actuels de Bioéthique," *Revue Théologique de Louvain*, 6 (1975), 436.

be established, of course, to what is legitimate after our social insertion; but Ramsey's position denies such insertion altogether in his definition of rights and claims. Here I believe we should pause to "stifle our amazement."

In conclusion, then, Ramsey's first objection (that *ought* language involves small-sized participation in adulthood) seems to me to be without foundation. Indeed, if the objection is telling, it tells equally against Ramsey, for after denying any "shoulding" on the part of the child, he gives his account of proxy consent. "He (the parent, proxy) rather 'construes,' 'constructs,' 'infers' what the child would consent to, *if he could,* from the child's needs alone."

Ramsey realizes that "woulding"—on his terms—must impute adulthood and moral agency just as much as "shoulding." Any objection based on the imputation of adulthood loses its teeth as soon as one starts "woulding" the child—and claims that this is not adulthood, whereas "shoulding" is. So Ramsey beats a quick retreat and argues, lamely, I believe, that "it is clear, in any case, that the substantive positions are May/Ramsey vs. McCormick, so far as legitimate parental authorization is concerned," to which I must respond that this is true with regard to the position Ramsey adopts, but not to the rationale or the analysis. In the therapeutic situation Ramsey legitimates proxy consent on the basis of a construction of what the child *would* do. That is reasonable, I think—that is, it is language that attempts to construe the reasonable. But if "should" language imputes adulthood, then so does "would" language, for the child is no more capable of "woulding" than he is of "shoulding."

My contention, of course, is that neither usage implies moral agency. They are devices to get at the reasonable. And "should" constructions, I argue, are much more adequate because they explain many things more adequately (for example, they provide rational limits)—especially in terms of what the child (or anyone) would *not* choose to do, because in the circumstances (by construction) he *need not.*

Ramsey's second concern is with the ceiling I put on the reasonableness of nontherapeutic experimentation with children. I used phrases such as "minimal risk," "no discernible risk," and "no notable inconvenience." He sees this as "wavering" and argues that we moralists should provide "real standards" and "not an accordion that can be expanded and contracted according to the need for results."

Several things ought to be said here. First, the language used is necessarily *somewhat* flexible because what we are seeking is a human judgment or assessment, not a mathematical one. Ramsey implies that the inability to specify exactly what minimal risk is leaves us not with real standards, but with an expandable accordion. In moral judgments, that is erroneous. It says if we cannot mathematicize norms, they are unavoidably expandable.

What is wrong with that? Several things. First, it reveals, I think, a basic mistrust of human judgments. Furthermore, at some point it is inconsistent; for while demanding from the moralist exact determinations of what "discernible risk" and "no discernible risk" mean, Ramsey agrees with me that the value judgment in question "is the heavy responsibility of the medical profession (*not the moral theologian*) to make."

Second, to illustrate the "accordion character" of the term "minimal risk," Ramsey cites my distinction between a buccal smear and a kidney transplant. Unaccountably he then asks: "Is it not possible for moral theologians to close that gap somewhat more by further discussion of cases, without usurping the proper discussion of physicians?"

Who said anything about a gap? The gap is of Ramsey's making. I used the example of a buccal smear as one of insignificant (in human judgment) risk. Of course, there are many procedures beyond this ("in the gap") before one gets to kidney transplants. But they are scarcely my problem. The very point of using a buccal smear as an example was to indicate that anything beyond this was no longer insignificant. Anything beyond the insignificant risk (if indeed it is insignificant—I am open to medical correction in that judgment) of such a smear should not be allowed. There is no question of a "gap" where further, more dangerous procedures might be considered. And I have no idea of why Ramsey conceived that there is a gap problem here. Once it is agreed that a buccal smear constitutes an insignificant risk, it is the task of the scientific community to tell us what other procedures are equivalent to such a smear in human judgments of risk. It is an abuse of this responsibility to extend the example into some "gap" where procedures get increasingly dangerous.

In pursuit of this matter, Ramsey put a question to me. It is the example of a Pap test. He agrees that a nontherapeutic Pap test on an infant with no body consciousness would not be *harmful*. (He holds, however, that it would be "offensive" touching and morally wrong.) He then asks: "Would McCormick agree that no parent ought to consent to a Pap test solely for research purposes on their girl children who are approaching puberty or in early puberty *when body consciousness may be a problem?*" (emphasis added).

Of course, I would agree that if there are associated psychological dangers, they must be weighed. And if they are significant, they interdict the procedure. Nothing in what I have written implies anything else.

The medical profession—in spite of some abuses in the past—can be trusted to make equivalent judgments. Thus Ramsey's statement that "further exemplification in terms of cases is needed if McCormick's position is to instruct" and not simply legitimate current trends manifests a basic distrust of the profession that my experience would not support.

Behind Ramsey's concern with "closing the gap" is fear that my "strict sounding limitations" will be abused and used as the bases for exposing children to truly wrongful risks. After insisting that the possibility of abuse does not invalidate a principle, I should further add that any strict rule can be abused, such as the just-war theory.

In conclusion, then, I do not find Ramsey's two objections persuasive. Proxy consent—or perhaps, better, vicarious consent—I am convinced, can be morally legitimate where nontherapeutic experimentation on infants and children is concerned, providing the strict limits I suggested are observed.

But the further question remains: What precisely is the function of this proxy consent? It is not, in my judgment, *constitutive* of the legitimacy of these experimental procedures. It is merely *protective*—that is, the basic moral legitimacy must be argued from the sociality of all of us, infants and children included. My *ought* language was an attempt to state this. I remain persuaded of its legitimacy, not because it responds to any alleged *research*

imperative (Ramsey's words),[4] but because it corresponds to the
stirrings of common sense where infant and child-health care are
concerned and does so in a way that rigorously protects the child.
Ramsey's position protects the child, but so absolutely that it
offers no account at all of the child's sociality and in the process
all too easily undermines not only the over-all good of children,
but even and eventually of the individual child. The child, when
she becomes an adult with children of her own, will—if she has
the good of her own children at heart—look back with regret on
the *trivial* experiments that could have been done on her but were
not, and that could have improved the lot of her own present children. Speaking to herself and of herself as a child, that child-
become-parent would, I judge, say: "I *would* have consented because I *ought* to have." Saying this, she would mean only that she
was as a child a sharer in a common and social human nature, and
that it was proper to take that into account in deciding what was
and was not reasonable to do medically.

---

[4] Ramsey repeatedly refers to the "research imperative" as if it were some
great beast ready to devour us all. His point is valid—but, as not infrequently,
overstated; that is, he plays upon it to defend a position rather than to arrive
at one. "Research imperative" can mean at least two things: (1) an *excessive*
zeal on the part of researchers, a zeal ready and eager to achieve its purposes
at any cost (and this is Ramsey's sinister suggestion); (2) an urgent concern
to prevent, or alleviate disease, especially crippling disease. I would argue that
(1) if it is right and charitable to heal the wounds of the wounded (as in
the case of the Good Samaritan), (2) then it is at least as right and charitable
to *prevent* them, (3) and that if research is a necessary means in our time to
prevent them (as, on all accounts, it seems to be), (4) then research (experimental procedures) is an imperative and indeed a Christian one. The imperative
is not concerned with some vague, impersonal "medical progress." It is rather
closely—inseparably, really—tied to the health and sufferings of individuals—
here and now, and in the immediate years to come. If this is what "research
imperative" means, I am all for it, as I think all should be. If it means, as
Ramsey's usage too easily connotes, results *at any cost*, then clearly no one
ought to be for it. Should not Ramsey stop using the phrase in order to get
leverage out of its ambiguity? I think so; for in doing so, he indulges in
hortatory discourse but at a possibly frightful cost to all of us—as scientists,
ethicists, and, above all, as human beings.

7. The Rights of the Voiceless

In Chapters 4 to 6 I have argued a position that would allow minimal-risk nontherapeutic experimentation on the incompetent (children and fetuses). I have argued this on the basis of a construction of what the child would do because he "ought" to do so. Clearly this is a construction, for the child is incapable of moral obligation (ought). But by using "would" and "ought," I am clearly appealing to two tests: the hypothetical test (what the child would do), and the best-interests test (because it is not opposed to his best interests). Put in this way, it is clear that the two tests seem related to each other. This has not gone without challenge, perhaps very legitimate. But I want to explore the matter further using one of my critics, Benjamin Freedman, as the occasion for my reflections. In his thoughtful essay, Benjamin Freedman continues the discussion of incompetents and argues that there are only two tests for determining the content of the rights of the voiceless: the hypothetical test and the best-interests test.[1] He further argues that these are totally different tests that yield different content conclusions. He finally rejects the hypothetical test on practical and theoretical grounds, and concludes that the best-interests test is the one that ought to be used where giving content to the rights of the voiceless is concerned. In the process of arriving at this conclusion, he asserts that the two tests have been "confused" through the use of the reasonable-man standard —the reasonable man being one who would, it is assumed, choose reasonably and in his best interests.

Freedman's conclusion (that it is the best-interests test we ought to use) rests on two arguments: (1) the two tests are "entirely distinct" conceptually and in practice can yield different

[1] Benjamin Freedman, "On the Rights of the Voiceless," *Journal of Medicine and Philosophy*, 3 (Sept. 1978), 196–210.

content conclusions; (2) there are grave practical and theoretical difficulties with the hypothetical test. As support for the first statement, he cites the instance adduced in *Strunk* v. *Strunk* (1969) of an incompetent's estate being diminished in favor of a needy brother and in favor of an elderly servant—the court being "satisfied that the Earl of Carysforth would have approved if he had been capable of acting himself." This is clearly the hypothetical test. But, Freedman argues, in neither of these cases were the actions taken in the best interests of the incompetent. Therefore, clearly the two tests are different.

As support for the second assertion, he notes the grave difficulties and perils involved in attempting to determine what a person would do were he competent. While purporting to give empirical evidence, it is not clear that the hypothetical test does so. But beyond these problems, he wonders theoretically what is the point in doing what a person would have wanted. In doing what he would have wanted, we are not satisfying his right at all, since the value of that right is in the subject's freedom, his free exercise of the right. By doing what he would have wanted, we are not satisfying his freedom, nor his desire. The two arguments often used to give plausibility to the hypothetical test (similarity to wills, respect for persons—namely, honoring them by carrying on their projects) he finds unpersuasive. This is how I read Freedman.

In this brief chapter, I want to argue that Freedman has unduly separated the two tests. While they are distinct schemata or formulations, they are, I believe, closely interrelated. And notwithstanding Freedman, I believe the "reasonable man" (in the normative sense) is precisely the mediating vehicle of this relationship. Those who acknowledge this interrelationship and its bases Freedman accuses of "confusing" the two, and even of "blatant" confusion. We shall have to see about that, but for now let it be said that a close relationship within a distinction is not necessarily a confusion. Second, I want to point to the reasons why he unduly separated the two. And finally, I want to suggest that my own attempt at a normative statement (what they would choose because they ought) of the hypothetical test was precisely an effort to relate these two formulations (hypothetical test, best-interests test). In brief, I want to suggest that it remains appropriate to approach the voiceless in terms of what they would choose because it is in their best interests. This unified formulation attempts to show the close relationship between the hypothetical test and the best-interests test. In the course of making these points, I shall make reference to arguments and analyses where I believe Freedman is incomplete and even inaccurate.

Freedman's undue separation of the two tests: As I read him, Freedman offers several reasons for these two tests being "entirely distinct." The first is practical—that is, they can and do lead to different content conclusions. *Strunk v. Strunk* is his example. In that case, the majority supported its use of the hypothetical test (what the incompetent would have consented to) by citing cases involving diminution of the estate of an incompetent to aid an indigent and, in another instance, an elderly servant. In both instances an annuity was allowed on the grounds that the incompetent would have approved (hypothetical test-substituted judgment). Yet in these cases Freedman argues that the actions were not in the best interests of the incompetent. Therefore, since the tests yield different conclusions, they are "entirely distinct."

I have several problems with this analysis. First, it patently equates "best interests" with "getting or keeping something for oneself" or, more generally, with "deriving personal benefit." That equation, when unpacked, is a highly individualistic one and a subtle attack on the social dimension of our persons. As social beings, our good, our flourishing (therefore, our best interests) is inextricably bound up with the well-being of others. That is one reason why, for instance, a long Christian (in this case Catholic) tradition has held it to be morally acceptable for an individual to forego expensive life-saving medical treatment if such treatment would exhaust family savings, plunge the family into poverty, and deprive other members of the family of, for example, educational opportunity. In such an instance, it would not be in the best interests of the ill individual because his best interests include his family.

Something can be, therefore, in our best interests without we ourselves, precisely as isolated individuals, deriving any benefit or gain in the sense that Freedman uses that term. Another modest example of this is the case where one individual (1) can provide considerable benefit to another or others (2) at no cost to himself. I believe that if one considers our social being, it is legitimate to say that such provision is in the best interests of the individual. Indeed, that is exactly how I argued when attempting to justify nontherapeutic experimentation on those children incapable of consent. In brief, then, it is only by assuming a very individualistic (and inaccurate) notion of best interests that these interests are different from "what he would have chosen" in the cases cited. I shall return to Freedman's individualism because it surfaces later in dealing with freedom and respect for persons and their projects.

Second, the verdict of the majority in *Strunk v. Strunk* (that the incompetent would have consented to kidney donation had he been competent and that it was in the best interests of the incompetent to donate a kidney) is highly questionable. Indeed, I would agree with the minority that it was not in the best interests of the child. But I would similarly argue that the child would not have consented. So the fact that the minority found it sufficient to rebut the claim that the operation would be in the best interests of the incompetent does not mean that the two tests were confused by the court, or that they are "entirely distinct." It simply suggests that the majority was wrong in its application of both interrelated test schemata.

In this context, Freedman has argued that the court used two different tests in *Strunk v. Strunk* (hypothetical, best-interests). That is not a necessary reading of that decision. Indeed, in a recent decision, the Massachusetts Supreme Court reads the matter differently (*Superintendent of Belchertown State School et al.* v. *Joseph Saikewicz* [1977]). In reporting *Strunk v. Strunk* (1969)[2] the court stated: "The court concluded that, due to the nature of their relationship, both parties would benefit from the completion of the procedure, and hence the court could presume that the prospective donor would, if competent, assent to the procedure." Here we see not two different tests, but two interrelated formulations: He would assent because it is in his best interests (benefit).

The Massachusetts Supreme Court adopted this reasoning in deciding the Saikewicz case. It accepted the doctrine of substituted judgment, but insisted that this judgment must be determined by and brought into step with "the wants and needs of the

---

[2] *Strunk v. Strunk*, Ky., 445 S.W. 2d 145 (1969), and *Superintendent of Belchertown State School et al.* v. *Joseph Saikewicz*, Mass., 370 N.E. 2d 417 (1977).

individual involved . . . the values and desires of the affected individual . . . the incompetent person's actual interests and preferences." "Needs, interests, preferences, wants" are all ways of saying "best interests," as is clear from the Massachusetts Supreme Court's repeated reference to "best interests" when defining the jurisdiction of the probate court in such cases. Thus, in actually deciding the case, the Supreme Court of Massachusetts decided that it was not in Saikewicz's best interests, to his benefit, to get chemotherapy, and that therefore he would not have wanted it. In other words, it related the test schemata.

Somewhat similarly, Freedman tries to get leverage against the hypothetical test in the case of the reckless spender declared incompetent. By citing an abusive application of the hypothetical test, or at least a highly questionable one (the questions Freedman raises are legitimate), he attempts to invalidate or at least weaken the test itself—thus further separating it from the best-interests test. But rather than arguing a separation of the tests, the case only illustrates the possible abuse of both interrelated tests.

Therefore, I do not find Freedman's reasons for the total distinction of the tests persuasive. And if they are not distinct as he asserts, but interrelated, then those who acknowledge this close relationship, and use the tests somewhat interchangeably, are hardly "confusing" the two, a claim Freedman repeatedly makes.

If the test schemata are really closely related, as I argue, then I must deal with the grave difficulties, both practical and theoretical, Freedman adduces against the hypothetical test; for if his objections against the hypothetical test are valid, they would argue powerfully against the close relationship I assert between the two.

The first difficulty Freedman asserts against the hypothetical test is practical. "We do not," he says, "in general, have any reason for assuming that we know what he [an incompetent] would have wanted." Written declarations can help, but they do not fall under the hypothetical test. Lacking such a declaration, the "determination of what a person would have wanted is difficult, obscure, and, in fact, fraught with peril."[3]

Since these perils and difficulties apply as well to the best-interests test as he interprets it, they are no reason for separating the

---

[3] Freedman, "On the Rights of the Voiceless," 205.

two tests or of preferring one test over the other, for in determining what best interests are, it is always a question of our judgment as to what they are. Mysteriously, however, Freedman asserts that the best-interests test is more easily determinable and less given to abuse than the hypothetical test, whose perils and difficulties apply also to the best-interests test, as he admits. I say "mysteriously" because he offers no reasons for this statement, and it is crucial if the practical difficulties he raises against the hypothetical test are to count at all toward a separation or preference.

That being said, let me turn to the problems he raises. First, I believe we do have reasons for assuming we know in many cases what an incompetent would want. We may assume that most people are reasonable, and that being such they would choose what is in their best interest. At least this is a safe and protective guideline to follow in structuring our conduct toward them when they cannot speak. The assumption may be factually and *per accidens* incorrect. But I am convinced that it will not often be. In discussing the Karen Ann Quinlan case throughout the country, I have found a virtual consensus of people on what it would have been morally proper to do once the facts became clear (remove Karen from the respirator). This tells us a good deal about what these people would want were they in the same condition. The court, in the Saikewicz case, admitted that this type of evidence is valuable even if only indirect—that is, it is valuable in pointing to what Karen would want were she competent. For this reason, I believe I would simply have to deny Freedman's statement that "we do not, in general, have any reason for assuming that we know what he would have wanted." In general we have some fairly good reasons for this assumption.

Evidence such as this removes much (but not all) of the bite in Freedman's practical problem with the hypothetical test (that is, that while purporting to give empirical guidance, it is not clear that it is successful). This test should be approached as an approximation only. The question to be put to the test is not whether it is empirically accurate in all cases, but whether it is sufficiently accurate in most cases to provide the basis for a prudent and protective rule of practice. In brief, in the vast majority of cases, the test will not be falsified, and that is sufficient for guidance.

As an example of the practical difficulty in applying the hypothetical test, Freedman gives the case of the reckless spender who is found incompetent. He asks, "How do we judge what he would have wanted in his right mind?"[4] I would answer: by consulting reasonable people. For Freedman, because there is leeway within the reasonable, the very concept seems to be invalidated. We may grant the difficulty in drawing the line distinguishing reasonable from unreasonable spending (indicative of incompetence). But the very fact that one can appeal to incompetence at some point because of spending shows that there is a line we admit between the reasonable and the unreasonable in this area. That should be the criterion for both the hypothetical-test formulation and the best-interests formulation.

Freedman then argues against the hypothetical test on theoretical grounds. "What is the point," he asks, "of doing what a person would have done? . . . What purpose does this serve?" His answer: none, because in option rights it is the freedom itself that is the value, not the use to which it is put. "There is nothing sacred about the use to which one puts . . . option rights." Furthermore, in acting toward a person as we believe he would have wanted us to act, we are not preserving his freedom.

I think this has to be denied outright. For example, by protecting a dying incompetent person from months on a respirator, I am protecting him against those who would take advantage of his incompetence. I am substituting my judgment and freedom for his and thus supplying for his lack thereof to act in his best interests.

Therefore, to Freedman's question ("What purpose does it serve?") I would say that the closer we can construct their reasonable wishes, the better we protect the dignity of persons. By negating their reasonable wishes, we tend to treat persons as things, and hence, by extrapolation, we render ourselves vulnerable to treating others (even competents) arbitrarily and as objects. But Freedman would object: What has reasonableness to do with it? You have intruded the notion. I think not. Perhaps I have more normative instincts than Freedman, but I believe most of us want to act reasonably within parameters that are objective in character, even though we do not always do so. Or at least I think it good protective policy to assume this.

4 Ibid.

Behind and beneath our disagreement here is Freedman's total separation of human freedom from the object of its exercise. For Freedman, freedom as a pure and arbitrary power is a value in itself, an end value, a value independent of the task to which it turns or of the rightness or wrongness of its exercise. I cannot accept that (and that is why he is at best a reluctantly normative thinker). It unduly exalts mere nondetermination (freedom *from*). There is a long and honored philosophical and theological tradition that values self-determination above all in terms of the goods or values encompassable by free choice (freedom *to*). Misuse of that freedom is not a value in itself, as Freedman's perspective implies; indeed, it is a disvalue. Whenever human beings misuse their freedom, they suffer and visit suffering. The capacity to misuse freedom is but the unavoidable condition of its proper use. In this perspective, the right is to be free in order to do something. In doing that something for someone and letting him know in advance of his death or incompetence that I will, I am expanding his freedom by rendering more secure the good for which his freedom exists. But an exchange longer than possible here would be required to expose Freedman's philosophical assumptions about freedom, assumptions with which I almost certainly would disagree.

Freedman's second theoretical problem with the hypothetical test is the ultimate unpersuasiveness of the "whole-life view" of rights—the notion that respect for persons demands of us that once they become incompetent, we carry forth their project. He rejects this on the grounds that "it is engaging in the project, and not the project itself, which respect for persons enjoins us to support."[5]

Once again we have projects unduly separated from engaging in them—a kind of canonization of mere engagement, just as we saw a purely formal notion of freedom canonized. Actually, respect for persons must encompass both the person's engagement and the project itself. That is why, I submit, it makes sense for families to specify the charity favored by the deceased as an appropriate manifestation of solidarity. That is why caring for the children of the

[5] Ibid., 209–10.

deceased is not simply an act of beneficence to the children, but also an act of respect for the deceased.

Furthermore, and practically, if one knew that others need not further one's projects after one's death (on the grounds that only his personal engagement, not his project, is of value), one would resent this as denigrating him by denigrating one's projects after death. It would equivalently say that one's projects—the objects of one's care and love—did not matter. There is a radical individualism at work in Freedman's analysis—namely, the idea that what concerns me, interests me, is my doing of the charitable work, not the fact that others whom I love are bettered as a result. For instance, if I am devoted to my mother, I certainly wish (now) that after my death others continue to benefit her. If I do not so wish now, then I am interested only in myself. And if others tell me that respect for my person involves their support only of my engagement in my care and love for my mother, not her care after my incompetence, then I now experience their lack of respect for me. Freedman's undue separation of project from personal engagement leads to this kind of individualism. Contrarily, I want to know now that others will care for the persons I love, and the assurance that gives me this knowledge is an act of respect for me. Its fulfillment, as completion of a consoling promise, is no less.

The reasons for Freedman's undue separation of the two tests. We turn now to the second point. Why does Freedman unduly separate the two test schemata ("entirely distinct")? I have already suggested above why this is the case—for example, his individualistic notion of best interests, of freedom, etc. Here I should like to concentrate more specifically on these reasons, especially his notion of best interests. "How are we to determine," he asks, "what is in his best interest? Through determining his idiosyncratic notion of what is in his best interest, or through some community standard of what is good for a person—and if the latter, which of the communities in which he partakes is relevant?"[6] Here we see Freedman having difficulty in determining what is in a person's best interests by giving equal valence to two criteria: (1) one's own idiosyncratic notion of best interest; and (2) some community standard. Most people, I believe, would have no such difficulty. They would think that what is actually in a person's best interests ought to prevail over what the deluded or misguided person thinks is in his best interests. In this sense, again, most people would be objective or normative in determining best interests, for best interests are best interests, not putative best interests. Furthermore, most people would accept "some community standard of what is good for a person." Freedman's reluctance to do this underlines either of two facets of his thought: (1) his skepticism about our ability to determine what is truly for the good of persons, or (2) his reluctance to use such standards in cases of incompetence once we have discovered them.

In contrast to this, I believe the broad lines of what is in our best interests as persons is available to human insight and reasoning—that is, there are certain actions objectively destructive or promotive of us as persons. Furthermore, I believe that such perceptions should form the basis on which we build our judgments about what is in the best interests of incompetent persons. It is possible that behind Freedman's skepticism is the lack of a normative theory of man, of those goods that define our flourishing as persons. It is also possible that he has such a theory but is reluctant to use it in this context. I just do not know. At any rate, best interests seem to be in his thought what any individual judges them to be, however idiosyncratically.

Let me detail this in another way. I find five factors converging in Freedman's presentation—five factors that are responsible for his total separation of the two test schemata. (1) There is a lack of any normative anthropology whereby we know what goods are the source of our well-being (best interests). (2) Desires and wants are purely arbitrary (and they are the foundation of rights, and therefore of duties with regard to rights). There is no way of adjudicating between reasonable and unreasonable, and even if there were, it is not clear how these notions are relevant to decisions for the incompetent. (3) He is unduly skeptical about our ability to know what a person would want. (4) Best interests are narrowly identified with getting or keeping something for myself (an insensitivity to our social nature and the conclusions we might draw from this). (5) There is a failure to distinguish the occasional difficulty we experience in applying a test with its general validity.

For these reasons, what a person would want, as we construe it, can be entirely different from what is in his best interests. Therefore, the tests are "entirely distinct." Or, as Freedman words it, "there is not much conceptually in common between what someone wants with what is best for him." Of course, that is true. We are all inconsistent; we are even sinners. But here we are trying to construct what is in the best interests of an individual, what the reasonable person would desire or want. Therefore, we do not and need not take as our guide in some area what some eccentric desires, or what we desire when we commit sin (that is, act against our best interests and those of our neighbor). There is at least an area of the objectively reasonable; otherwise there would be no standard against which we could identify the eccentric, the idiosyncratic, the wrongful. Or again, without an area of the reasonable, judicial reversal of parental refusal of treatment for a child would be utterly arbitrary. Relating desires to reasonable desires is not "confusing" the two. It is rather insisting that the normative in our conduct is related to available insights about what is good and bad for us as persons and is the basis for safe and respectful (of persons) judgments.

In summary, then, I cannot agree with Freedman that the hypothetical test and the best-interests test are "entirely distinct." Rather, the hypothetical test is a way of formulating, of getting at the best-interests test, this latter being the basic test. That is why it is legitimate and meaningful to say that "he would want it that way were he competent because it is in his best interests." The vehicle that helps to keep these tests closely related is the reasonable-person test—that is, the reasonable-person test is a way of saying that best interests ought to be interpreted normatively, not just according to arbitrary wishes, if we are truly seeking best interests.

In the light of this, let us return to the Swiss Academy. In November 1976, the Swiss Academy of Medical Sciences issued guidelines for the care of the dying. The guidelines concerned with the comatose made the presumed current wish of the comatose patient the decisive factor. In other words, the physician is to act as he presumes the patient would now act. Freedman sees their approach as problematic because it creates the possibility of disregarding the living will when the physician feels this is not in the best interests of the person. The academy, he argues, has made the mistake of thinking the living will is a "means to determining what a person would have wanted." Actually, I do not believe this is a mistake. If the best interests are truly determinative, and the circumstances determining this have substantially changed, then what the person would want now is clearly a useful way of getting his best interests cared for.

In other words, what the person would want can at times better protect his interests than a living will. If so, it is reasonable to think a living will can above all serve the purpose of a general pointer toward best interests. It is not, therefore, the academy's position that is problematic. It is first written living wills that are problematic. They cannot foresee all circumstances and hence cannot be written in such a way as to guarantee the best interests of the patient. The academy is right, I think, to believe that these interests ought ultimately to be controlling, and that therefore wills are not always binding. This is admittedly a sensitive and difficult area, but where incompetents are concerned (with competents the physician can always withdraw from the case where he feels the patient is frivolously endangering his best interests), the problems and dangers of overriding a will in certain cases are less than those associated with unquestioning adherence to it, for this latter policy could involve us (and the medical profession) in responding to a person's incompetence in ways we all admit are genuinely opposed to his best interests. I see that as an assault on our integrity and that of the medical profession.

Freedman's treatment of my use of the reasonable-man standard. I turn now to my third point, Freedman's treatment of my use of the reasonable-man (I prefer "person") standard. He sees this use as a normatively based test "rather than" an empirically grounded one. The emphasis is correct, but the contrast ("rather than") is too sharp, as are most of Freedman's distinctions and separations. I simply have more confidence than Freedman in the fact that most people would choose (empirical) in the direction of their objective best interests (normative).

Be that as it may, Freedman has difficulties with the normative sense of the hypothetical test. He believes it abounds in confusions ("blatant" is his rendering). He cites two: (1) material goods for the child with moral goods, and (2) "what the child would choose with what the child would reasonably choose with what the child, if moral, would choose." A word about each.

First, it is not clear to me what Freedman means by attributing to me a confusion of material and moral goods. The argument I had made in attempting to justify minimal-risk nontherapeutic experimentation on incompetents (children) is that a good (material) is procured for others at no cost to the child (*parum pro nihil reputatur* [very little counts for nothing] in moral estimates). If I had argued that the child benefits by practicing virtue, I would indeed be commensurating material and moral goods. But that is not the heart of the argument. However, I will concede that my wording could have misled Freedman, for, in analogy with the therapeutic situation, where the fetus or child could be construed (substituted judgment) as choosing for his own best interests, I stated: "Are there other things that the child *ought*, as a human being, to choose precisely because and insofar as they are goods definitive of his growth and flourishing? . . . If we can argue that a certain level of involvement in nontherapeutic experimentation is good for the child and therefore that he *ought* to choose it, then there are grounds for saying that parental consent for this is morally legitimate. . . ."[7]

That phraseology ("good for the child") is misleading because it leads too many to interpret it as a moral good. The phrase was actually meant to convey the idea of "not opposed to the child's best interests." I used the wording "good for the child" to keep the thought continuous with the general theory I was proposing.

If something is not opposed to a child's best interests and simultaneously offers great hope of benefit to others, then there is legitimacy in saying (by obvious construction) that the child "ought" to do it. This by no means implies that the child is a moral agent. It is simply a way of formulating what we may do with a child short of violating his or her integrity. However, if too many readers are perplexed by the strong formulation "the fetus/child *ought* reasonably to consent to," I am perfectly willing to accept Stephen Toulmin's emendation, what he calls "one small modification." It reads as follows: "What may it be pre-

[7] Richard A. McCormick, S.J., "Proxy Consent in the Experimentation Situation," *Perspectives in Biology and Medicine*, 18 (Autumn 1974), 2–20.

sumed that the fetus *could not reasonably object to*, if it were capable . . . ?"[8]

I accept that emendation, but would note several things. (1) It does not alter the substance of my position, as Toulmin notes. (2) It is a clear instance of substituted consent (hypothetical test). (3) It has normative roots—that is, the fetus could not reasonably object because a potentially great good is supplied to others at no cost to the fetus/child—hence, by construction, the fetus "ought" to choose it. (4) What one "ought" to do (that is, cannot reasonably be opposed to) is at least not opposed to his best interests; or, more positively, is compatible with his best interests. This reveals the complementarity of the hypothetical and the best-interests tests.

I would conclude, therefore, that the position I attempted to propose supports, as I think it should, the close relationship between the hypothetical test and the best-interests test. Concretely, the fetus/child would choose his share in nontherapeutic experimentation because—to adapt from Toulmin—it is compatible with and not opposed to his best interests.

The second "confusion" Freedman believes he finds (between what the child would choose, would reasonably choose, would choose if moral) is not a confusion at all. It is simply an attempt to interrelate the hypothetical and best-interests tests. It is a "confusion" only if these tests are "entirely distinct," as Freedman claims. They are not.

In summary, then, I agree with Freedman that there are only two test formulations for determining the content of the rights of the incompetent: the hypothetical test and the best-interests test. The reasonable-person test is a vehicle for the interpretation of either of them.

I disagree with him on three major points. First, he conceives these tests as "entirely distinct," as two different ways of concretizing the right of the incompetent. I do not. They are interrelated. Indeed, in a sense, there is only one basic test: the best-interests test. The hypothetical test is subordinated to, is a proximate formulation of, the best-interests test: He would choose because it is in his best interests.

[8] Stephen Toulmin, "Exploring the Moderate Consensus," *Hastings Center Report*, 5 (June 1975), 31–35.

Second, I believe my own analysis is precisely at root and in substance a best-interests test: The fetus/child would choose nontherapeutic experimentation of minimal risk because it is compatible with and not opposed to his best interests.

Third, I suspect (but only that) that we have substantial disagreements about how normative the determination of the rights of the incompetent should be. Of the three assertions (what the child would choose, would reasonably choose, would choose if moral), Freedman says: "Each of these steps is logically illegitimate." He will have to explain this more than he has. If he means that we cannot deduce one step from the other without some normative anthropology, he is certainly correct. If he means, however, that such an anthropology has no place in determining the best interests and rights of the incompetent, then our disagreement is profound indeed, for in my judgment the best interests of a person, if they are truly to remain *best* interests, must root in the very notion of who the person is.

SECTION III

ABORTION, MORALITY, AND PUBLIC POLICY

8. The Abortion Dossier

On January 22, 1973, the U. S. Supreme Court handed down its historic decisions on abortion (*Roe* v. *Wade*, *Doe* v. *Bolton*). The reactions to these decisions were swift and predictable. Paul Blanshard and Edd Doerr, apostles of a rather tedious and faded anti-Catholicism,[1] exulted that "we felt like a champagne dinner in honor of the United States."[2] Flushed with victory, they were in a "festive mood" and called the Court's action "the most direct defeat for the Catholic hierarchy in the history of American law." J. Claude Evans regarded the decision as "a beautifully accurate balancing of individual rights gradually giving way to community rights as pregnancy progresses. It is a decision both pro-abortionists and anti-abortionists can live with, as it leaves the decision up to the individuals most closely involved. . . ."[3] Lawrence Lader, chairman of the National Association for the Repeal of Abortion Laws, spoke of "a stunning document . . . a humanitarian revolution of staggering dimensions."[4]

On the other hand, the Administrative Committee of the National Conference of Catholic Bishops rejected the opinion as "erroneous, unjust, and immoral."[5] Similarly, the episcopal Committee for Pro-Life Affairs branded the Court's action as "bad

[1] See Paul Blanshard and Edd Doerr, "Parochaid, Abortion, School Prayer," *Humanist*, 33 (1973), 34–35. The authors refer to "Pope Paul . . . their antisexual chieftain." They note that "the hierarchy is doubly embarrassed because celibate bishops are not recognized as the most natural guardians of a woman's womb."

[2] Paul Blanshard and Edd Doerr, "A Glorious Victory," *Humanist*, 33 (1973), 5.

[3] J. Claude Evans, "The Abortion Decision: A Balancing of Rights," *Christian Century*, 90 (1973), 195–97.

[4] Lawrence Lader, "The Abortion Revolution," *Humanist*, 33 (1973), 4.

[5] See NCCB Pastoral Message, *Hospital Progress*, 54 (Mar. 1973), 83 ff.

morality, bad medicine, and bad public policy."[6] John Cardinal Krol, president of the National Conference of Catholic Bishops, referred to the decision as "an unspeakable tragedy" and added that "it is hard to think of any decision in the two hundred years of our history which has had more disastrous implications for our stability as a civilized society."[7] For Most Reverend Edward D. Head, chairman of the Committee on Health Affairs (USCC), it was a "frightening decision."[8] *Christianity Today* editorialized that the decision "runs counter . . . to the moral sense of the American people . . . (and) reveals a callous utilitarianism about children in the womb that harmonizes little with the extreme delicacy of its conscience regarding the imposition of capital punishment."[9] And so on.

Whatever one's opinion of the Court's action, one thing is clear: in *Wade* and *Bolton* we are dealing with "one of the most controversial decisions of the century," as the Hastings Report phrased it.[10] With other nations contemplating or having completed similar liberalization, it is understandable that the literature on abortion in the past months has been enormous. In the many years that I have followed the literature in moral theology, I have never seen so much writing in so concentrated a period of time on a single subject. Since that time the literature reviewed here has, by and large, remained the focus of attention and reference.

Abortion is a matter that is morally problematic, pastorally delicate, legislatively thorny, constitutionally insecure, ecumenically divisive, medically normless, humanly anguishing, racially provocative, journalistically abused, personally biased, and widely performed. It demands a most extraordinary discipline of moral thought, one that is penetrating without being impenetrable, humanly compassionate without being morally compromising, legally realistic without being legally positivistic, instructed by cognate disciplines without being determined by them, informed by tradition without being enslaved by it, etc. Abortion, therefore, is

6 See "Statement of the Committee for Pro-Life Affairs, NCCB, January 24, 1973," *Catholic Lawyer*, 19 (1973), 31–33.
7 Ibid., 33.
8 See "Commentary: Bishop Head," *Hospital Progress*, 54 (Mar. 1974), 96a.
9 "Abortion and the Court," *Christianity Today*, 17 (1973), 502–3.
10 "Abortion: The New Ruling," *Hastings Center Report*, 3 (Apr. 1973), 4.

a severe testing ground for moral reflection. It is transparent of the rigor, fullness, and balance (or lack thereof) that one brings to moral problems and is therefore probably a paradigm of the way we will face other human problems in the future. Many of us are bone-weary of the subject, but we cannot afford to indulge this fatigue, much as the inherent risks of the subject might be added incentive for doing so. Thus these "Notes" will be devoted entirely to this single issue.[11]

To order this review, four subdivisions may prove of use: (1) critiques of the Court's decision; (2) legality and morality; (3) moral writings on abortion; (4) personal reflections.

Critiques of the Court's Decision

I shall limit this overview to seven or eight critiques, since it is fair to say that they raise most of the substantial issues. David Goldenberg, in a good review of the legal trends leading to *Wade* and *Bolton*, takes no moral position but faults the Court on legal grounds.[12] For instance, on the basis of lack of direct reference to the unborn in the Constitution, the Court asserts that the fetus is not protected by constitutional guarantees. "If this is so, how could a state satisfy the compelling-interest test in purporting to protect the fetus at the stage of viability?" A similar criticism of the Court's consistency is made by Emily C. Moore of the International Institute for the Study of Reproduction.[13] After saying that "person" does not cover the unborn, how can the Court segment pregnancy by trimesters and permit the state a controlling interest in the third trimester? This point is repeated throughout the literature.

Daniel Callahan rightly contends that the Court did for all practical purposes decide when life begins: not in the first two trimesters, possibly in the third.[14] He scores the Court for making it impossible to act in the future even if a consensus on this point

[11] Much interesting and important literature must be overlooked at this point.

[12] David Goldenberg, "The Right to Abortion: Expansion of the Right to Privacy Through the Fourteenth Amendment," *Catholic Lawyer*, 19 (1973), 36–57.

[13] "Abortion: The New Ruling," 4.

[14] Ibid., 7.

were achieved. He shrewdly notes that there is a hidden presumption that when the state withdraws from resolving "speculative" questions, freedom is somehow served. If this were true, all decisions touching equality and justice would be up to the individual conscience, for these notions are highly speculative in their final meaning. Callahan argues that the entire matter should have been left to state legislatures. I agree and will return to this point.

Dr. André Hellegers (Kennedy Institute for the Study of Reproduction and Bioethics) resents in the entire debate the falsification of embryology for the purpose of avoiding the fundamental question: "When shall we attach value to human life?"[15] Hellegers, therefore, argues that the basic question is not: When does life begin? It is: When does dignity begin? The Court fudged this. "They have used terms like 'potential life' trying to say that life wasn't there, when the reason for saying that life wasn't there was because they didn't attach any value to it. The abortion issue is fundamentally a value issue, not a biological one."[16] If the Court is to be truly consistent, Hellegers contends, there is no reason to worry about the health of the fetus. This implies that experimentation on the fetus *in utero* is perfectly acceptable. It also renders uncomfortably inconsistent the FDA's strict rules about drugs during pregnancy.

Several longer critiques round out this review. In a stinging but cogent rebuttal to the Court, John Noonan raises several serious questions.[17] First, if the liberty to procure termination of pregnancy is "fundamental" and "implicit in the concept of ordered liberty," how is it that this liberty has been consistently and unanimously denied by the people of the United States? Second, with many commentators, Noonan argues that the Court, in spite of its contrary allegations, allowed abortion on request; for the viable fetus was denied personhood, and the state was granted the right to proscribe abortion in the third trimester "except when it is necessary to preserve the life or health of the mother." Then the Court describes "health" as involving a medical judgment to be

15 André Hellegers, "Amazing Historical and Biological Errors in Abortion Decision," *Hospital Progress*, 54 (May 1973), 16–17.

16 Ibid., 16.

17 John Noonan, "Raw Judicial Power," *National Review* (Mar. 2, 1973), 260–64.

made "in light of all the factors—physical, emotional, psychological, familial, and the woman's age—relevant to the well-being
of the patient. All these factors may relate to health." Briefly, in
the third trimester a child may be aborted for the mother's well-
being. As Noonan reasonably notes: "What physician could now
be shown to have performed an abortion, at any time in the pregnancy, which was not intended to be for the well-being of the
mother?"

Noonan's next objection is aimed at the Court's schizoid style
of judicial interpretation—that is, the Court was evolutionary in
its reading of the notion of liberty, but utterly static and con-
structionist in its interpretation of the term "person." Finally,
Noonan, with Callahan, argues that the Court was inconsistent
on its own competence. "[T]he judiciary," Wade reads, ". . . is
not in a position to speculate as to the answer [as to when life
begins]."[18] Yet Texas is said to be wrong in "adopting one theory
of life." Clearly, if Texas is wrong, then the Court does indeed
know when life begins, especially "meaningful life."

Underlying this decision Noonan sees a whole new ethic of life
wherein it is appropriate for the state to protect beings with the
"capability of meaningful life." We used to contend that all life is
a sacred trust. Now, however, only "persons in the whole sense"
are protected. Noonan warns that the mentally deficient, the retarded, the senile, etc., are now exposed, for each could be described as lacking "the capability of meaningful life."

P. T. Conley and Robert J. McKenna accuse the Court of a
"foray into the legislative domain."[19] After confessing its own incompetence about life, the Court should have, on this basis, declared the matter nonjusticiable. Furthermore, they argue that the
Court has failed to practice what it preaches. In several recent decisions it had decided that the more fundamental the right, the
more compelling must be the state or government interest in excluding certain groups from enjoyment of the right. After criticizing the Court's utilitarian valuation of life, its inconsistencies
and intellectual sloth, they contend that while the unborn's right
to life is not explicit in the Constitution, still, unlike the right to

[18] Roe v. Wade, 410 U.S. 113, 159 (1973).
[19] P. T. Conley and Robert J. McKenna, "The Supreme Court on Abortion
—a Dissenting Opinion," Catholic Lawyer, 19 (1973), 19–28.

abort, it is recognized by law, custom, and majority opinion, and could rather easily be inferred from the Declaration of Independence. There it is stated that "all men are created equal and endowed with inalienable rights." But creation is traditionally associated with conception. They conclude that "the decision was patently unsound from either a logical, biomedical, moral, or legal perspective."

Many of the points raised by Noonan and others are covered by Edward Gaffney in a devastating critique of the Court's use of history and of its defective anthropology.[20] For instance, using three of Lonergan's imperatives for the operations of human consciousness (be attentive, be intelligent, be reasonable), he finds the Court's use of history in violation of all three.

Blanshard and Doerr state that "the Court proved in long and scholarly footnotes that the Church had permitted abortion for centuries."[21] Footnotes may be lengthy, but whether they are scholarly is another question. The footnoting in *Wade* does, indeed, appear imposing and could be very deceptive. But John R. Connery, S.J., in a careful study of the animation-nonanimation debate, notes that from the beginning of Christianity abortion has been condemned as morally wrong. The only issue was one of classification.[22]

Finally, Robert M. Byrn accuses the Court of inartistic and unpersuasive historical revisionism "before it could administer the fatal blow."[23] The controversy is about the value of human life, and the Court refused to protect unborn children "because there is a controversy over whether their lives are of value—whether they are 'meaningful.'" Social convenience and utility decided the day. If there is any doubt about the Court's shabby utilitarianism, Byrn acidly reminds the justices of William O. Douglas' dissent in *Sierra Club* v. *Morton*. In this dissent Douglas urged that "swamps and woodpeckers should be considered legal persons entitled to due process of law." Douglas continued: "The problem is

20 Edward M. Gaffney, "Law and Theology: A Dialogue on the Abortion Decisions," *Jurist*, 33 (1973), 134–52.

21 Blanshard and Doerr, "A Glorious Victory," 5.

22 See John R. Connery, S.J., *Abortion: The Development of the Roman Catholic Perspective* (Chicago: Loyola University Press, 1977).

23 Robert M. Byrn, "Goodbye to the Judaeo-Christian Era in Law," *America*, 128 (1973), 511–14.

to make certain that the inanimate objects, which are the very core of America's beauty, have spokesmen before they are destroyed."[24]

In summary, the critiques available thus far attack the Court's reasoning from almost every conceivable point of view: logic, use of history, anthropology. As William J. Curran, J.D., of the Harvard Medical School, notes, "The abortion decisions are already under a good deal of attack by constitutional lawyers, not so much for their result as for their reasoning."[25] At some point there must be a relationship of dependency between conclusion and reasoning; otherwise the conclusion is simply arbitrary. Whether another form of reasoning is available to support the Court's conclusion is, of course, what the legal discussion is all about.

From the point of view of the Christian ethician, what is most interesting (and appalling) is the utilitarian form of argument adopted by the Court and its one-dimensional value scale within the utilitarian calculus. For the Court, the overriding value is privacy. Three points here. First, if traditional attitudes toward abortion have been one-dimensional in their deafness to the resonances of other (than the sacredness of fetal life) values, the Court is no less one-dimensional. Second, one may legitimately ask with Albert Outler "just how private an affair is pregnancy, after all—since, from time immemorial, it has been the primal social event in most human communities?"[26] This is not to negate the value of privacy; it is merely an attempt to hierarchize it. Finally, the Court's reasoning on privacy raises a much broader cultural issue. Are *Wade* and *Bolton* simply symptoms of a highly individualized and ultimately antisocial notion of rights? There are many other indications in American life that such a notion of rights does indeed dominate our cultural and legal consciousness. If this is the case, there is much in the Catholic tradition, particularly in the recent social encyclicals, to redress the imbalance.

The discussion of *Wade* and *Bolton* will continue for years to come. And as with so many other profoundly divisive issues, it will

[24] Cited in Byrn, "Goodbye to the Judaeo-Christian Era in Law," 514.

[25] William J. Curran, "The Abortion Decisions: The Supreme Court as Moralist, Scientist, Historian, and Legislator," *New England Journal of Medicine,* 288 (1973), 950–51.

[26] Albert C. Outler, "The Beginnings of Personhood: Theological Considerations," *Perkins Journal,* 27 (1973), 28.

inevitably be boxed and labeled with the misleading terms "liberal" and "conservative." For this reason Donald Nugent is right on target when he lobs a few mortars into the so-called liberal camp.[27] In an amusing but dead-serious essay he argues that, even if we do not know when human life begins, "in a matter of life and death the only humane position is to give life the benefit of any doubt." Liberalism's cozying to the abortion cause is, he believes, symptomatic of a more general disenchantment with liberalism. Anglo-Saxon liberalism is a tradition of rationalized self-interest. "Abortion is in a tradition of interests, and it is inapposite that its exponents present themselves as the paladins of human values."

Legality and Morality

The Court's decision opens on the larger question of the relationship between morality and law, or what may be called the morality of law. More specifically: What is the responsibility of law where abortion is concerned? What is the appropriate strategy, what the criteria, when moral sensitivity attempts to translate itself into social policy in a pluralistic society? These questions have been approached in a variety of ways in recent literature.

Gabriel Fackre approaches the question as an ecumenical peacemaker and suggests that three "perceptions" must be shaken and mixed if the Protestant and Catholic communities are to cease casting glances of hostility across an abyss.[28] The first is the dignity of fetal life. "The central thrust of this perception is the weightiness of any aggression against fetal life with its incarnationally derived dignity." The second is a certain sobriety or realism that realizes the need to translate visionary commitments into norms that take account of our sinfulness and temporality. Thus, just as we have a just-war doctrine to qualify our eschatological moral expectations, so too we need a doctrine of "just abortion." Finally, there is the perception of liberation, the movement from necessity to self-determination.

27 Donald Nugent, "Abortion: An Aquarian Perspective," *Critic*, 31 (1973), 32–36.
28 Gabriel Fackre, "The Ethics of Abortion in Theological Perspective," *Andover Newton Quarterly*, 13 (1973), 222–26.

On the basis of these "perceptions," Fackre proposes a doctrine of just abortion with the following motifs. (1) The dignity of the fetus is to be honored and protected with a zeal commensurate with its development toward fullness of time. (2) The limits of that protection are determined by fetal peril to others who live in the land of ripened humanity, *plene esse*. (3) The definition of that peril should be worked out in each case by those affected by it: personal (mother, father), medical (physician, psychiatrist), social (moral resource or community representative). (4) The final decision about the future of fetal life rests with the one most intimately involved, the mother. (5) The dignity of the fetus and the stake of society are so great as to necessitate fetal law. The law should require the consultative process of No. 3, guarantee self-determination of No. 4, and assure the best medical care. (6) Fetal dignity is best served through raising the consciousness of society about that dignity and attacking the social and educational conditions that nourish the abortion problem.

Briefly, then, Fackre endorses a law that requires and supports the constraints of a consultative process. Fackre was writing before the Court's decision, and when compared to that decision his proposals look downright stringent. Ultimately, however, Fackre's doctrine of just abortion contains both moral and legal ingredients. Whether the legal constraints he proposes (consultative process) are sufficient will depend to some extent on his moral position. For instance, the retarded and the aged certainly would not be reassured if their dignity were acknowledged by policy proposals similar to Fackre's. He might respond that fetuses are not the aged and retarded. Correct. But what are they? Here I find Fackre evasive. His "to be honored and protected with a zeal commensurate with its development toward fullness of time" is just vague enough to be comfortable with almost any legal implementation. And that eventually is the weakness of the legal conclusion. It is proposed as a doctrine of "just abortion" without a rigorous exposition of the claims that allow us to decide the issue of justice-injustice. In other words, it builds on and reflects an uncertain or at least undeveloped moral position. And therefore his conclusions lack the lively sense of being accommodations to our sinfulness and temporality. When this sense of tension is lacking, legal tolerance tends to get simply identified with moral propriety.

J. Claude Evans seeks to defuse what he calls "Protestant and Catholic polarities" on abortion by "taking abortion out of the statute books altogether, a position earlier endorsed by Robert Drinan, S.J."[29] He believes that pro-abortionists and anti-abortionists could unite on this point. Somewhat unaccountably, then, he adds that all we need is some limiting law "perhaps stating that no abortions are permitted beyond eighteen-week gestation" and guaranteeing personal and institutional protection against abortion on demand. Evans' suggestion that the disputants can unite by taking abortion off the statutes is another example of an invitation to unity by unilateral surrender. The precise contention of very many disputants is that the state has the duty to protect infant life, both before and after birth, with legal sanctions.

This is the very point made by C. Eric Lincoln as he recounts his remarkable change of mind on abortion away from a position based rather exclusively on a woman's autonomy over her own body.[30] Without detailing what the law should be, Lincoln insists that the state, as party to every marriage contract or implied contract[31] (and therefore burdened with certain responsibilities), does have something to say about the interruption of pregnancy. The state is the guardian of the public welfare and in that capacity exercises control over our bodies in many areas (for example, drug and beverage control, medical practice, seat belts, inoculations, water treatment, helmets, etc.). The desire to privatize and individualize the abortion decision totally Lincoln sees as a retreat from personal and social accountability. He makes no secret that he is appalled at the present levels of bloodletting.

This same point is underscored by A. Jousten as he discusses the situation in Belgium.[32] The law, he argues, acts as a support for morality in order to guide the exercise of liberty and responsibility to the common good. Not all men are saints who spontaneously seek the good of others. However, the more complex and

[29] J. Claude Evans, "Defusing the Abortion Debate," *Christian Century*, 90 (1973), 117–18.

[30] C. Eric Lincoln, "Why I Reversed My Stand on Laissez-Faire Abortion," *Christian Century*, 90 (1973), 477–79.

[31] By "implied contract" Lincoln refers to the situation of an unmarried woman consenting to intercourse. In this instance the partner may be liable for support, etc. Since in reasonable societies rights and responsibilities go in tandem, the consenting woman is involved in an implied contract.

[32] A. Jousten, "La réforme de la législation sur l'avortement," *La foi et le temps*, 3 (1973), 47–73.

pluralized a society is, the more distinction there is between law and morality, without there being separation. And with distinction comes tension. Concretely, in the definition of the rights and duties of each, it is not always possible to take account of the individual interest. If the state tries to satisfy every individual interest, it renounces certain socially useful values in the process. In explanation of this, Jousten agrees with M. T. M. Meulders: "In the case where two individuals are at stake, and where one risks causing a grave harm to another, there is no longer question of a 'private' matter and the law may not turn away from this situation."[33]

After reviewing the pros and cons of liberalization, Jousten tends to side with those authors who oppose liberalization and believe the situation is best handled by trusting the honesty of physicians and the jurisprudential process without trying to codify all tolerable indications.

Harvard's Arthur J. Dyck argues that one who is for civil rights, sound population policy, and compassion for unwanted children need not be committed to a policy of abortion on request.[34] Quite the contrary. Where civil rights are concerned, Dyck notes that women's rights encounter an evolution in property, tort, and constitutional law favoring the recognition of the fetus as a living entity. It is now clearly recognized, for example, that the "unborn child in the path of an automobile is as much a person in the street as the mother."[35] Dyck is convinced that it would be a considerable step backward "if governments, which had acknowledged all of these rights, were now to deprive the fetus of any legal protection of its most fundamental right—that is, its right to life."[36] As for population growth, permissive laws do not significantly affect this in the long run, since population growth

[33] Cited in Jousten, "La réforme de la législation," 54. See M. T. Meulders, "Considérations sur les problèmes juridiques de l'avortement," *Annales de droit,* 31 (1971), 507–19.

[34] Arthur J. Dyck, "Perplexities for the Would-be Liberal in Abortion," *Journal of Reproductive Medicine,* 8 (1972), 351–54.

[35] Here Dyck is citing William Prosser, *The Law of Torts,* 3d ed. (St. Paul, Minn.: West Publishing Company, 1964), Sec. 56.

[36] In support of this, see "Declaration of the Rights of the Child," proclaimed by the General Assembly of the United Nations (Nov. 20, 1959). It states: "Whereas the child, by reason of his physical and mental immaturity, needs special safeguards and care, including appropriate legal protection, before as well as after birth." See T. W. Hilgers and D. J. Horan, *Abortion and Social Justice* (New York: Sheed & Ward, 1972), 133.

depends upon the number of children people want. For these and
other reasons, Dyck favors laws that would permit abortion only
where the life or the physical and mental health of the pregnant
woman are seriously threatened.

The editors of *America*, obviously convinced that whatever the
law ought to be, it should not be the simple abortion-on-request
policy adopted in *Wade*, discuss resistance through amendment.[37]
Two amendments are possible. First, the absolutist type resem-
bling the Thirteenth Amendment's prohibition of slavery: "No
abortion—period." The difficulty here is that such an amendment
goes beyond even Catholic formulations. And if "our" exceptions
are written into law, then why not the exceptions of other groups?
Second, there is the state's-rights type of amendment that leaves
regulation to the individual states. The difficulty here is that the
fight to preserve the sanctity of fetal life would have to be waged
in fifty states. *America* asks: "Why should an enormous national
effort be made to secure a constitutional amendment, the only result of which will be to guarantee fifty-one more struggles?" The
most immediate answer to that question would be simply: It is
worth it.

But is it really? Albert Broderick, O.P., constitutional lawyer at
Catholic University, has his doubts. In a very interesting article
Broderick argues that the Court was simply substituting its own
moral values for those of the community. In justifying its un-
dervaluation of life, "the Court scorned current medical and biological evidence . . . distorted history, distorted or misconstrued
contemporary social and professional morality as represented in
legislation of every state and the medical associations, positioned
itself again as supreme arbiter of a nation's social ethics and
theology. . . ."[38] How are we to face this revival of judicial supremacy? Broderick sees the amendment route as the "byway of
frustration," because an amendment is practically impossible of
enactment. Instead he discusses two alternative strategies. First,
the very internal defectiveness of the decisions provides some
hope that the Court will reverse itself. Therefore, the first strategy

[37] "Abortion: Deterrence, Facilitation, Resistance," *America*, 128 (1973),
506–7.
[38] Albert Broderick, O.P., "A Constitutional Lawyer Looks at the *Roe-Doe*
Decisions," *Jurist*, 33 (1973), 123–33.

is to provide it with every opportunity for doing so. Broderick is not optimistic here, but more so than he is about the heavily loaded amendment process. Second, he argues that if a constitutional amendment is indicated, it ought to move in on judicial supremacy. An example he gives: Allow Congress (through a majority of both houses) to override any decision of the Supreme Court that declares unconstitutional on Fourteenth Amendment grounds legislation of the several states.

The Supreme Court's reasoning in *Wade* relied heavily on the right of privacy. Indeed, much prior campaigning had emphasized the abortion decision as private, and therefore not a matter for legislative regulation. Behind these and similar assertions is an entire philosophy of law. Paul J. Micallef traces two different approaches to the relation of law and morality, the positivistic and the Thomistic.[39] The former found its champions in Bentham and Mill and surfaced practically in the Wolfenden Report. It is clear that Micallef is unhappy with the distinction established—indeed, almost canonized—by Wolfenden between crime and sin and then raised "to the compendious sphere of the relationship between law and morality." The relationship of human actions to criminal law, he argues, is not to be determined simply on the basis of the distinction between "the private act" and "its public manifestation."

In contrast to this analysis, Micallef carefully and thoroughly exposes Thomas' theory of law based on the common good of all persons. For Thomas, though law and morality are distinct, law has an inherently moral character due to its rootage in existential human ends. Once this has been said, the one criterion of legislation is feasibility, "that quality whereby a proposed course of action is not merely possible but practicable, adaptable, depending on the circumstances, cultural ways, attitudes, traditions of a people, etc. . . . Any proposal of social legislation which is not feasible in terms of the people who are to adopt it is simply not a plan that fits man's nature as concretely experienced."[40]

Therefore, within Thomas' perspectives, all acts, whatever their nature, whether private or public, moral or immoral, if they have

[39] Paul J. Micallef, "Abortion and the Principles of Legislation," *Laval théologique et philosophique*, 28 (1972), 267–303.
[40] Ibid., 294.

ascertainable public consequences on the maintenance and stability of society, are legitimate matters of concern to society, and consequently fit subjects for the criminal code. But it is feasibility that determines whether they *should be* in the penal code, and this cannot be collapsed into the private-public distinction. Therefore, while Thomas does not tell us whether abortion ought to be in the criminal code, his philosophy of law tells us what questions to ask. These questions were put very helpfully by the late John Courtney Murray. He wrote:

> A moral condemnation regards only the evil itself, in itself. A legal ban on an evil must consider what St. Thomas calls its own "possibility." That is, will the ban be obeyed, at least by the generality? Is it enforceable against the disobedient? Is it prudent to undertake the enforcement of this or that ban, in view of the possibility of harmful effects in other areas of social life? Is the instrumentality of coercive law a good means for the eradication of this or that social vice? And, since a means is not a good means if it fails to work in most cases, what are the lessons of experience in the matter?[41]

Micallef and Murray present a tidy account of Thomistic perspectives on law and morality. What makes the matter so terribly complicated is that at the heart of the feasibility test is the fact that there is basic disagreement to start with on the moral character of abortion.

Charles Curran faces these complications with insight and restraint. He summarizes very well the relationship of law and morality in pluralistic societies by walking a middle path between the "idealist" tradition (wherein the natural law simply translates into civil law and merely tolerates deviations) and the purely pragmatic tradition (wherein law merely reflects the mores of a particular society).[42] Laws must root in both prophetic ideal and pragmatic reality. Thus in pluralistic societies government will

---

[41] J. C. Murray, S.J., *We Hold These Truths* (New York: Sheed & Ward, 1960), 166–67.

[42] Charles E. Curran, "Abortion: Law and Morality in Contemporary Catholic Theology," *Jurist*, 33 (1973), 162–83.

acknowledge the right of the individual to act in accord with the dictates of his conscience, but "the limiting principle justifying the intervention of government is based on the need to protect other innocent persons and the public order." In determining what this means concretely, especially with regard to innocent persons, Curran adduces other important factors: enforceability and equity. Laws that are unenforceable or have discriminatory effects compromise their contribution to the over-all good of a society.

On the basis of this understanding of the relationship of law and morality, Curran believes that those who hold strongly anti-abortion moral positions could arrive at any of three possible legal positions on abortion: almost absolute condemnation, modified regulation, no law at all. His own legal position, in light of the factors adduced above, is close to that proposed in 1961 in the Model Penal Code drafted by the American Law Institute. The ALI proposed that abortion be exempted from the penal code in certain tragic instances such as life threats to the mother, rape, and incest.

Roger Shinn, in a painstakingly fair article, attempts to relate social policies to personal decisions in a pluralistic society.[43] Shinn first asks: What morality is it *right* to legislate? Behind the question is, of course, Shinn's realistic thesis that it is both possible and desirable to legislate and enforce *some* morality. The crucial question concerns only *what* morality to legislate where abortion is concerned. Both opposing positions on this question (legal freedom of abortion, legal constraints) root their case in moral convictions. Shinn discusses these with remarkable objectivity and concludes that we have a profound conflict of convictions and values and that the most we can do is learn to live with these conflicts.

He then turns to the second question: What is it *possible* to legislate? Here Shinn emphasizes the fact that law must rest on a fairly broad shared conviction or, if there is not such consensus, on a very fundamental moral or constitutional principle that people are reluctant to deny. Without these broad bases—which do not exist in our society on the immorality of abortion—prohibitive laws will be futile. For this reason Shinn argues that the Court's decision is a reasonably adequate framework for this society at this

[43] Roger L. Shinn, "Personal Decisions and Social Policies in a Pluralist Society," *Perkins Journal,* 27 (1973), 58–63.

point in history. Shinn is not arguing that the decision was good history, good logic, or good judicial practice; he suggests only that "the decision offers a better way of living with a profound conflict of moral convictions than most alternatives."

Perhaps Shinn is right. Perhaps the Court's decision is a better way of living with a profound conflict of values. But before this is too readily concluded, two cautions seem in place. First, what represents a better way of living with a profound conflict will depend to some rather intangible extent on what one supports as the direction of the solution of this conflict. And this gets us right back to moral positions. For instance, if I grant that there is presently conflict in moral positions rendering strongly prohibitive laws impracticable, but if I believe (as a moral position) that nascent life is human life deserving of protection and possessed of the rights we attribute to other human beings, and if I hope that others will eventually share this conviction, then I might easily believe that the Court's decision simply deepens the difficulty of ever arriving at this conclusion. Thus the decision is, in some sense, calculated to freeze the situation of present conflict, to settle for it without providing any hope of a resolution.

If, on the other hand, my moral position were that of Shinn, I would more readily see the Court's conclusion as the best oasis during moral conflict. What is his position? Shinn believes that "the fetus has *some* rights, especially in the later stages of pregnancy, but that the woman also has rights to freedom. . . ." On this basis he states his own preference for weighting the law on the side of the woman's rights, not because fetal rights are insignificant but because the "problems of defining the health of the mother are extremely difficult." If I held that moral position, then I might conclude with Shinn that the Court's "decision offers a better way of living with a profound conflict of moral convictions than most alternatives."

My point is that Shinn's acquiescence in the Court's decision traces back, to some extent, to his moral position. Therefore, in these terms, whether one can agree with this acquiescence depends on whether one is satisfied with Shinn's moral position. Shinn has not argued this position sufficiently to invite agreement. To say that the fetus has *some* rights—without explaining

what these are, how strong they are, why, etc.—and then to weight
the law in favor of a woman's rights, leaves many unanswered
questions. Until Shinn has argued his moral position more thoroughly and persuasively (which he professedly did not want to undertake in this essay), his conclusion about the Court's decision as
a way of living with conflict remains moot if not arbitrary. What
Shinn should have said is that for those who hold his moral position the Court's decision "offers the better way of living with a
profound conflict of moral values."

The second caution is closely connected with the first. What is
the best way of accommodating legally to moral conflict should
hardly be left exclusively to those who obviously side with one
side of the conflict. This is as true of the Court's decision as it is
of the traditional prohibitive legal stands. The reasoning of the
majority of the Court left little doubt where this majority stood
on the substantive issue of fetal value. For such a group to determine what is most equitable for the country is at least as objectionable as allowing the classical prohibitionist to make this determination. The better way of discovering the appropriate legal
position at the present time of moral pluralism is to leave the matter to the state legislatures, even though this procedure itself is
not without problems.

Papal and episcopal statements on abortion have abounded in
the recent past, and since their context has been that of threatened or actual liberalization of abortion law, there is a decided,
though far from exclusive, emphasis on the relation of morality
and law. Pope Paul VI, in an allocution to Italian jurists, noted
that the state's protection of human life should begin at conception, "this being the beginning of a new human being."[44] This is
an emphasis that reappears in nearly all the national episcopal
statements.

When relating abortion to women's liberation, Pope Paul insists that true liberation is found in the vocational fulfillment of
motherhood. There follows an extremely interesting analysis of
the pertinence of relationships to human dignity and rights, an

[44] Pope Paul VI, "Pourquois l'église ne peut accepter l'avortement," *Documentation catholique*, 70 (1973), 4–5; *The Pope Speaks*, 17 (1973), 333–35.

analysis that in its way anticipates some of the theology to be reported below (especially the *Études* dossier). The Pope notes:

> In such a vocation there is implicit and called to concretization the first and most fundamental of the relations constitutive of the personality—the relation between this determined new human being and this determined woman, as its mother. But he who says *relation* says *right*; he who says fundamental relation says *correlation between a right and an equally fundamental duty*; he who says fundamental human relationship says a universal human value, worthy of protection as pertaining to the universal common good, since every individual is before all else and constitutively *born of a woman.*[45]

If I read him correctly, Paul VI is insisting that the relationship constitutive of the personality and generative of rights and duties is not basically and primarily at the psychological or experienced level—a point I shall touch on later.

The Belgian bishops make this very same point.[46] Relationships —and by this they obviously mean experienced relationships—important as they are, are not the sources of the dignity and rights of the nascent child. Rather, the source is the personality in the process of becoming. They cite *Abortus Provocatus*, a study issued by the Center of Demographic and Family Studies of the Belgian Ministry of Health: "There is no objective criterion for establishing, in the gradual process of development, a limit between 'nonhuman' life and 'human' life. In this process each stage is the necessary condition for the following and no moment is 'more important,' 'more decisive,' or 'more essential' than another."[47] Therefore they are puzzled at the fact that at the very time we are eliminating discrimination between sexes and among races and social classes, we are admitting at the legal level another form of discrimination based on the moment, more or less advanced, of life.

As for the law itself, the Belgian hierarchy is convinced that lib-

---

45 Pope Paul VI, "Pourquois l'église," 5.
46 "Declaration des évêques belges sur l'avortement," *Documentation catholique*, 70 (1973), 432–38.
47 Ibid., 434.

eralized abortion law does not solve the real problems. Indeed, by seeming to, it leads society to neglect efforts on other fronts to get at the causes of abortion. Therefore they are opposed to removal of abortion from the penal code, because such removal would, among other things, imply the right to practice abortion and put in question one of the essential foundations of our civilization: respect for human life in all forms.

The Swiss bishops, after noting with other national hierarchies that God alone is the judge of consciences and that no one has the right to judge other persons, put great emphasis on corporate responsibility for the abortion situation.[48] Those who neglect the social measures for family protection, for aid to single women, etc., are more culpable than those who have abortions.

The Italian hierarchy sees abortion as part of a general trend of violence against man.[49] Its legalization will not only not eliminate the personal and social evils by getting at their causes, it will also augment the harm in many ways—for example, by misshaping our moral judgments. The bishops of Quebec echo many of these same points and make it clear that what is at stake is the very idea on which our civilization is built: the conviction that all men are equal, whether young or old, rich or poor, sick or well, etc.[50] They associate themselves with all men who seek truly human solutions through establishment of a more just and humane society.

The German episcopate, after noting that protection of human life is an "absolutely fundamental principle," registers its opposition to the liberalization before the Bundestag.[51] Not only is the legislation morally unacceptable, but also it will not solve the alleged difficulties it is supposed to solve. In the course of this interesting statement, the bishops turn to the relation of morality and law. Clearly, not every moral imperative should be in the penal code (for example, envy, ingratitude, egoism). But where the rights of others are at stake, the state cannot remain in-

---

[48] "Déclaration des évêques suisses sur l'avortement," *Documentation catholique*, 70 (1973), 381.

[49] "Déclaration des évêques italiens sur l'avortement et la violence," *Documentation catholique*, 70 (1973), 245.

[50] "Déclaration des évêques du Québec," *Documentation catholique*, 70 (1973), 382–84.

[51] "Le problème de l'avortement: Lettre pastorale des évêques allemands," *Documentation catholique*, 70 (1973), 626–29.

different. "Its primordial duty is to protect the right of the individual, to assure the common good, to take measures against the transgressions of right and violations of the common good, if necessary by means of penal law." In doing this, the state becomes a *constitutional* state.

But legislation is not enough. The difficulties leading to abortion must be overcome by other measures. It is here that genuine reform ought to occur. And in undertaking these reforms, the federal republic becomes a *social* state. "It is only when the state is disposed to recognize the principle according to which no social need, whatever it be, can justify the killing of a human being before birth, that it merits the name of social state. It is only when the state is disposed to protect the right to life of a human being before birth and to punish violations of this right, that it merits the name of constitutional state."[52] Only within these parameters and on these conditions should legislators withhold penal sanctions for conflict cases—cases that ought to be precisely determined in law.

More recently the Conference of German Bishops (Catholic) and the Council of the Evangelical Church (EKD, Protestant) produced a common statement on abortion.[53] The most remarkable thing about the document is its common endorsement by the leadership of the vast majority of Christians, Catholic and non-Catholic, in Germany. Once again there is insistence on the fact that a social state will approach abortion reform positively—to wit, in terms that attempt to reorder social relationships in such a way that pregnant women receive the type of support that will prevent their seeing abortion as the only way out of difficult situations. The bishops underscore the fact that no society can long exist when the right to life is not acknowledged and protected. "The right to life must not be diminished, neither by a judgment on the value or lack thereof of an individual life, nor by a decision on when life begins or ends. All decisions that touch human life can only be oriented to the service of life."

The document resolutely rejects simply legalization of abortion in the first three months (*Fristenregelung*) as a form of abortion reform. Rather, the task of the lawgiver is to identify those

---

[52] Ibid., 628.
[53] " 'Fristenregelung' entschieden abgelehnt," *Ruhrwort* (Dec. 8, 1973), p. 6.

conflict situations in which interruption of pregnancy will not be punished (*straflos lassen*). By this wording the document insists that the moral law is not abrogated by legal tolerance but it remains to guide individual decisions in exceptional situations where the state decides not to punish abortion. Throughout, the document lays emphasis on the fact that positive law regulating abortion roots not merely in considerations of utility and party politics, but also in basic human values (*Grundwerte menschlichen Zusammenlebens*). An excellent pastoral statement on all counts.

The Permanent Council of the French Episcopate calls attention to the difference between legislation and morality.[54] The task of the legislator is to see how the common good is best preserved in the circumstances. But in drawing up legislation, the government will necessarily express a certain concept of man; for this reason the bishops feel impelled to speak up. Recalling that abortion, no matter how safe and clean it is, always represents a personal and collective human defeat, the bishops remind the legislators that in widening the possibilities for abortion they risk respect for human life, open the door for further extensions, and consecrate radical ruptures among sexuality, love, and fecundity. Ultimately, the remedy for the problem of widespread clandestine abortions in France is neither legal constraints nor liberalization. Women tempted to abortion must experience, really and personally, the fact that they are not alone in their distress. Any reform of abortion law must provide for this.

The statement of the Administrative Committee of the National Conference of Catholic Bishops of the United States in response to the Supreme Court's *Wade* and *Bolton* decisions is the strongest, and in this sense most radical, episcopal statement I have ever encountered.[55] After detailing the Court's assignation of prenatal life to nonpersonhood, the pastoral states: "We find that this majority opinion of the Court is wrong and is entirely contrary to the fundamental principles of morality." The document continues: "Laws that conform to the opinion of the Court are immoral laws, in opposition to God's plan of creation. . . ."

[54] "Déclaration du Conseil permanent de l'épiscopat français sur l'avortement," *Documentation catholique*, 70 (1973), 676–79.
[55] NCCB Pastoral Message, 83.

After citing the fundamental character of the right to life as guaranteed in the Declaration of Independence and buttressed in the Preamble to the Constitution, the bishops conclude that "in light of these reasons, we reject the opinion of the U. S. Supreme Court as erroneous, unjust, and immoral." While the statement contains no protracted discussion on the relation of law and morality, it is clear that the American bishops utterly reject the implied doctrine of the Court on the question.

Even this brief roundup probably justifies the conclusion of Michael J. Walsh, S.J., that we have here an "impressive example of the Magisterium in action."[56] It would be useful to list the common and dominant themes of this sprawling papal and episcopal literature. I see them as follows:

1. There is total unanimity in the recent teaching of the Pope and bishops on the right to life from conception. Furthermore, as Ph. Delhaye points out,[57] there is the pronounced consciousness that this teaching is the fulfillment of the commission received by Christ to teach and witness to the constant teaching of the Church.

2. There is repeated emphasis on the fact that we are dealing with a fundamental value, one at the very heart of civilization. The documents generally place the fight against abortion in the larger context of respect for life at all stages and in all areas.

3. It is the task of civil society to protect human life from the very beginning.

4. Human life is a continuum from the beginning. As Walsh puts it, "Essential continuity of a human being from conception to death is the presupposition of every episcopal argument."[58] In light of this we encounter terms such as "person in the process of becoming." And to this individual there is repeatedly ascribed the *droit de naître*, as Pope Paul puts it, a relatively recent rendering of the more classical right to life.

5. The protection provided for this *personne en devenir* must be both legal and social. With regard to the law, there is the practi-

[56] Michael J. Walsh, S.J., "What the Bishops Say," *Month*, 234 (1973), 172–75.
[57] Ph. Delhaye, "Le magistère catholique et l'avortement," *Esprit et vie*, 83 (1973), 449–57 and 434–46. The first part of this two-part article contains a rather full dossier of papal and episcopal statements on abortion.
[58] Walsh, "What the Bishops Say," 174.

cally unanimous conviction that legalization of abortion on a broad scale will not solve the many problems associated with abortion, but will rather bring further devastating personal and social evils, particularly through miseducation of consciences. Beyond that, the pastorals are rather reserved in their demands about legislation, except for the American statement, which Delhaye regards as *assez dur*. By "social protection" I refer to the unanimous and strongly stated conviction of the episcopates that we must do much more, personally and societally, to get at the causes of abortion. If there is a single major emphasis in all of the documents, it is this.

6. In arguing their case for respect for nascent life and for its protection through public policy, the hierarchies suit the argument to the local situation, as Walsh notes.[59] For instance, the Americans appeal to American legal traditions and the declaration of the United Nations. The Scandinavians, in opposing further liberalization, are deeply concerned to protect individuals against pressurization.

7. The statements generally note that their teaching is not specifically Catholic, though the Church has always upheld it and though it can be illumined, enriched, and strengthened by theological sources.

8. While urging the teaching clearly and unflinchingly, the bishops manifest a great compassion for individuals in tragic circumstances and a refusal to judge these individuals. On the other hand, there is a rather persistent severity with society in general, whose conditions so often render new births difficult or psychologically insupportable.

In the finest piece of writing I have seen on abortion in some time, the editors of *Month* propose a new strategy on abortion.[60] It is simply this: Make abortion as unnecessary as possible. "If one assumes that in a pluralist society the law cannot be repealed, then all recommendations will be designed to mitigate the evil rather than eliminate it." This duty to ensure the conditions for humanized life falls in a special way on those who have refused the facility of abortion. It involves two steps, one short-term, the other long-term. The immediate response envisages practical care

[59] Ibid., 173–74.
[60] "A New Catholic Strategy on Abortion," *Month*, 234 (1973), 163–71.

for mother-to-be. The editors cite the remarkable pastoral of Bishops Eric Grasar and John Brewer (Diocese of Shrewsbury) as an
example. It deserves quoting.

> We recognize that, for one reason or another, a preg-
> nancy can cause a problem, distress, shame, despair to
> some mothers. Perhaps, in our concern to uphold the
> sanctity of life, we have failed to show sufficient practical
> concern for the mother-to-be who feels herself in an in-
> tolerable situation. That is all over. The Diocese of
> Shrewsbury publicly declares its solemn guarantee. It is
> this: Any mother-to-be, Catholic or non-Catholic, is
> guaranteed immediate and practical help, if, faced with
> the dilemma of an unwanted pregnancy, she is prepared
> to allow the baby to be born and not aborted. This help
> includes, if she wishes, the care for her baby after birth.
> All the resources of the diocese are placed behind this
> pledge.[61]

As for long-term measures, the editors note that the motivations
behind most abortion requests are social and economic. This
being the case, it is absolutely essential that we so modify the social and economic conditions that these motivations will disappear. "Society should treat these requests as a *symptom of its own
sickness*" (emphasis added).

In developing their presentation, the *Month* authors have an
excellent treatment of fetal personhood as stemming from social
interaction, from relationships. In this view humanity is an
achievement, not an endowment. Thus the justification of abortion has reshaped the definition of what it means to be human.
The authors reject the idea that achievement is to be preferred to
potentiality, and for two reasons. First, no one believes this and
no one acts on it, facts evidenced in our treatment of children.
They are prized and valued for their potentiality. Second, the
preference of achievement over potentiality affirms the rights of
the big battalions over the defenseless. "To weight the debate a
priori in favor of the mother who can then deal with the fetus as

61 Ibid., 169–70.

though it were a malignant growth is to sanction a drastic exercise of power. In all other fields, we would recognize this and stop it at once. But here, and for most of us, the victims die unseen, and so consciences are easily tranquillised."[62] The authors see this as an unevangelical failure to rise to the love of the intruder, the unwelcome guest—as a racism of the adult world. If one decides to read but a single article on abortion, this is in my judgment the one to read.

The realistic, temperate, and persuasive study by the editors of *Month* contrasts with Rachel Wahlberg's brief report of a conference on abortion held at Southern Methodist University.[63] Distinguishing between the abstract and the personal, she concludes that those not involved with a specific unwanted pregnancy tend to discuss the philosophical, medical, or moral questions. Abortion debates must move from the "ivory-tower formulations to the gut-level issues." This fairly common attitude, while it does contain an obvious truth, is, I believe, ultimately mischievous. It opposes the "person" and "immediate crisis" to moral discourse—as if morality had nothing to do with the personal dimensions of problem pregnancies and were unrelated to immediate crises. Morality is, more than inferentially, associated with ivory-towerism. Ms. Wahlberg has not really abandoned morality to deal with the "gut" issues. She has rather collapsed morality into the "gut" issues and thereby opted for her own form of morality, and one with enough only half-hidden assumptions to rock many a tower into response. But that brings us to the recent work on the morality of abortion.

The Morality of Abortion

The study that has provoked the most interest on the Continent in many a year is the *Études* dossier.[64] It is a summary of the deliberations of a pluricompetent group gathered by Bruno Ribes, S.J., editor of *Études*. The report delves into many aspects of the

[62] Ibid., 167.

[63] Rachel C. Wahlberg, "Abortion: Decisions to Live with," *Christian Century*, 90 (1973), 691–93.

[64] "Pour une réforme de la législation française relative à l'avortement," *Études* (Jan. 1973), 55–84.

abortion question. For instance, with regard to a desirable law, they recommend that the French law bear essentially on the objectivization and maturation of the decision, on "conscientization" of the responsibility involved. A permissive law will not lead to a collapse of public morality, if the experience of other countries is any indication.

But it is their moral probing that is especially interesting. Noting that the two positions on the humanity of the embryo (developmental vs. one continued vital process) have led to a dialogue of the deaf, they propose their own solution. It is based on a distinction between "human life" and "humanized life." Since we are essentially relational beings, it is in relation to others that we discover, exercise, and receive our singularity and proper being. The very existence of the fetus is a kind of injunction to the parents. Their recognition of fetal life gathers this injunction into a new call. The parents call the child to be born. It is this recognition and call of the parents (and beyond them, of society) that *humanizes*. Prior to this event the fetus is a "human being" but is not humanized.

Refusal to humanize, the group argues, is intolerable; for it dissociates the biological from the human, the generating function from the humanizing. However, interruption of pregnancy is "socially justifiable" if it represents the refusal to bring about a dehumanization; for there are instances where genuine humanization is impossible. The terms "dehumanization" and "inhuman situation" are not definable or codifiable except for the obvious cases— for instance, of fetal deformity that will deprive the fetus of all social relations. The authors conclude that no abortion situation is "socially justifiable" unless accompanied by an attestation of the impossibility for the parents to give birth without creating an inhuman situation.

Reactions to this study were many and swift. The Belgian bishops, as noted above, explicitly rejected such a distinction.[65] A subsequent issue of *Études* published the interesting reader response, especially on the distinction between *vie humaine* and *vie humanisé*.[66] Bruno Ribes repeated once again the contention

---

[65] "Déclaration des évêques belges," 434 ff.
[66] Bruno Ribes, S.J., "Dossier sur l'avortement: L'apport de nos lecteurs," *Études* (Apr. 1973), 511–34.

that, while a person certainly cannot exist without the individuality he has prior to humanization, this individuality does not suffice to specify him. Ph. Delhaye regards the *Études* distinction as only the clearest formulation of an objection against which the episcopal texts are aimed.[67] He cites the archbishop of Rouen as branding the distinction "inadmissible casuistry," as at once "subtle and coarse." Cardinal Renard, adverting to the distinction in a speech to journalists, noted that if the fetus can be humanized, it is because it is fundamentally human to start with.[68]

R. P. Corvez, O.P., believes that the thought of the *Études* group is clearly insufficient on the key point;[69] for human life is present in its essentials even without "recognition" of the parents. "The child is really man, even in the womb of his mother, sharing human nature before receiving a humanizing formation. It is humanity which humanizes. It is [human] nature which humanizes."

Michel Schooyans rightly claims that abortion discussions faithfully reflect the cultural climate in which they occur, and in the West they reflect the axioms and ideology of a consumer culture.[70] In this light he sees liberalization of abortion as a form of "the medicine of luxury." He then turns to the human being vs. humanized being of the *Études* study. After granting the importance of relationships as constitutive of personality, Schooyans accuses the authors of a surreptitious slip from a distinction to a division. The distinction, valid enough in itself, results from an analysis of a unique process, an integral one. But a corresponding *division* lacks any foundation, for in concrete reality there is no stage marking the passage from one mode of being to another. This point is repeated by Outler (below).

Schooyans should have stopped there, for his final reflections represent a painful collapse of theological courtesy. He accuses these attempts of sterilizing the gospel of its intransigence. "The premises," he contends, "are forged for the needs of the

[67] Delhaye, "Le magistère catholique et l'avortement," 449–57.
[68] Alexandre C. Renard, "Allocution prononcée par le Cardinal Renard," *Documentation catholique*, 70 (1973), 183–84.
[69] R. P. Corvez, O.P., "Sur l'avortement," *Esprit et vie*, 83 (1973), 97–101.
[70] Michel Schooyans, "La libéralisation de l'avortement," *Esprit et vie*, 83 (1973), 241–48.

cause." There are references to theologians in the service of princes, and so on. In this instance, to illustrate is to deplore.

That being said, I believe Schooyans is correct in asserting that a distinction is not a division. Furthermore, it seems that the notion "humanize" is being used in two different senses by the *Études* group. First, it refers to a recognition and call by the parents. As a first relation, that recognition is said to humanize. Second, there is reference to the "impossibility to humanize." Here "humanize" implies something more than the first relation of recognition and call. It refers to a quality of life after birth.

Ribes returned to the abortion discussion later and took a somewhat different approach.[71] The thought of some Catholics is changing on abortion because the context (cultural, political, sociological) is changing. He describes the situation in terms of a thesis (the classical position) and a growing antithesis (an ensemble of affirmations that modify or move away from the classical position). At the heart of the thought of many contemporaries, Ribes argues, is the refusal of undue generalization, a rejection of moral norms that seem independent of scientific, sociological, and political data. The good is ultimately the function of many approaches and currents; therefore the moral act must integrate diverse and sometimes contradictory principles.

Concretely, where abortion is concerned, it is obviously necessary to insist on the principle of respect for nascent life. But Ribes contends that this principle must be proposed along with others that are equally valid. His chief complaint is against "the enunciation of a principle while appearing to neglect another *equally valuable* (emphasis added) principle."[72] It is the responsibility of the individual to balance and compose the various competitive principles in the situation. And when he does so, his decision is not simply the choice of the lesser evil; it relates to what is more human, therefore to the order of duties. This latter assertion is targeted at Gustave Martelet, S.J., who in interpreting *Humanae vitae* had argued that the choice of the lesser evil, while tolerable and un-

[71] Bruno Ribes, S.J., "Les chrétiens face à l'avortement," *Études* (Oct. 1973), 405–23.
[72] Ibid., 420.

derstandable at times, never pertains to the order of objective values and hence to the order of duties.[73]

Ribes is, I believe, correct in his criticism of Martelet. Martelet's delineation of "objective values" pertains to an unreal, almost platonic world. Nevertheless, my impression is that Ribes has confused two things: motivation and justification. Motivation refers to the perception of a person about why an abortion is necessary or desirable. In our insistence on the immorality of abortion, we may well have tended to overlook these perceptions and their underlying causes. Justification refers to an assessment of the perception of the person in light of a value scale that transcends and challenges individual perceptions.

The confusion of motivation and justification reflects an inadequate distinction between the pastoral and the moral—a point to which I shall return below. In pursuit of this point, Ribes could be confronted with two alternatives. (1) The respect for nascent life prevails over other values in most situations—as the classical tradition maintains. (2) The respect for nascent life does not prevail over other values in most situations. These are moral statements. If Ribes denies the first statement, as he seems to, then he must hold the second. But if he does want to endorse the second statement, he should get into a thorough discussion about the relationships of values, not about the complex web of motivations and perceptions that are the personal filters for the assimilation of values. These latter are basically pastoral concerns. Contrarily, if Ribes accepts the first statement, then why all the tortured concern about "other principles" of equal value that can only be composed by the individuals? Briefly, what Ribes has failed to argue convincingly is that other principles are of *equal* value. He has shown only that they are perceived as such by many of our contemporaries.

In a long study Bernard Quelquejeu proposes that a change in method is called for in facing the contemporary abortion situation.[74] If we consult the concrete perplexed conscience, we may discover there a new principle, not yet perceived and formulated. This would provide the basis for a new attitude toward abortion.

[73] Cited in Ribes, "Les chrétiens face à l'avortement," 414.
[74] Bernard Quelquejeu, O.P., "La volonté de procréer," *Lumière et vie*, 21 (1972), 57–71.

Quelquejeu then argues that any judgment that prescinds from the right to exercise one's sexuality isolates the problem out of context. Concretely, if the preceding will not to conceive was reasonable and responsible, then interruption of pregnancy is justifiable. "To affirm that an accidental conception, not desired, is in itself enough to cancel out in every case, the will not to conceive—to the point of constituting an unconditioned obligation of procreation and education—is equivalent to denying this antecedent will, in its reasonable freedom. . . ." A biological fact is allowed to prevail over a reasonable will, a felt and well-founded freedom.

V. Fagone, S.J., will have none of this.[75] He admits that a concrete solution to an abortion problem has to be found in the general context of responsible procreation. However, equating an accidental pregnancy with a biological fact rests on a false supposition and vitiates the whole argument. Quelquejeu holds that if the will to procreate is absent, the fetus is merely a biological fact. Against this Fagone urges that the will not to procreate can claim rights after conception "only if the intention to procreate is required, ontologically, for the fruit of conception to be truly human." The ontological status of a being cannot depend on a subjective decision exterior to its being. Therefore Fagone contends that two things have been confused by Quelquejeu: the legitimacy of the will to procreate or not to procreate (a *moral* question), and the relationship of parental will and intent to the constitution of fetal humanity (an *ontological* question). Furthermore, how in consistency could Quelquejeu rebut the contention that even a born child is only a "biological fact" as long as the will not to procreate still persists?

Bernard Häring evaluates the main theories about the moment of hominization and concludes that each of them has some probability.[76] He grants that the data of embryology seem to buttress the position of biologists, philosophers, and moralists who view the moment of fertilization as the most decisive moment in the transmission of human life. "They are convinced that every-

---

[75] V. Fagone, S.J., "Il problema dell'inizio della vita dell'uomo," *Civiltà cattolica*, 124 (1973), 531–46.
[76] Bernard Häring, *Medical Ethics* (Notre Dame, Ind.: Fides, 1973), 81 ff.

thing is directed by a typically human life principle which we may call 'soul' or the life-breath of the person."

Häring believes, however, that the theories that give prime importance to implantation and/or to the final establishment of individualization cannot be simply ignored. When does this individualization occur? Häring discusses at length the theory favored by Teilhard de Chardin, Karl Rahner, and P. Overhage,[77] and strongly advocated by Wilfried Ruff, S.J., physician and professor of bioethics.[78] They believe that hominization of nascent life should be related to the development of the cerebral cortex; for it is the cerebral cortex that constitutes the biological substratum for personal life. Since, Häring argues, a considerable percentage of embryos turn out anencephalic (characterized by lack of essential parts of the typically human brain) and therefore simply incapable of any personal activity, and since the maternal organism automatically rejects nearly all cases of such embryos, it seems to follow that before the formation of the cerebral cortex "there exists merely a biological center of life bereft yet of the substratum of a personal principle." The basic structure of the cerebral cortex is outlined between the fifteenth and twenty-fifth day, or, as Häring notes, "at least after the fortieth."

What does Häring make of all this? First, he grants that the theory "which presents hominization as dependent on the development of the cerebral cortex has its own probability"—that is, "before the twenty-fifth to fortieth day, the embryo cannot yet (with certainty) be considered as a human person." Second, Häring proposes this as a theory or opinion only, and not something that can be acted on until it gains greater acceptance by "those in the field." Or, as he puts it, "the theory . . . does not provide sufficient ground for depriving the embryo of the basic human right to life."[79] In other words, Häring believes that at present the fetus enjoys the favor of doubt and that fetal life must be protected *ab initio*, but that the uncertainties surrounding the very early stages of embryonic development "could contribute

[77] Karl Rahner and P. Overhage, *Das Problem der Hominisation* (Freiburg: 1961).

[78] Wilfried Ruff, S.J., "Individualität und Personalität im embryonalen Werden," *Theologie und Philosophie*, 45 (1970), 24–59; "Das embryonale Werden des Menschen," *Stimmen der Zeit*, 181 (1968), 331–55.

[79] Häring, *Medical Ethics*, 84.

greatly to the resolution of those difficult cases involving conflict of conscience or conflict of duties."

Kevin O'Rourke, O.P., regards this opinion as "outmoded."[80] Whether or not that judgment is too strong depends on one's assessment of the development of the cerebral cortex. If cortical development is viewed as a qualitative leap determinative of *personal* existence, then the theory does indeed have its probability. If it is not viewed in this way, then another conclusion is warranted. On the basis of the evidence I have seen (though I have not seen it all, by any means), I am inclined to see individualization as the crucial developmental stage—and individualization seems to occur prior to the development of the cerebral cortex. Be that as it may, what calls for our protection is *personne en devenir,* a contemporary rendering of Tertullian's "he is a man who will become a man." To this Häring would certainly agree.

In a good review, Charles Curran ultimately rejects delayed hominization based on either relational analyses (Pohier, Quelquejeu, Beirnaert, Ribes' earlier writing) or cortical development (Ruff).[81] Against the relational school, Curran argues that there is no reason to draw the line, for example, at birth. "After birth these relationships could so deteriorate that one could judge there was not enough of a relationship for truly human existence." Furthermore, he contends, the relational criterion proposed does not accept a full mutuality of relationships. For instance, why not press the argument and say that before a truly human relationship constituting "humanized life" is present, the child must acknowledge and recognize the parents? Finally, the exclusively relational account of the origin of life encounters problems when dealing with the other end of the cycle: death. Has death occurred when relationships deteriorate or cease?

Against Ruff and Häring, Curran argues that the *basis* for personal relations and spiritual activity (which admittedly occur only after birth, and considerably thereafter) "is not qualitatively that much more present because there is now a cortex in the brain."

[80] Kevin O'Rourke, O.P., "Häring on Medical Ethics," *Hospital Progress,* 54 (July 1973), 24–28.
[81] Charles E. Curran, "Abortion: Law and Morality in Contemporary Catholic Theology," *Jurist,* 33 (1973), 162–83.

Therefore the emergence of these organs is not a threshold that can divide human life from nonhuman life.

I find Curran's objections very persuasive. As for his own position, Curran argues that individual human life does not begin until after the possibility of twinning and recombination has been concluded.[82] Thereafter life may be taken only if necessary "to protect life or other values proportionate to life." Curran argues, and I agree, that this phrase ("other values proportionate to life") must be interpreted in a way consistent with our assessment of the values justifying the taking of extrauterine life. In summary: This is a useful survey and a carefully argued statement of his own position—one I find very close to my own.

In an excellent[83] article, Albert Outler also rejects as arbitrary all "magic-moment theories" as to when the defenseless deserve to be defended.[84] Such magic moments, whether they be ensoulment, cortical development, viability, birth, achievement of rationality, or acquisition of language, are merely prolongations of the body-soul dualism that has caused so much mischief. Outler grants that the distinctions are sometimes illuminating but that the radical disjunctions built on them do not make sense. In this he agrees with Schooyans.

From a theological perspective Outler sees terms such as "person," "personality," "personhood," and "self" as code words for a transempirical or self-transcending reality. This self-transcendence has been valued as a sign of life's sacredness in Christian tradition. It is not a *part* of the human organism nor is it inserted into a process of organic development at some magic moment. "It *is* the human organism oriented toward its transcendental matrix." Therefore Outler sees personhood as "a divine intention operating in a lifelong process that runs from nidification to death." For this reason abortion must be seen as "a tragic option of what has been judged to be the lesser of two real evils."

[82] See André E. Hellegers, "Fetal Development," *Theological Studies*, 31 (1970), 3–9.

[83] I realize that terms of approval such as "excellent," especially in this context, very often betray the fact that the article in question corresponds to or reinforces the position of the commentator. Whether this is the case here, one will know only if he tests the essay, and I urge such testing.

[84] Albert C. Outler, "The Beginnings of Personhood: Theological Considerations," *Perkins Journal*, 27 (1973), 28–34.

Since abortion is now legal, the moral issue is more urgent and agonizing than ever. This shift from legal to moral grounds might be an advance, according to Outler, "*if* the value-shaping agencies in our society were agreed that abortion is a life-and-death choice; *if* there were legal and social supports for conscientious doctors in their newly appointed roles as killers as well as healers; *if* we had a general will in our society to extend our collective commitments to the unborn and the newly born; and *if*, above all, there were any prospects in our time for higher standards of responsible sexuality. What has actually happened, however, is that in our liberation from abortion as a 'crime,' many of us have also rejected any assessment of it as a *moral evil*—and this will further hasten the disintegration of our communal morality."[85]

Notre Dame's Stanley Hauerwas studies three questions that enlighten the abortion issue: When does life begin? When may life be taken legitimately? What does the agent understand to be happening?[86] Having answered in rather classical terms the first two, Hauerwas turns to the third question, which is at the heart of his interesting article. He contends that there is more "in an agent's deliberation and decisions that is morally important than is in the spectator's judgment." What is this more? Briefly, the agent's perspective. To illustrate how this perspective functions, he takes a situation earlier presented by James Gustafson.[87] It is a very tragic instance of pregnancy resulting from multiple rape in a situation of poverty, illness, and lack of employment. After very sensitively describing the values involved, Gustafson had concluded that abortion could be morally justified—or, more accurately (for Gustafson strongly resists being a spectator-judge), that if he were in the woman's position, he could see how it would be morally justified.

The special warrants for this exception Gustafson stated as follows: (1) pregnancy resulted from a sex crime; (2) the social and

[85] Ibid., 32.

[86] Stanley Hauerwas, "Abortion: The Agent's Perspective," *American Ecclesiastical Review*, 167 (1973), 102–20.

[87] James M. Gustafson, "A Protestant Ethical Approach," in John T. Noonan (ed.), *The Morality of Abortion* (Cambridge, Mass.: Harvard University Press, 1970), 101–22. For a different perspective on Gustafson's essay, see Frederick Carney, "The Virtue-Obligation Controversy," *Journal of Religious Ethics*, 1 (1973), 5–19.

emotional conditions for the well-being of mother and child are not advantageous.

Hauerwas defends Gustafson's approach, not on the basis that abortion is a good thing, but rather because "abortion morally is justified under an ethical perspective that tries to pull as much good as possible from the situation." It might be a different thing if societal conditions and the woman's biography favored and supported carrying the pregnancy to term. "Yet Gustafson does not think such moral possibilities are present in this girl, at least not at this time." Behind this Hauerwas sees Gustafson's conviction that "the good and the right are found within the conditions of limitations. Present acts respond to the conditions of past actions, conditions which are usually irrevocable and unalterable."[88] Hauerwas agrees and states that our moral choices do not occur in ideal conditions where right and wrong are apparent, but rather the right must be wrenched from less than ideal alternatives.

I wish to pursue this point with Gustafson and Hauerwas, because further clarification may allow us to turn an ecumenical corner on the matter by bringing together two traditions that look rather sharply different but perhaps are really not. The point of concentration will be the phrase "moral justification." I would suggest that Gustafson has not "morally justified" abortion if we press that wording; for to do that he would, on his own terms, have to show what values are "higher in order to warrant the taking of life." I do not believe this has been shown. Gustafson-Hauerwas have rather shown that this girl in a real and understandable sense can do nothing else—that is, she has not (in her personal and societal situation) the resources to do what might in other conditions be the good thing to do. I should like to suggest that, if the emphasis falls on the woman's personal perspectives, strengths, and biography, then we are dealing with pastoral understanding or tolerance, not precisely with moral justification.

It is precisely in dealing with Gustafson's approach to abortion that Bernard Häring explains very well the distinction between moral theology and pastoral counseling.[89] Moral theology, he states, operates on a level "where questions are raised about general rules or considerations that would justify a particular moral

---

[88] Gustafson, "A Protestant Ethical Approach," 115.
[89] Häring, *Medical Ethics*, 112 ff.

judgment." Pastoral prudence, however, looks to the art of the possible. Catholic tradition has always been familiar with the notion of "invincible ignorance" (surely a poor term because of its one-sidedly intellectual connotations and its aroma of arrogance). Häring rightly notes that this term refers to the existential wholeness of the person, the over-all inability to cope with a certain moral imperative. This inability can exist not only with regard to the highest ideals of the gospel, but also with regard to a particular prohibitive norm. On this basis Häring concludes that he would "not pursue the question once it had become evident that the woman could not bear the burden of the pregnancy."

Gustafson is thoroughly familiar with this discussion; for that reason it would be illuminating to have his further reflections on the point. In the altogether worthy cause of eliciting these reflections, I would like to continue to suggest, as a basis for discussion, that it seems more accurate to refer to Gustafson's conclusion in the case described not as "moral justification" but as "pastoral justification," for in dealing with concrete instances, are we not at the level where inprincipled values are assimilated by the individual in her situation, with her background, etc.? Behind Gustafson's use of "moral justification" is, perhaps, his strong reluctance to be a judge. But here I believe a distinction is called for. The moralist is a judge of necessity, a point made excellently by Hauerwas. But a moralist is not only a moralist in dealing with concrete situations. He is also a pastoral counselor, and *as such* is not a judge, if by "judge" we mean one who dictates what must be done regardless of a person's capacities and situation.[90] Could it be that because of his remarkable pastoral instincts Gustafson too quickly identifies the moral and pastoral role and therefore uses the term "moral justification" where something else is involved? Possibly.

Every priest who has heard confessions knows the difference between moral judgment and pastoral compassion, between the good that ought to be and the good that cannot be as yet, between aspiration and achievement. When some segments of the

[90] A balanced presentation of the counseling approach to abortion is that of Harry E. Hoewischer, S.J., "A Counseling Approach to the Problems of the Unwanted Pregnancy," *Inquiry* (Regis College) (Oct. 1973), no pagination given.

Protestant community say that every human choice stands in need of forgiveness, they are saying something unfamiliar to Catholic *moral* tradition (especially the manualist moral tradition) but not to Catholic *pastoral* practice. If Gustafson would speak more of the good that ought to be, and his Catholic counterpart would speak (as well he can) more of what cannot yet be and why, the twain could easily mate into a position identifiable as catholic, because humanly compassionate, yet evangelically uncompromising and radical.

J. Robert Nelson writes that discussion of abortion among Christians would be considerably helped if "sanctity of life" were understood as including both *bios* (mere sustenance for mortal existence) and *zoe* (the qualitative dimension of life).[91] According to Nelson, *zoe* always has the higher value. If this is remembered, "Christians would never think of the fetus, at whatever stage of development, as a disposable 'thing'; nor would they have so strong a fixation on the preservation of the fetus 'at all costs' that they would be callous to either the pregnant woman's *zoe* or to the well-being of society."

Nelson's elaboration of "sanctity of life" is shot through with Christian insight and common sense. However, two points deserve comment. First, there is the meaning, or rather the implications, of the contention that *zoe* always has the higher value. Physical life is, to be sure, not the highest good for man, if one can use such language without plunging into dualism. But it is, as Schüller has recently insisted,[92] the most fundamental, and as such it is to be preferred over other conflicting goods which, even though they rank higher on a scale, are less fundamental.

Second, in terms of the basic moral issue, Nelson's treatment leaves the matter pretty much where it was; for the issue is precisely: How much *bios* can be sacrificed to *zoe* without undermining *zoe* itself? And on what warrants, with what controls, developed out of what form of moral reasoning? Nelson does not help here.

[91] J. Robert Nelson, "What Does Theology Say About Abortion?" *Christian Century*, 90 (1973), 124–28.

[92] Bruno Schüller, S.J., "Zur Problematik allgemein verbindlicher ethischer Grundsätze," *Theologie und Philosophie*, 45 (1970), 1–23; "Typen ethischer Argumentation in der katholischen Moraltheologie," *Theologie und Philosophie*, 45 (1970), 526–50.

In a long and rather strange article, Judith Jarvis Thomson tries to establish the moral justification for abortion by assimilating the procedure to a situation where one need not continue to provide his body as a source of life-saving sustenance to someone who cannot be saved without it.[93] Thus, refusing to allow a pregnancy to continue can be the moral equivalent of refusing to be a Good Samaritan. If there are times when one may legitimately argue that the cost is too great to demand that one be a Good Samaritan, so too with continuing the pregnancy. "I have been arguing," she writes, "that no person is morally required to make larger sacrifices to sustain the life of another who has no right to demand them, and this even where the sacrifices do not include life itself."

To the objection that the mother has special responsibilities and obligations to the child and that the child has certain rights, Thomson argues that we do not have special responsibilities for a person unless we have assumed them, explicitly or implicitly. This means that "if a set of parents do not try to prevent pregnancy, do not obtain an abortion, and then at the time of birth of the child do not put it out for adoption, but rather take it home with them, then they have assumed responsibility for it, they have given it rights, and they cannot now withdraw support from it. . . ."[94] Contrarily, "if they have taken all reasonable precautions against having a child, they do not simply by virtue of their biological relationship to the child . . . have a special responsibility for it." They may wish to assume this responsibility, but "if assuming responsibility for it would require large sacrifices, then they may refuse."

Thomson's essay stirred two formidable combatants into activity. Baruch Brody (MIT) replies that Thomson has overlooked the distinction between our duty to save a life and our duty not to take a life.[95] The former duty is much weaker than the latter. In another article Brody sets out his own understanding of when it is legitimate to abort.[96] Hypothesizing that the fetus is a human

[93] Judith Jarvis Thomson, "A Defense of Abortion," *Philosophy and Public Affairs*, 1 (1971), 47–66.

[94] Ibid., 65.

[95] Baruch Brody, "Thomson on Abortion," *Philosophy and Public Affairs*, 1 (1972), 335–40.

[96] Baruch Brody, "Abortion and the Sanctity of Human Life," *American Philosophical Quarterly*, 10 (1973), 133–40.

being whose life may not be taken except in the most extreme circumstances, he seeks a rule that would best state what these circumstances are. After rejecting any justification based on fetal aggression, Brody concludes with a norm that states that it is permissible to abort to save the mother's life if the fetus is going to die anyway in a relatively short time and taking its life is the only way to save the mother. The whole rationale for taking some life to save others "is that he whose life will be taken loses nothing of significance and [he] is not therefore being treated unfairly." But he insists on tightening this rule by adding the requirement that taking the mother's life will not save the child, or even if it will, it has been determined by a fair random method that the mother, not the child, ought to be saved.

While Brody's reasoning will appear quaint to a world whose attitudes toward abortion have been profoundly influenced by a variety of pressure groups (sexual freedom, population control, women's liberation, etc.[97]), it strikes me as being a very useful attempt to deal with the morality of conflict situations in a disciplined and controlled way without falling into the standard traps of utilitarian analysis. Unfortunately, however, the whole thing looks a bit too much like an academic game, since Brody begins by admitting that there are "others who claim, *with equally good reason* (emphasis added), that a fetus is not a human being. . . ."[98] His study would be much more persuasive if he had explored and validated that judgment.

Philosopher John Finnis also takes on Thomson.[99] Finnis claims that Thomson has muddied the discussion by conducting it in terms of rights. The dispute is properly about what one "must" do, is "morally required" to do. After such determinations have been made, we will be able, by a convenient locution, to assert the child's right. Furthermore, Thomson's constant appeal to rights obscures the weak point in her defense of abortion. That point is seen in her contentions that (1) rights typically or essentially depend on grants, concessions, etc.; (2) special responsibilities

[97] See David R. Mace, *Abortion: The Agonizing Decision* (Nashville, Tenn.: Abingdon, 1972), 60–62.

[98] Brody, "Abortion and the Sanctity of Human Life," 133.

[99] John Finnis, "The Rights and Wrongs of Abortion," *Philosophy and Public Affairs*, 2 (1973), 117–45.

likewise depend on grants, concessions, etc.; (3) therefore the
whole moral problem here concerns one's *special* responsibilities.
Finnis rejects utterly the idea that the mother's duty not to abort
is an incident of a special responsibility she undertook. It is rather
a straightforward incident of an ordinary duty everyone owes to
his neighbor.

Finnis then sets out his own understanding of the morality of
abortion, the moral "musts" and "mays." It builds along the lines
of the analysis elaborated by Germain Grisez that there are basic
goods that demand, among other things, that we never choose
directly against them. Finnis spends the rest of the article lifting
up the considerations that reveal whether and when our choices
must be characterized as directly against a basic good. His answer
is that destruction of life is inescapably antilife and against a basic
good when it is intended.

Finnis has scored some telling points against Thomson, a judgment I would defend in spite of a subtle response-article in which
she attempts again to equate not saving with killing.[100] However,
two points merit notice here. First, Finnis refers to "traditional
nonconsequentialist ethics which has gained explicit ecclesiastical
approval in the Roman Church these last ninety years. . . ." This
overstates the matter, I believe. The moral formulations of the
Church are, above all, practical guides for the formation of conscience and direction of the faithful. Since they are teaching statements, moral reasoning and various forms of persuasion will be—
indeed, must be—used. And moral reasoning does imply ethical
structure. But because a structure or system may be implicit in the
way a teaching is formulated, this should not be taken to mean
that this system is being taught or approved. It remains, as did
scholastic language in the past, a vehicle only more or less inseparable from the substance of the teaching. In this sense it is incorrect to refer to nonconsequentialist ethics as gaining "explicit ecclesiastical approval." Furthermore, there are those who would
argue that if there are practical absolutes in the moral domain,
their absoluteness can be argued precisely on consequentialist
grounds.

Second and very substantially, in discussing those actions that

[100] Judith Jarvis Thomson, "Rights and Deaths," *Philosophy and Public
Affairs*, 2 (1973), 146–59.

must be seen as choices against a basic good, Finnis notes that "the 'innocence' of the victim whose life is taken makes a difference to the characterizing of an action as open to and respectful of the good of human life, and as an intentional killing. *Just how and why it makes a difference is difficult to unravel* (emphasis added); I shall not attempt an unraveling here."[101] This is a crucial point. If Finnis were to attempt to unravel this—as applied, for example, to capital punishment in the past—he would encounter a consequentialist calculus at work in creating this exception, one that ultimately allows for the destruction of an individual's life if it is a threat to the common good and there is no other way of preventing this threat. On the basis of this and other forms of exception-making in the development of traditional norms, one has to conclude that a form of consequentialism cannot be excluded.

In a tortuous and ultimately very vulnerable study, Michael Tooley rejects both the "liberal" position of Judith Thomson and the more classical views of Finnis and Brody.[102] The former position is weak because of the impossibility of establishing any cutoff points that are acceptable. The classical position is rejected because it rests on the "potentiality principle" (the fetus deserves protection not for what it is physiologically but because this physiology will lead to psychological differences later that are morally relevant).

Tooley attacks this principle through a strange analogy. Suppose it might be possible at some future date to inject kittens with a chemical that would cause them to develop into cats possessing a brain similar to that of humans (with psychological capabilities, thought, language, etc.). One would not argue that they have a right to life just because of this potentiality. "But if it is not seriously wrong to destroy an injected kitten which will naturally develop the properties that bestow a right to life, neither can it be seriously wrong to destroy a member of *Homo sapiens* which lacks such properties, but will naturally come to have them."

Tooley then elaborates his own position. Briefly, it contends that "an organism possesses a serious right to life only if it

[101] Finnis, "Rights and Wrongs of Abortion," 141.
[102] Michael Tooley, "Abortion and Infanticide," *Philosophy and Public Affairs*, 2 (1972), 37–65.

possesses the concept of self as a continuing subject of experiences and other mental states, and believes that it is itself such a continuing entity." This concept of self is required by Tooley because right is defined in terms of a desire—and desires are limited by the concepts one possesses. Thus "an entity cannot desire that it itself *continue* existing as a subject of experience and other mental states unless it believes that it is now such a subject." On this basis Tooley accepts not only all abortions but even infanticide.

What is wrong with all this? Several things. First, a simple test of an analysis is the fit of its conclusions with the moral convictions of civilized men. To the best of my knowledge, most civilized men would recoil in sheer horror at the wholesale infanticide justified by Tooley's analysis. Second, in his animal analogy, Tooley has doubled his middle term ("potentiality"), well, monstrously. Finally, Tooley's key mistake is connecting inseparably rights and desires. He correctly notes that to ascribe a right is to assert something about the *prima facie* obligations of other individuals to act or to refrain from acting. But he then asserts that "the obligations in question are conditional ones, being dependent upon the existence of certain desires of the individual to whom this right is ascribed." Thus, he continues, if an individual asks me to destroy something to which he has a right, one does not violate his right to that thing if one proceeds to destroy it; for the owner no longer *desires* the object. On this basis desire, and therefore the capacity to desire, are said to be essential to the possession of rights.

Here Tooley has forgotten that the notion of right is an analogous one, not a univocal one. Basically this analogy traces to one's understanding of moral obligation, its source and meaning. Here Finnis is absolutely correct. Before one can move securely within the vocabulary of rights and their limits, he must return to their source; for rights are convenient locutions for the existence of obligation. At the level of moral obligation, Tooley must examine why it is wrong to kill a person. To say that it is wrong because it is in violation of a person's right is patent circularity. In his deliberations I believe Tooley will soon discover two things: (1) Any viable analysis will apply to all men, neonates and uterine babies not excluded. (2) Material goods (as goods that are subordinate to persons and can become one's *property*) generate different moral assertions than human life itself. It is these different moral assertions that are the basis for the analogy of rights. For example, we speak of *jus connaturale* (a right natural to man—for example, to his life) and *jus adventitium* (a right that arises from some positive event—for example, from buying, selling, finding, etc.). There are other such distinctions. Tooley treats them as if they were all the same, and basically because he has not traced their origin to a systematic theory of moral obligation.

Therefore, when he says that the obligations connoted by the term "right" are dependent upon the existence of certain desires of the individual to whom the right is ascribed, he is guilty of confusing apples and oranges, or better, of reducing all of them to prunes. One cannot, in other words, argue that what is true of one right is true of all rights. Tooley is correct in saying that I violate no right of ownership when I destroy property the owner desires destroyed. Scholastic philosophy has long been familiar with the axiom *consentienti non fit injuria* (no injustice is done to one who consents or waives his right). However, scholastic tradition has, no less than the Declaration of Independence, regarded certain rights as inalienable. If certain rights are alienable, others inalienable, then clearly one must return to the drawing boards if he treats them as all the same.

In a long and closely argued review article, Paul Ramsey takes up the books of Daniel Callahan and Germain Grisez.[103] Ramsey criticizes as "idiosyncratic" Callahan's use of the notion of sanctity of life and his espousal of the developmental school's answer to the question about the beginning of life. Callahan's analysis, Ramsey argues, has eroded the notion of equal justice. Behind it all Ramsey sees an incorrect premise—to wit, the idea that there can be inequality between life sanctities pitted against one another in conflict. Ramsey regards this as the major flaw in Callahan's defense of a legal policy of abortion on demand. Noting that Callahan regards the use made of his book on abortion as a "personal disaster," Ramsey contends that the book can and should be read in this abusive way and calls for a retraction of the structure of Callahan's moral argument.

I share Ramsey's discomfort with Callahan's analysis, an analy-

[103] Paul Ramsey, "Abortion: A Review Article," *Thomist*, 37 (1973), 174–226.

sis to which he recently returned.[104] As I read his book (*Abortion: Law, Choice and Morality*), it seems that Callahan is still trying to have it both ways. His sanctity-of-life principle yields a "strong bias against abortion," instills "an overwhelming bias in favor of human life." One "bends over backward not to eliminate human life." Abortion is the last resort of a woman, "to be avoided if at all possible." And this is a *moral* position. And yet we find him saying that it is "possible to imagine a *huge* [my emphasis] number of situations where a woman could, in good and sensitive conscience, choose abortion as a moral solution to her personal and social difficulties." In other words, Callahan feels the wrong of abortion; yet he feels the desperation of its need. Armed with these, he states in his recent essay that the moral problem is *balancing* the right of the fetus with the right of the mother. However, his ultimate moral position is hardly a balance; it comes close to eliminating one right altogether. Therefore Callahan ends up (since he cannot divest himself of his knowledge of and deep sensitivity to what is going on) cursing the rotten decisions imposed by a world most of us never made or chose.

What I miss here, then, is not sensitivity. Callahan's writings on abortion are utterly honest, appropriately corrective, and profoundly sensitive. I miss the moral reasoning that would explain his phrase "often necessary" choice. Something is necessary, first of all, in terms of competitive values and available alternatives. But, unless I have misunderstood him, Callahan explains this necessity almost exclusively in terms of the woman's perception of it. Important as these perceptions are, they do not constitute the heart of an ethical or moral position on abortion. Rather, I believe that they pertain to an ethics of an individual's response to a morality of abortion—what above was called pastoral counseling. Does not a true morality of abortion have to provide the possibility for expansion of an individual's perspectives and value commitments? I think so.

Ramsey next turns to Germain Grisez. Grisez, it will be recalled, argued that the traditional understanding of the principle of the twofold effect was too restrictive. It demanded that in the order of physical causality the evil effect not precede the good.

---

[104] Daniel Callahan, "Abortion: Thinking and Experiencing," *Christianity and Crisis*, 32 (1973), 295–98.

Grisez proposed that the intention of the agent remains upright (not choosing directly against a basic good) as long as the evil aspect is part of an indivisible process. The test of this indivisibility is whether no other human act need intervene to bring about the good effect.

Thus, as Ramsey interprets him, Grisez would allow abortion in a case of primary pulmonary hypertension where the woman could not oxygenate both herself and the fetus. However, in the instance of aneurysm of the aorta in which the wall of the aorta is so weakened that it balloons out behind the pregnant uterus, the physician must first kill the fetus (in a separable act) to get at the aneurysm. On Grisez's criterion, this second procedure would not be allowed. Ramsey sees this as too restrictive and not "confirmed by common sense or intuitive moral judgment."

The crucial question, Ramsey believes, is whether the target of the deadly deed is upon fetal life or upon what that life is doing to another life. "While the life is taken with observable directness, the intention of the action is directed against the lethal process or function of that life." Thus, in terms of its meaning, the action is describable as "removal," not precisely as "death-dealing." But Ramsey limits this to situations where both lives cannot be saved but only the mother's. "My view," he writes, "is that 'removal' is what *is done* and is justified in all cases where 'necessity' foredooms that only one life can be saved. . . ."[105]

Ramsey contends that Grisez's analysis would afford little or no guidance "where there is no necessity to do the intended action"; for every abortion could be arguably concerned with the removal of the child, not its death. Therefore he equates Grisez's view to that of Judith Thomson, of all people. Here I think he has misread Grisez. Grisez insists throughout that indirectness is but a single condition of the twofold effect; proportion is another. For instance, Grisez repeatedly asserts that we do not take life for the sake of health.

Ramsey's limitation of his analysis to instances where only one life can be saved (the mother's) leads one to ask whether the really operative factor is the intention of the action as he has struggled to analyze it. Is it not more broadly the proportionate reason?

[105] Ramsey, "Abortion: A Review Article," 223.

That is, it seems better to sound reasoning to save one life than to lose two in a situation where the fetus cannot be saved anyway.

I am not contesting Ramsey's conclusions; that is not the point here. It is the form of moral reasoning that deserves attention. Ramsey argues that interruption of pregnancy, *direct* in its external observableness, is aimed at stopping the fetus from doing what it is doing to the mother. He is inclined to call this a justifiable direct abortion, but presumably an indirect killing. And he explicitly rejects the idea that fetal death must be indirect in Grisez's sense —an inseparable aspect of a single act. Fetal death could be, in other words, the result of a prior separable action.

Actually, it seems clear that directness and indirectness do not really function critically in Ramsey's analysis, though he continues to use the distinction;[106] for Ramsey repeatedly restricts abortion to those instances where only one (the mother) can be saved. This suggests that what is really the justification in the case under discussion is the broader principle of doing the lesser evil in a tragic conflict situation, the principle of proportionate reason. This has to be the meaning of Ramsey's phrase "what the fetus is doing to the mother." Otherwise why could we not extend this to other cases short of life threats where pregnancy is a hardship (psychological, physical, economic), where the fetus is indeed "doing something to the mother" but something far short of a life threat?

In this connection the Belgian bishops have an extremely interesting but somewhat ambiguous paragraph on the moral principles governing abortion situations.[107] They write:

> In the case—today fortunately quite rare due to the progress of science—where the life of the mother and that of the child are in danger, the Church, concerned to meet this situation of distress, has always recognized the legitimacy of an intervention, even if it involves the indirect loss of one of the two lives one is attempting to save. In medical practice it is sometimes difficult to determine whether this misfortune results directly or indirectly

---

[106] Ibid., 220. "I agree with Grisez that any killing of man by man must be 'indirect.'"

[107] "Déclaration des évêques belges sur l'avortement," 443.

from the intervention. This latter intervention, from the point of view of morality, can be considered as a whole. The moral principle which ought to govern the intervention can be formulated as follows: Since two lives are at stake, one will, while doing everything possible to save both, attempt to save one rather than to allow two to perish.

I say the paragraph is ambiguous because there are at least two ways of reading it. (1) Intervention in these desperate instances is legitimate *providing it is indirect in character*. Its indirectness is determined by viewing it "as a whole." (2) Intervention to save one where the alternative is to lose two is *for this very reason* (the desperate alternatives) *indirect*. The first rendering is close to that of Grisez. If the second is the proper reading, it comes very close to the analysis of Peter Knauer. One can only ask what meaning the terms "direct" and "indirect" have if the crucial moral principle is to be formulated as in the last sentence of the episcopal statement; for what seems obviously at the heart of this principle is the conflict model of human choice, a model ultimately governed by the principle of the lesser evil. I have tried elsewhere, though with considerably less than total satisfaction, to explore the very thorny problem of the moral relevance of the direct-indirect distinction.[108]

In discussing this very question, William May appeals to the writings of Joseph Fuchs, S.J.[109] After pointing out that a person becomes morally good when he intends and effects premoral good (life, health, culture, etc.), Fuchs asks: "What if he intends and effects good, but this necessarily involves effecting evil also?" The answer given by Fuchs is: "We answer, if the realization of the evil through the intended realization of good is justified as a proportionately related cause, then in this case only good was intended."

As a gloss on this citation May states: "At first it might seem

108 Richard A. McCormick, S.J., *Ambiguity in Moral Choice* (Milwaukee, Wis.: Marquette University Press, 1973); McCormick and Paul Ramsey, *Doing Evil to Achieve Good* (Chicago: Loyola University Press, 1978).

109 William E. May, "Abortion as Indicative of Personal and Social Identity," *Jurist*, 33 (1973), 199–217.

(and unfortunately has so seemed to Richard McCormick . . .)
that Fuchs is saying that we may rightfully intend and effect a
premoral evil (for example, death) provided there is some proportionate good that will be achieved." May denies that this is the
way Fuchs is to be read, and for two reasons. First, Fuchs insists
that *only* good is intended in an act that has evil effects as well as
good consequences. "He refuses to say that the evil effected was
properly intended in the moral sense." Second, May points out
that Fuchs insists that the evil must be a part or element of *one*
human act. "He is saying, in short, that the act in question must
be describable as one ordered of itself to the good and that the act
in question is itself the means to the end."

Here two points. First, Fuchs is saying, I believe, that premoral
evil may indeed be intended—as the word "intend" has been used
traditionally in applications of the twofold effect—to wit, in a psychological sense. He is saying it is not intended "in the moral
sense." At this point, however, one must ask what it means to intend something "in the moral sense." It seems to be nothing more
than a convenient and *postfactum* way of saying that the good
pursued was fully proportionate to the evil effected within the
choice. If there is true proportion, then, as Fuchs notes, "only
good was intended." This is much more a *postfactum* ascription
than an analysis of human intending.

Second, there is question of what is meant by saying that the
evil must be a part or element of *one* human act. When I criticized Fuchs on this very point,[110] he answered[111] that an action
can be taken in three ways: physically, psychologically, humano-
morally. This last is the only description of an action that suffices
for its moral assessment. But taken in a humanomoral sense, the
one choice or action includes also its intended results and foreseen
circumstances. What is intended in a choice (not necessarily
achieved) pertains to the *oneness* of that action. Thus, in the famous case of Mrs. Bergmeier, the action was not simply adultery,
as a means to a good end. Rather, it was sexual union with a certain intended effect and in certain circumstances. Viewed in this
way, the extramarital intercourse was a part of *one* action that in-

---

[110] Richard A. McCormick, S.J., "Notes on Moral Theology," *Theological
Studies*, 33 (1972), 72 ff.
[111] Personal communication.

cluded the intended good also. I have some problems, or at least further questions, about this; but it is what Fuchs means; and it is a bit different from the interpretation given Fuchs by May.

In an interesting article Louis Dupré grapples with this very problem.[112] He first argues that inchoate personhood is present in fetal life from the beginning but that it must be evaluated differently according to a developmental scale. He then rejects the direct-indirect analysis as a "purely verbal solution" to the abortion problem. "I prefer," he writes, "to consider abortion always a direct killing of human life and then to ask under which circumstances it could be licit." What are these circumstances? As a general rule, Dupré seems satisfied with the norm that it is permissible to kill "only to prevent a person from inflicting a *comparable* type of harm to others." However, the implications of that norm depend on one's reading of "comparable." What values are comparable to life? In making this assessment, he contends that "the degree of development inevitably enters into the evaluation of the life value." He then goes on to suggest that personal liberty is a value comparable to that of life to many people and that a minimum degree of mental health is a condition for personal liberty. Thus he moves away from the traditional position.

I find Dupré undecided and ambiguous about what is the really decisive norm in abortion decisions. He presents two considerations as central: the developmental evaluation of personhood, and the values comparable to life itself. But what constitutes the heart of his opening of perspectives is not clear. At one point he states that "an identical risk to a woman's health decreases in moral weight as the pregnancy progresses. What would constitute a sufficient factor during the first two days after conception no longer does so after two months." This suggests that what justifies the abortion is a sliding scale of evaluation of fetal life. But then he immediately adds that "no abortive action, early or late, becomes ever permissible under our principles *unless* (emphasis added) a value comparable to life itself is at stake." This means that *any* abortion is justified because the competitive value is comparable to life itself. Which of these two considerations is decisive?

[112] Louis Dupré, "A New Approach to the Abortion Problem," *Theological Studies*, 34 (1973), 481–88.

Dupré's own example illustrates this unclarity. He notes: "In cases of rape of an adolescent, the presumption of serious mental damage appears strong enough to warrant the general use of an abortifacient at least during several hours following the coitus. But the same presumption cannot be taken for granted at a later stage of development. . . ." Now the problem here is that according to Dupré "serious mental damage" can qualify as justifying abortion only because it is a value comparable to life itself. That point can be defended, and perhaps successfully. But then, why relate it to a stage in fetal growth? An equivalence is, after all, an equivalence—unless serious mental damage is a value comparable to life when compared to some lives but not to others. This seems to be what Dupré would have to hold, but I fail to see how this avoids eroding the notion of equal rights, an erosion Dupré wants desperately to avoid.

Frederick Carney (Perkins School of Theology) believes that Dupré has confused two concepts of person, concepts that lead to unacceptable results when substituted for each other.[113] The first concept centers in the attribution of rights and responsibilities. When this notion of person is used, we are speaking of a few basic concerns common to all men, such as life and liberty, and the relation of individuals to each other in respect to these concerns is one of moral and legal equality.

The second concept of person describes the development of individuals and highlights special competencies or achievements. Here the relationship of individuals is one of disequality. Carney believes that Dupré's approach makes the abortion decision hinge on the second concept of person (personality development) rather than on the first.

> There are other problems in which the second concept of person is very appropriate, for example, admission to a college, or the assignment of awards for some achievement. For these problems Dupré's concept of person seems to me to be the central one. But in the consideration of the basic protections of social life the second concept just cannot function in any appropriate way. In

[113] See Donald G. McCarthy (ed.), *Beginning of Personhood* (Houston: Institute of Religion and Human Development), 36–40.

fact, I would say it will undermine our social life to try to substitute that concept as Dupré apparently wishes to do.

There are, Carney argues, instances within the first concept of personhood when it is legitimate to take life, but these are never instances of a balancing of capacities, merits, or achievements over against basic rights.

Carney then proposes his own approach. Rather than beginning with biological facts (for example, conception, quickening, viability, birth) to which we assign decisive importance for personhood, he suggests that we begin with moral theory—that is, rather than first defining personhood and then attributing rights, he wants first to attribute rights and then assign personhood to those to whom rights are attributed.

What are the reasons for wanting to put anybody within the category of individuals possessing rights? Carney finds three types of reasons for such attribution. First, there is the notion of fairness. If "x" is a rightholder and "y" is like "x" in all relevant characteristics, why should "y" not be a rightholder? This is a kind of deontological argument. Second, there is a teleological argument, one concerned with ends. What individuals fundamentally are or are destined to be cannot be fully acknowledged and enhanced without the attribution of basic rights. The third reason is a form of revelation, a theological argument. One believes that God wills that certain beings be protected in this fundamental way and therefore assigns basic rights to these beings.

Carney's suggestion is extremely interesting. Starting with biological fact is quite legitimate, as he notes. But it has not proved very helpful in achieving acceptable clarification and consensus in the body politic. If clarification and consensus in the body politic is what Carney wants from a switch in approach, then I seriously doubt that he is going to get it; for the supposition underlying such a switch is that people come out this way or that on abortion because of the rational persuasiveness of the arguments made. That can be doubted.

At any rate, a reading of recent episcopal and theological literature will lead to the conclusion that both approaches suggested by Carney are used, both by those who support the classical position on abortion and by those who would modify it. For instance, Pohier attempts to move away from the traditional position by showing two things:[114] first, that there are reasons in reproductive biology—for example, the number of spontaneous miscarriages— for saying that the fertilized ovum is not *être humain déjà*; second, that God's providential concern for life and man's share in this responsibility are not necessarily best described and supported by an absolute position on abortion.

If one impression is inseparable from this interesting literature, it is that abortion is a moral problem far more complex and anguishing than any one-dimensional approach (for example, right to privacy, woman's right to dispose of her body, absolute prohibition of abortion, etc.) would suggest.

Personal Reflections

Exposure to such a rich and varied literature inevitably leaves one with some more or less settled reactions and opinions, which I would order as follows.

Moral Position

Human life, as a basic good and the foundation for the enjoyment of other goods and rights, should be taken only when doing so is the lesser of two evils, all things considered. In this Outler is, I believe, correct. "Human life" refers to individual life from conception, or at least from "the time at or after which it is settled whether there will be one or two or more distinct human individuals" (Ramsey). As this qualifier receives the continued discussion by theologians that it deserves, the benefit of the doubt should ordinarily be given to the fetus. To qualify as the lesser of two evils there is required, among other things, that there be at stake a human life or its moral equivalent. "Moral equivalent" refers to a good or a value that is, in Christian assessment, comparable to life itself (compare Dupré and Curran). This is the *substance* of the Christian tradition if our best casuistry in other areas (for example, just warfare) is carefully weighed and sifted; for the permis-

---

[114] Jacques-Marie Pohier, O.P., "Réflexions théologiques sur la position de l'église catholique," *Lumière et vie*, 21 (1972), 73–107.

sible exceptions with regard to life-taking (self-defense, just war, capital punishment, indirect killing) are all formulations and con- cretizations of what is viewed in the situation as the lesser human evil.

This position represents an achievement that, in terms of exist- ing evidence, it would be unscientific to deny and uncivilized to abandon. I am comfortable with it as a normative statement. Re- cent attempts to extend exceptions through notions of delayed hominization and gradual personhood are, it seems, but contem- porary analogues of the earlier theories about delayed animation. To this commentator they appear strained, though continued dis- cussion is certainly called for. On this matter I am in agreement with Curran.

The determination of the moral equivalent of life is both difficult and dangerous.[115] It is difficult because it is very difficult to compare basic human values. Furthermore, such comparisons are shifting things, reflecting our change in value perceptions.

It is dangerous for several reasons. First, because such evalua- tion is vulnerable to unrecognized, cultural biases. Cultures are more or less civilized, more or less violent, more or less hedonistic, etc., and hence will be more or less human in their value judg- ments. We can never completely transcend the distorting influences embedded in our culture. Second, it is dangerous be- cause such formulations are hard put to resist abusive inter- pretation. In general, it can be said that while the casuistry of the tradition shows that there are other values comparable to human life, the thrust of the tradition supports an inclination (and only that) to narrow rather than to broaden the comparable values. To make this comparison with prudence in our time calls not only for honesty and openness within a process of communal discernment, but also for further careful studies of past conclusions and present evaluations.

[115] For some extremely interesting suggestions on comparable values where abortion is concerned, see James J. Diamond, "Pro-Life Amendments and Due Process," *America*, 130 (1974), 27–29.

Pastoral Care

The position thus delineated is a *moral* position, to be equated neither with pastoral care nor with a legal position, but to be totally dissociated from neither. Pastoral care deals with an individual where that person is (compare Häring) in terms of his perceptions and strengths. Although it attempts to expand perspectives and maximize strengths, it recognizes the limits of these attempts.

There are two aspects profoundly affecting the determination of where many people are. First, we live in a society with structures that often do not support and aid women with unwanted pregnancies, a society that heavily contributes to the factors that make pregnancies unwanted—a society with not only broad areas of structural poverty, repression, and injustice, but also with subtle escalating pressures against childbearing. Second, perception of the existence and value of fetal life differs. Wertheimer is probably right when he notes that it is the severely limited possibilities of natural relationships with the fetus that generate the unlimited possibility of natural responses to it.[116] In combination, these facts mean that many people will perceive the abortion problem above all in terms of the inconvenience, hardship, or suffering a prohibitive position involves, and will tend to find that position unacceptable *for that reason.*

Since the sum total of these influences, then, is an attitude that increasingly tends to frame the moral question almost exclusively in terms of the sufferings resultant on a prohibitive moral position, it is important to distinguish two things: (a) whether a moral position is right and truly embodies the good; (b) whether standing by it and proposing it as the object of aspiration, both personal and societal, entails hardships and difficulties. In a highly pragmatic, technologically sophisticated, and thoroughly pampered culture, the latter point (certainly a fact) could lead many to conclude that the moral position is erroneous. This must be taken into account in any sound pastoral procedure.

Abortion, like any humanly caused disvalue, is sought not only for a reason, but also within a culture that either sanctions or not

[116] Roger Wertheimer, "Understanding the Abortion Argument," *Philosophy and Public Affairs*, 1 (1971), 67–95.

the reason and alters or not the conditions that give rise to the abortion. One of the most important functions of morality is to provide to a culture the ongoing possibility of criticizing and transcending itself and its limitations. Thus genuine morality, while always compassionate and understanding in its meeting with individual distress (pastoral), must remain prophetic and demanding in the norms through which it invites to a better humanity (moral); for if it ceases to do this, it simply collapses the pastoral and moral, and in so doing ceases to be truly human, because it barters the good that will liberate and humanize for the compromise that will merely comfort.

Legal Regulation

Law is analogous to pastoral practice in that it must look not merely to the good, but also to the good that is possible and feasible in a particular society at a particular time. However, just as sound pastoral care takes account of individual strength and limitation ("invincible ignorance") without ceasing to invite and challenge the individual beyond his present perspectives, so the law, while taking account of the possible and feasible at a particular time, must do so without simply settling for it. Simple accommodation to cultural "realities" not only forfeits altogether the educative function of law, but also could leave an enormous number of people without legal protection. For this reason I find the legal positions of both Grisez and Callahan unpersuasive. Grisez has not sufficiently attended to the feasibility dimension of legislation, and therefore his position seems to represent a confusion of morality with legislation. Callahan, on the other hand, has by implication weighed only this dimension and therefore his position seems to represent a total dissociation of the moral and the legal, and an ultimate undermining of the moral by the legal, as the statement of the German bishops (both Catholic and Evangelical) notes.

Thus there is and probably must be this side of eternity a constant tension between the good and the feasible. A healthy society attempts to reduce this tension as much as possible. But it is only more or less successful. This leads me to three observations where abortion law is concerned.

First, the feasibility test (of law) is particularly difficult in our

society. Ideally, of course, where we are concerned with the rights
of others and especially the most fundamental right (right to
life), the more easily should morality simply translate into law.
But the easier this translation, the less necessary is law. In other
words, if this represents the ideal, it also presupposes the ideal.
And we do not have that, above all because the moral assessment
of fetal life differs. And ultimately law must find a basis in the
deepest moral perceptions of the majority or in principles the majority is reluctant to modify (Shinn). This means that it is especially difficult to apply the test of feasibility to an abortion law,
for the good itself whose legal possibility is under discussion is an
object of doubt and controversy. Given this situation, a totally
permissive law in the present circumstances would tend only to
deepen further the doubt and confusion, and in the process to risk
unjustifiably further erosion of respect for human life. On the
other hand, a stringent prohibitive law (such as the Texas law declared unconstitutional in *Wade*) in our circumstances would
have enormous social costs in terms of other important values.

Second, no law will appear to be or actually be adequate
(whether permissive or prohibitive) if it does not simultaneously
contain provisions that attack the problems that tempt to abortion. Our mistake as a nation and that of many countries has been
just that: to leave relatively untouched the societal conditions and
circumstances that lead to abortion, and to legislate permissively,
usually on the basis of transparently fragile slogans created by a
variety of pressure groups. This has been shown to be destructive
in every other area of human planning. It can be no less so here.

Third, and as a consequence of the above considerations, in
designing present legislation we are confronted at the present time
with a choice of two legal evils. No choice is going to be very satisfactory, because the underlying conditions for truly good legislation are lacking. What is to be done when one is dealing with
evils? Clearly the lesser evil should be chosen while attempts are
made to alter the circumstances that allow only such a destructive
choice. How one compares and weighs the evils, where he sees the
greater evil, will depend on many factors, not excluding fetal life.
That is why a moral position on fetal life, while distinguishable
from a legal position, will have a good deal to say about what one
regards as a good or a tolerable legal position, at least at the pres-

ent time. But here again we reach an impasse, for there is profound disagreement at the moral level. For instance, given the moral position I find persuasive, I believe that the most equitable law would be one that protects fetal life but exempts abortion done in certain specified conflict situations from legal sanctions (compare the joint Catholic-Protestant statement from Germany). In other words, I believe that the social disvalues associated with such a law (a degree of unenforceability, clandestine abortions, less than total control over fertility) are lesser evils than the enormous bloodletting both allowed and, in some real and destructive sense, inescapably encouraged (*teste experientia*) by excessively permissive laws. However, I realize that very many of my fellow citizens do not share this judgment.

What, then, is to be done? In our pluralistic atmosphere, legal provisions tracing back to almost *any* moral position (whether it be that of Vatican II or that of the U. S. Supreme Court—this latter I use deliberately because the legal conclusions so obviously reflect a moral position, though they need not do so) are going to be seen and experienced as impositions of one view on another group. In such an impasse, the only way out seems to be procedural. Two procedures recommend themselves. First, the matter should be decided for the present through the state legislatures, where all of us have an opportunity to share in the democratic process. We have learned in our history that while this process is often halting and frustrating, sometimes even corrupt, still it provides us with our most adequate way of living with our differences —a way certainly more adequate than a decision framed by a Supreme Court that imposes its own poorly researched and shabbily reasoned moral values as the basis for the law of the land.[117]

Second, I used above the phrase "for the present." It is meant to suggest that our societal situation is such (both in terms of the conditions provoking abortion and in terms of the pluralism about its moral character) that any legal disposition of the question now must be accompanied by hesitation and a large dose of dissat-

---

[117] Philip B. Kurland, professor in the law school at the University of Chicago, wrote recently: "The primary defect of the Burger Court so far revealed is the same defect that was observed in the Warren Court. It has failed to account properly for its judgments. It has issued decrees but it has not afforded adequate rationales for them; it has attempted to rule by fiat rather than reason" (*University of Chicago Magazine* [July/Aug. 1973], 9).

isfaction. This means that it is the right and the duty of conscientious citizens to continue to debate this matter in the public forum. The values at stake are fundamental to the continuance of civilized society. For this reason, to settle for the status quo is to settle for societal sickness. Much as we are individually and corporately tired of this subject, continued rational discussion is essential. It is one means—but only one—that will allow us, as a nation, to arrive at a position that is compatible with the fundamental moral principles undergirding our republic.

Whatever the proper answer to the legal question, one final point must be made. We sometimes think of certain problems like abortion as pertaining to individual morality, and others like poverty and racism as being social morality. The Supreme Court decision only reinforced this perspective. The contemporary emphasis is on the need to solve the "bigger" and "less domestic" problems. Catholics, it is averred, have for too long been fascinated by and preoccupied with micromorality.

The matter is far more complex than this. As the literature brought under review here has shown, economic insecurity, racism, oppression, and abortion share a common root: the quality of the society in which we live. In this perspective abortion is a *social* problem of the first magnitude insofar as the factors so often involved in abortion decisions are societal in character. Similarly, poverty and racism are *individual* problems insofar as we bear as individuals responsibility for their existence and continuation. To say anything else would be un-Christian; for it would deny that we are, by our Christian being, *individual members of a community* who have, as a community, responsibilities toward individuals and who have, as individuals, responsibilities toward the community. These responsibilities, while distinguishable, are continuous. Abortion exists because of a cluster of factors that make up the quality of a society. It will disappear only when that quality is changed. Hence true abortion reform must begin here. Unless and until it does, any law on abortion will be more or less inhumane.[118]

[118] In a review such as this a good deal of literature is necessarily overlooked. Instances are Sissela Bok, "Ethical Problems of Abortion," *Hastings Center Studies,* 2 (Jan. 1974), 33–52; John T. Noonan, "Responding to Persons: Methods of Moral Argument in Debate over Abortion," *Theology Digest,* 21

(1973), 291–307; Peter A. Facione, "Callahan on Abortion," *American Ecclesiastical Review*, 167 (1973), 291–301; G. Caprile, "Il magistero della Chiesa sull'aborto," *Civiltà cattolica* (May 1973), 359–62; "Déclaration des juristes de France sur l'avortement," *Documentation catholique*, 70 (1973), 749; Francis Dardot, "L'adoption, une alternative méconnue à l'avortement," *Études* (May 1973), 701–14; A. Théry, "L'Avortement dans la législation française," *Esprit et vie*, 83 (1973), 293–95; Michael Alsopp, "Abortion—the Theological Argument," *Furrow*, 24 (1973), 202–6; Stefano Tumbas, S.J., "Ci sarà anche un aborto 'cattolico'?" *Palestra del clero*, 52 (1973), 662–71.

9. Rules for Abortion Debate

There are a million legal abortions done annually in the United States. If this is what many people think it is (unjustified killing of human beings, in most cases), then it certainly constitutes the major moral tragedy of our country. In contrast, over many years fifty thousand Americans were lost in Vietnam. About the problem of abortion and its regulation, however, Americans are profoundly polarized, and there seems little hope of unlocking deeply protected positions to reach any kind of national consensus. Yet surely that is desirable on an issue so grave.

I have been professionally involved in this problem for well over twenty years, on podium and in print, and above all in many hundreds of hours of conversation. Such experiences do not necessarily increase wisdom. But they do generate some rather clear impressions about the quality of discourse on the problem of abortion. I have to conclude, regrettably, that the level of conversation is deplorably low. On both sides, slogans are used as if they were arguments; the sound level rises as verbal bludgeoning and interruptions multiply; the dialogue of the deaf continues. Some of the most prestigious organizations of the news media (for example, the New York *Times*, the Washington *Post*) support policies that stem from moral positions whose premises and assumptions they have not sufficiently examined, let alone argued. The same can be said of some anti-abortionists in the policies they propose. An executive assistant in the Senate told me recently that the two most obnoxious lobbies on the Hill are the anti-abortionists and the pro-abortionists. Briefly, civil conversation on this subject has all but disappeared. Perhaps that is as it should be. Perhaps now is the time for camping in abortion clinics or beneath Joseph Califano's office windows. But I think not, at least in the sense that such tactics should not replace disciplined argument.

Many of us have become bone weary of this discussion. But to yield to such fatigue would be to run from a problem, not wrestle with it. If stay we ought and must, then it may be of help to propose a set of "rules for conversation," the observance of which could nudge us toward more communicative conversation. That is surely a modest achievement, but where the level of discourse is as chaotic and sclerotic as it is, modesty recommends itself, especially when so many begged questions and *non sequiturs* are traceable to violations of some of the fundamental points raised below. I do not believe these guidelines call for compromise or abandonment of anyone's moral conviction. At least they are not deliberately calculated to do this. Basic moral convictions have roots, after all, in some rather nonrational (which is not to say irrational) layers of our being. Rather, these suggestions are but attempts to vent and circumvent the frustrations that cling to bad arguments. In qualifying certain arguments as "bad," one unavoidably gives his position away at some point. But that is neither here nor there if the points made have independent validity. Perhaps the following can be helpful.

Attempt to identify areas of agreement. Where issues are urgent and disputants have enormous personal stakes and investments, there is a tendency to draw sharp lines very quickly and begin the shootout. Anything else strikes the frank, let-it-hang-out American mind as hypocrisy. We have, it is argued, seen too many instances where a spade is called a shovel. Serious moral issues only get postponed by such politesse. Well and good. But this misses an important point: There are broad areas of agreement in this matter, and explicitly speaking of them at times will at least soften the din of conversation and soundproof the atmosphere. Some of those areas are the following.

Both those who find abortion morally repugnant and those who do not would agree that abortion is, in most cases, a tragic thing, an undesirable thing. It is not a tooth extraction, though some heavy doses of wishful thinking and sanitized language ("the procedure") sometimes present it this way. Therefore, all discussants should be clear-headedly and wholeheartedly behind policies that attempt to frustrate the personal and social causes of abortion.

One thinks immediately of better sex education (which is not equivalent to so-called plumbing instructions), better prenatal and perinatal care, reduced poverty, various forms of family support, more adequate institutional care of developmentally disabled children, etc. Furthermore, anyone who sees abortion as a sometimes tragic necessity should in consistency be practically supportive of alternatives to this procedure. While these two areas of agreement will not eliminate differences, they will—especially in combination with an over-all concern for the quality of life at all stages—inspire the stirrings of mutual respect that improve the climate of discussion. That is no little achievement in this area.

Avoid the use of slogans. Slogans are the weapons of the crusader, one who sees his role as warfare, generally against those sharply defined as "the enemy." Fighting for good causes clearly has its place, as do slogans. The political rally or the protest demonstration are good examples. But slogans are not very enlightening conversational tools, simply because they bypass and effectively subvert the process of communication.

I have in mind two current examples. The first is the use of the term "murder" to describe abortion. "Murder" is a composite value term that means (morally) unjustified killing of another person. There are also legal qualifiers to what is to count as murder. To use that term does not clarify an argument if the very issue at stake is justifiability. Rather it brands a position and, incidentally, those who hold it. It is a conversation stopper. Moreover, the term "murder" is absolutely unnecessary in the defense of the traditional Christian position on abortion.

On the other hand, "a woman has a right to her own body" is not an argument. It is the conclusion of an often unexamined argument and therefore a slogan with some highly questionable assumptions. For instance: that the fetus is, for these purposes, a part of the woman's body; that rights over one's body are absolute; that abortion has nothing to do with a husband, etc. To rattle some of these assumptions, it is sufficient to point out that few would grant that a woman's rights over her own body include the right to take thalidomide during pregnancy. The Supreme Court of our nation has gone pretty far in endorsing some of these assumptions. But even justices not above the use of a little "raw judicial power" would choke, I think, on the above slogan as an apt way to summarize the issue.

Represent the opposing position accurately and fairly. Even to mention this seems something of an insult. It contains an implied accusation. Unfortunately, the accusation is too often on target. For instance, those opposed to abortion sometimes argue that the woman who has an abortion is "antilife" or has no concern for her fetus. This may be the case sometimes, but I believe it does not take sufficient account of the sense of desperate conflict experienced by many women who seek abortions. A sense of tragedy would not exist if women had no concern for their intrauterine offspring.

On the other hand, those who disagree with a highly restrictive moral position on abortion sometimes describe this position as "absolutist" and say that it involves "total preoccupation with the status of the unborn." This is the wording of the unfortunate "Call to Concern," which was aimed explicitly at the American Catholic hierarchy.[1] The track record of the hierarchy on social concerns over a broad range of issues is enough to reveal the calumnious character of such protests. As Notre Dame's James Burtchaell wrote apropos of this manifesto: "Ethicians are expected to restrain themselves from misrepresenting positions with which they disagree."[2]

Distinguish the pairs right-wrong, good-bad. Repeatedly I have heard discussants say of a woman who has had an abortion: "She thought at the time and afterward that it was not morally wrong." Or: "She is convinced she made the right decision." It is then immediately added that the moral character of an action depends above all on the perceptions of the person performing it.

Indeed it does. But the term "moral character" needs a further distinction. One who desires to do and intends to do what is supportive and promotive of others (beneficence), performs a *good* act. That person may actually and mistakenly do what is unfortunately harmful, and then the action is morally *wrong*, but it is morally *good*. On the contrary, one who acts from motives of selfishness, hatred, envy, performs an evil, or *bad*, act. Thus a sur-

---

[1] "Call to Concern," *Christianity and Crisis*, 37 (1977), 222.
[2] J. Burtchaell, "A Call and a Reply," *Christianity and Crisis*, 37 (1977), 221–22.

geon may act out of the most selfish and despicable motives as he performs brilliant life-saving surgery. His action is morally *bad* but morally *right*. One's action can, therefore, be morally good, but still be morally wrong. It can be morally right, but morally bad.

The discussion about abortion concerns moral rightness and wrongness. This argument is not settled or even much enlightened by appealing to what a person thought of it at the time, or thinks of it afterward. Nor is it settled by the good and upright intentions of the woman or the physician. Those who destroyed villages in Vietnam to liberate them often undoubtedly acted from the best of intentions, but were morally wrong.

Not only is this distinction important in itself; beyond its own importance, it allows one to disagree agreeably—that is, without implying, suggesting, or predicating moral evil of the person one believes to be morally wrong. This would be a precious gain in a discussion that often witnesses this particular and serious collapse of courtesy.

Try to identify the core issue at stake. There are, of course, many issues that cluster around the subject of abortion. There are issues of health (fetal, maternal), family stability, justice (for example, rape), illegitimacy, etc. They are all genuine concerns and can represent sources of real hardship and suffering. Those who believe that abortion is sometimes justifiable have made a judgment that the hardships of the woman or family take precedence over nascent life in moral calculation. Those who take an opposing view weight the scales differently.

The core issue is, therefore, the evaluation of nascent life. By this I do not refer to the question about the beginning of personhood. That is a legitimate and important discussion. But the definition of "person" is often elaborated with a purpose in mind —that is, one defines and then grants or does not grant personhood in terms of what one wants to do and thinks it appropriate to do with nonpersons. That this can be a dog-chasing-tail definition is quite clear. As Princeton's Paul Ramsey is fond of saying: Does one really need a Ph.D. from Harvard to be a person, or is a functioning cerebral cortex quite sufficient?

The core issue, then, concerns the moral claims the nascent human being (what Pope Paul VI, in a brilliant finesse, referred to as *personne en devenir* [a person in the process of becoming])[3] makes on us. Do these frequently or only very rarely yield to what appear to be extremely difficult alternatives? And above all, why or why not? That is, in my judgment, the heart of the abortion debate. It must be met head on. It is illumined neither by flat statements about the inviolable rights of fetuses nor by assertions about a woman's freedom of choice. These promulgate a conclusion. They do not share with us how one arrived at it.

Admit doubts, difficulties, and weaknesses in one's own position. When people are passionately concerned with a subject, as they should be in this case, they tend to overlook or even closet their own doubts and problems. Understandable as this is—who will cast the first stone?—it is not a service to the truth or to good moral argument.

For instance, those with permissive views on abortion (who often favor Medicaid funding for it) sometimes argue that denial of Medicaid funding means a return to the back-alley butchers for many thousands of poor. This is deceptively appealing to a sensitive social conscience. But it fails to deal with the fact that in some, perhaps very many places, there is precious little price differential between the butchers and the clinics that now offer abortion services. So why go to the butchers? Furthermore, it conveniently overlooks the fact, noted by Daniel Callahan,[4] that the woman most commonly seeking an abortion is not the poor, overburdened mother of many children but "an unmarried, very young woman of modest, or relatively affluent means whose main 'indication' for abortion will be her expressed wish not to have a [this] child [now]."

Or, again, it is occasionally argued that in a pluralistic society we should refrain from imposing our moral views on others. This was the solution of the New York *Times*[5] when it welcomed the *Wade* and *Bolton* decisions of the Supreme Court. The *Times* stated: "Nothing in the Court's approach ought to give affront to persons who oppose all abortion for reasons of religion or individ-

---

[3] Pope Paul VI, "Pourquois l'église ne peut accepter l'avortement," *Documentation catholique*, 70 (1973), 4–5.

[4] Daniel Callahan, "Abortion: Thinking and Experiencing," *Christianity and Crisis*, 32 (1973), 295–98.

[5] New York *Times* (Jan. 23, 1973), editorial.

ual conviction. They can stand as firmly as ever for those principles, provided they do not seek to impede the freedom of those
with an opposite view."

I agree with Union Theological's Roger Shinn when he says
that this view is simplistic and disguises its own weaknesses. He
wrote: "If a person or group honestly believes that abortion is the
killing of persons, there is no moral comfort in being told, 'Nobody requires you to kill. We are only giving permission to others
to do what you consider killing.'" The protester ought surely to
reply that one key function of law is to protect minorities of all
types: political, racial, religious, and, as here, unborn.[6]

On the other hand, the traditional Christian view on abortion
(until recently, universally proposed by the Christian churches)
was that the fetus was inviolable from the moment of conception.
There are, I believe, certain phenomena in the preimplantation
period that raise doubts and questions about evaluation, and that
is all—namely, they do not yield certainties. I have in mind the
twinning process, the estimated number of spontaneous abortions
(thought to be huge), and, above all, the rare process of recombination of two fertilized ova into one. To admit that such phenomena raise serious evaluative problems is quite in place, if as a
matter of fact they do. Indeed, I would argue that it is a disservice to the over-all health and viability of the traditional Christian
evaluation to extend its clarity and certainty into areas where
there are grounds for residual and nagging doubts.

*Distinguish the formulation and the substance of a moral con-
viction.* This may seem a refined, even supertechnical and sophisticated guideline better left in the footnotes of the ethical elite.
Actually, I believe it is enormously important for bringing conver-
sationalists out of their trenches. And it applies to both sides of
the national debate.

For instance, not a few anti-abortionists appeal to the formulations of recent official Catholic leaders in stating their moral convictions. Specifically, Pius XI and Pius XII both stated (and, with
them, traditional Catholic ethical treatises on abortion) that direct abortion was never permissible, even to save the life of the

---

[6] Roger Shinn, "Personal Decisions and Social Policies in a Pluralist Society,"
Perkins Journal, 27 (1973), 58–63.

mother. As this was understood, it meant simply and drastically: Better two deaths than one murder. Concretely, if the only alternatives facing a woman and physician were either abort or lose both mother and child, the conclusion was drawn that even then the direct disposing of the fetus was morally wrong.

That is a formulation—and almost no one, whether liberal or conservative, endorses the conclusion as an adequate and accurate way of communicating the basic value judgment (substance) of the matter. Some moral theologians would say, in contrast to the Popes, that in this instance the abortion is indirect and permissible. Others would say, again in contrast to the Popes, that it is direct but still permissible. For instance, the Catholic bishop of Augsburg, Josef Stimpfle, recently stated: "He who performs an abortion, except to save the life of the mother, sins gravely and burdens his conscience with the killing of human life."[7] A similar statement was made by the entire Belgian hierarchy in its 1973 declaration on abortion. Of those very rare and desperate conflict instances, the Belgian bishops stated: "The moral principle which ought to govern the intervention can be formulated as follows: Since two lives are at stake, one will, while doing everything possible to save both, attempt to save one rather than to allow two to perish."[8] What is clear is that all would arrive at a conclusion different from the official one, even though the language might differ in each case.

The point here is, of course, that ethical formulations, being the product of human language, philosophy, and imperfection, are only more or less adequate to the substance of our moral convictions at a given time. Ethical formulations will always show the imprint of human handling. This was explicitly acknowledged by Pope John XXIII in his speech (October 11, 1962) opening the Second Vatican Council. It was echoed by Vatican II in *Gaudium et spes:* "Furthermore, while adhering to the methods and requirements proper to theology, theologians are invited to seek continually for more suitable ways of communicating doctrine to the

---

[7] This statement is cited in Franz Scholz, "Durch ethische Grenzsituationen aufgeworfene Normenprobleme," *Theologisch-praktische Quartalschrift,* 123 (1975), 342.

[8] "Déclaration des évêques belges sur l'avortement," *Documentation catholique,* 70 (1973), 432–38.

men of their times. For the deposit of faith or revealed truths are one thing; the manner in which they are formulated without violence to their meaning and significance is another."[9]

This statement must be properly understood. Otherwise theology could easily be reduced to word shuffling. If there is a distinction between substance and formulation, there is also an extremely close—indeed, inseparable—connection. One might say they are related as are body and soul. The connection is so intimate that it is difficult to know just what the substance is amid variation of formulation. The formulation can easily betray the substance. Furthermore, because of this close connection, it is frequently difficult to know just what is changeable, what permanent. Where abortion is concerned, one could argue that the Church's *substantial* conviction is that abortion is tolerable only when it is life-saving, therefore also life-serving, intervention. Be that as it may, to conduct discussion as if substance and formulation were identical is to get enslaved to formulations. Such captivity forecloses conversations.

On the other hand, something similar must be said of the 1973 abortion decisions of the U. S. Supreme Court. The Court was "evolutionary" in interpreting the notion of liberty enacted in 1868 as the Fourteenth Amendment to the Constitution. There is no evidence that the Congress and the states understood that amendment to include the liberty to abort. Yet the Court asserts that "liberty" there must be read in a way consistent with the demands of the present day. Therefore, it concluded that the right to terminate pregnancy is "implicit in the concept of ordered liberty."

That is but a formulation of the notion of constitutionally assured liberty, and to treat it as more than that, as an ironclad edict, is to pre-empt legal development. Indeed, the Court itself gives this away when it treats the term "person" in the Constitution in a very static and nondevelopmental way, as John Noonan has repeatedly pointed out. It looks at the meaning of the term at the time of the adoption of the Constitution and

___

[9] Vatican Council II, "Pastoral Constitution on the Church in the Modern World (Gaudium et spes)," translated from the Latin and reprinted in Walter M. Abbott, S.J. (ed.), *The Documents of Vatican II* (New York: Herder and Herder/Association Press, 1966), 199–308, No. 62.

freezes it there—just the opposite of what it does with the term "liberty." Such vagaries reveal that the Court's decisions and dicta are hardly identical with the substance of the Constitution. To argue as if they were is to confuse legal substance and legal formulations, and to choke off conversation. In brief, we must know and treasure our traditions without being enslaved by them.

Distinguish morality and public policy. It is the temptation of the Anglo-American tradition to identify these two. We are a pragmatic and litigious people for whom law is the answer to all problems, the only answer and a fully adequate answer. Thus many people confuse morality and public policy. If something is removed from the penal code, it is viewed as morally right and permissible. And if an act is seen as morally wrong, many want it made illegal. Behold the "there ought to be a law" syndrome.

This is not only conceptually wrong, it is also conversationally mischievous. It gets people with strong moral convictions locked into debates about public policy, as if only one public policy were possible given a certain moral position. That is simplistic. While morality and law are intimately related, they are obviously not identical. The closer we get to basic human rights, however, the closer the relationship ought to be in a well-ordered society. It is quite possible for those with permissive moral convictions on abortion to believe that more regulation is required than is presently provided in the *Wade* and *Bolton* decisions. Contrarily, it is possible for those with more stringent moral persuasions to argue that there are several ways in which these might be mirrored in public policy.

I am not arguing here for this or that public policy (though personally I am deeply dissatisfied with the present one on nearly all grounds). The point, rather, is that public discourse would be immeasurably purified if care were taken by disputants to relate morality and public policy in a more nuanced way than now prevails.

Distinguish morality and pastoral care or practice. A moral statement is one that attempts to summarize the moral right or wrong, and then invites to its realization in our conduct. As the well-known Redemptorist theologian Bernard Häring words it: Moral theology operates on a level "where questions are raised about general rules or considerations that would justify a particular moral judgment."[10] A moral statement is thus an abstract statement, not in the sense that it has nothing to do with real life, or with particular decisions, but in the sense that it abstracts or prescinds from the ability of this or that person to understand it and live it.

Pastoral care (and pastoral statements), by contrast, looks to the art of the possible. It deals with an individual where that person is in terms of his or her strengths, perceptions, biography, circumstances (financial, medical, educational, familial, psychological). Although pastoral care attempts to expand perspectives and maximize strengths, it recognizes at times the limits of these attempts.

Concretely, one with strong convictions about the moral wrongfulness of abortion could and should be one who realizes that there are many who by education, familial and religious background, economic circumstances, are, or appear to be, simply incapable in those circumstances of assimilating such convictions and living them out, at least here and now. This means that compassion and understanding extended to the woman who is contemplating an abortion or has had one need by no means require abandonment of one's moral convictions. Similarly, it means that a strong and unswerving adherence to a moral position need not connote the absence of pastoral compassion, and deafness to the resonances of tragic circumstances. I believe that if more people understood this, the abortion discussion would occur in an atmosphere of greater tranquillity, sensitivity, and humaneness—and therefore contain more genuine communication.

Incorporate the woman's perspective, or women's perspectives. I include this because, well, frankly, I have been told to. And I am sure that there are many who will complain: "Yes, and you put it last." To which a single response is appropriate: "Yes, for emphasis." In the many discussions I have had on abortion where women have been involved in the discussion, one thing is clear: Women feel they have been left out of the discussion. This seems true of both so-called prochoice women and so-called prolife adherents.

But being told to is hardly a decisive reason for urging this

10 Bernard Häring, *Medical Ethics* (Notre Dame, Ind.: Fides, 1973), 89.

point. And it is not my chief reason. Women rightly, if at times one-sidedly and abrasively, insist that they are the ones who carry pregnancies and sometimes feel all but compelled to have abortions. Thus they argue two things: (1) They ought to have an influential voice in this discussion. (2) Up to and including the present, they feel they have not had such a voice.

There are all kinds of shouts that will be heard when this suggestion is raised. We are familiar with most of them. For instance, some will argue paternal rights against the U. S. Supreme Court's 1976 *Planned Parenthood* v. *Danforth* decision. Others will ask: Which women are you talking about, prolife or prochoice? And then, of course, they will begin issuing passes to the discussion on the basis of predetermined positions. Still others will wonder why the fetus does not have a proxy with at least equal say. And so on. One can see and admit the point in all these ripostes. There is nothing in femaleness as such that makes women more or less vulnerable to error or bias in moral discourse than men, yet when all is shrieked and done, the basic point remains valid: The abortion discussion proceeds at its own peril if it ignores women's perspectives. As Martin I. Silvermann remarked in a recent issue of *Sh'ma*: "The arguments change when you must face the women."[11]

One need not make premature peace with radical feminists or knee-jerk pro-abortionists to say this. Quite the contrary. One need only be familiar with the growing body of literature on abortion by women (for example, Linda Bird Francke's *The Ambivalence of Abortion*,[12] or Sidney Callahan's essays on abortion) to believe that the woman's perspective is an important ingredient in this discussion. To those who believe that this is tantamount to conferring infallibility on Gloria Steinem, it must be pointed out that in nearly every national poll, women test out more conservatively than men on the morality of abortion.

These are but a few guidelines for discussion. I am sure that there are many more, perhaps some of even greater importance than the ones mentioned. Be that as it may, I am convinced that

[11] Martin Silvermann, *Sh'ma* (Jan. 20, 1978).
[12] Linda Bird Francke, *The Ambivalence of Abortion* (New York: Random House, 1978).

attention to these points cannot hurt the national debate. It may even help. Specifically, it may prevent good people from making bad arguments—chief of which, of course, is that it is only bad people who make bad ones.

10. Public Policy on Abortion

The present abortion situation is a major stain on the national conscience; and it is particularly upsetting during a time of cultural schizophrenia—that is, at a time when we rejoice in the production—at great cost and energy—of a test-tube baby.

One of the things that is particularly tiresome to a theologian is that the national debate on this utterly serious subject has collapsed into slogans. People feel deeply about this subject; and when they do, they are going to marshal every shred of evidence—questionable or not—and bend it to their purposes. As a theologian, I am committed to the thesis that emotions are excellent companions but not always good guides. It is essential, therefore, to submit one's loyalties and value judgments to constant scrutiny and questioning and to those theological criteria that make abortion also (though not only) a theological question, a task not without its risks. For instance, in a July issue of *America* I offered to both sides of this national discussion ten rules for debate (see previous chapter).[1] My own basic value commitments were, in my and almost everyone else's judgment, transparent—with one exception. In an August issue of the Steubenville *Register*, I was mildly shocked to read a column on the article entitled "How to Get Soft on Abortion."[2] I say that I was *mildly* shocked because it is well known that plenty of people in this debate are ready to excommunicate if one does not formulate matters exactly as they do.

In this chapter I want to discuss public policy on abortion. One cannot do that, of course, without discussing morality, for while public policy and morality are not identical necessarily, they are

[1] Richard A. McCormick, S.J., "Abortion: Rules for Debate," *America*, 139 (1978), 26–60.
[2] Steubenville *Register* (Aug. 11, 1978), p. 4.

intimately related—that is, if one regards fetal life as disposable tissue, clearly abortion ought not be on the penal code at all, except to protect women against bungling and incompetent tissue scrapers. If, however, fetal life is to be regarded as human life making claims on society's protection, then the possibility is that it ought to be protected by law.

Morality, then, concerns itself with rightness or wrongness of human conduct. Law, or public policy, on the other hand, is concerned with the common good, the welfare of the community. Clearly, morality and public policy are both related and distinct. They are related because law, or public policy, has an inherently moral character due to its rootage in existential human ends (goods). The welfare of the community cannot be unrelated to what is judged to be promotive or destructive to the individual. Morality and public policy are distinct because only when individual acts have ascertainable public consequences on the maintenance and stability of society (welfare of the community) are they the proper concern of society. Thus all civilized societies outlaw homicide.

What immoral or wrongful actions affect the welfare of the community in a way that demands legislation are subject to a further criterion: feasibility. Feasibility, as I noted earlier, is that quality whereby a proposed course of action is not merely possible but also practicable, adaptable, depending on the circumstances, cultural ways, attitudes, traditions of a people.

The criterion of feasibility, therefore, raises questions such as: Will the policy be obeyed? Is it enforceable? Is it prudent to undertake this or that ban in view of possibly harmful effects in other sectors of social life? Can control be achieved short of coercive measures? As John R. Connery, S.J., professor of moral theology, Loyola University of Chicago, words it: "One cannot conclude . . . that because the state does not penalize some action it is not morally wrong. All one can infer is that it was not judged to be harmful to the community, *or if it was judged harmful, the harm was less than that which would result from prohibitive legislation* [emphasis added]."[3]

What makes public policy on abortion such an intractable and

[3] John R. Connery, S.J., "Difference Between Law and Morality," *Catholic Standard* (Apr. 6, 1978), p. 10.

divisive issue is that the good (and evil) itself whose legal possibility is under discussion is an object of doubt and controversy—that is, the evaluation of fetal life differs in our society. Some persons see it as living, but disposable (worthless?) tissue. Others see the fetus as human life making claims, but claims that are overridden by a rather broad class of maternal or familial concerns. Still others see nascent life as something to be protected in all but a very few exceptional instances. In other words, some see permissive laws as injustice (and therefore clearly as things touching the welfare of the community). Others see restrictive laws as injustice to the woman. To complicate matters, all of these positions are enveloped in some highly questionable rhetoric and question begging. Given this disagreement, it is very difficult to arrive at acceptable or feasible policy, for ultimately public policy must find a basis in the deepest moral perception of the majority; or if not, at least in principles the majority is reluctant to modify.

The key issue—both morally and eventually legally—is the evaluation of nascent life, first in itself, then when set against competing claims. By this I do not mean, "Is the fetus a person?" That is a legitimate question and of no inconsiderable legal importance. But as pointed out earlier, the definition of person is often elaborated with a purpose in mind. One defines personhood and then grants or does not grant personhood according to what one wants to do or thinks it acceptable to do with nonpersons. That this can be a circular definition is quite clear. Nor do I mean, "When does human life begin?" Put a hundred biologists and geneticists in a room on that question, and you will get a single answer: at fertilization. What results from fertilization is living, not dead; is human, not a mouse.

So the question is one of evaluation of nascent life, of the moral claims that the nascent human being makes on us. This is a straightforward moral question, and we must turn to it if reflections on public policy are to be coherent. Daniel Callahan of the Hastings Center has caught this exactly when he says: "The essence of the moral problem in abortion is the proper way in which to balance the rights of the unborn . . . against the right of a woman not to have a child she does not want."[4]

---

[4] Daniel Callahan, "Abortion: Thinking and Experiencing," *Christianity and Crisis*, 32 (1973), 295-98.

The present public policy of this country in the *Wade* and *Bolton* decisions is that the nascent being has no rights. The underlying moral evaluation is quite clear: Whatever the fetus is, it is not to be evaluated as a higher priority than any competing concern of the woman. To be perfectly blunt, this means that the fetus is a nothing, a zero. Justice Harry Blackmun held that the fetus is only "potential life." Chief Judge Clement F. Haynsworth, Jr., of the U. S. Court of Appeals, Fourth Circuit, carried one step further what was implicit in Blackmun: "The Supreme Court decided that the fetus in the womb is neither alive nor a person within the meaning of the Fourteenth Amendment" (*Floyd* v. *Anders*, F. Supp. DSC 1977). Callahan is once again absolutely correct when he says: "Under permissive laws, any talk whatever of the 'sanctity of life' of the unborn becomes a legal fiction. By giving women the full and total right to determine whether such a sanctity exists, the fetus is, in fact, given no legal or socially established standing whatever."[5] Under such policy any talk of fetal sanctity is double-talk. Callahan continues: "The law forces a nasty either-or choice, devoid of a saving ethical ambiguity."

It is not surprising, then, that the ethical history of abortion is the history of an evaluation. What has that evaluation been? Over the centuries—as Connery has so painstakingly pointed out in his historical study of abortion—some theologians, because of the biological knowledge available to them, spoke of three types of abortion: prevention of conception, abortion of an inanimate fetus, and abortion of an animated fetus.[6] Still others felt that all interventions into the life-giving process were homicides. Others argued that evacuation of a nonanimated fetus was permissible to save the mother's life, for the inanimate fetus was not yet a human being. Some contended that abortion even of an inanimate fetus was immoral either as imperfect homicide or as misuse of *semen conceptum.*

As time went on, many of these qualifications vanished and obscurities diminished. Beneath these debates and developments, one finds an evaluation of fetal life that yielded it to very few compet-

5 Ibid.

6 John R. Connery, S.J., *Abortion: The Development of the Roman Catholic Perspective* (Chicago: Loyola University Press, 1977).

ing interests—what John Noonan of the University of California at Berkeley calls "an almost absolute value."

In recent years nearly every national Catholic episcopal conference has repeated some such evaluation. By noting this I do not mean that others than Catholics have not made similar statements, nor do I mean that the matter is a "Catholic question." Clearly it is not. For example, as noted above, the Belgian bishops, in their 1973 pastoral, cite approvingly *Abortus Provocatus*, a study issued by the Center of Demographic and Family Studies of the Ministry of Health: "There is no objective criterion for establishing, in the gradual process of development, a limit between the 'nonhuman' life and 'human' life. In this process each stage is the necessary condition for the following and no moment is 'more important,' 'more decisive,' or 'more essential' than another."[7] In a previous chapter I noted several of these attempts: Häring, *Études Dossier*, and Quelquejeu, for example. After considering these probes carefully it is my judgment that recent theological and philosophical studies have not made serious inroads on the substance of the classical position. I say "substance" deliberately because one must always distinguish the substance from its formulation at a given time. For this reason eminent theologian Karl Rahner correctly notes that the concrete ethical judgments of the Church's Magisterium are inherently "provisional." For instance, when one questions the crucial moral relevance of the direct/indirect distinction in this area—as one can and, I think, ought to do—one is questioning the formulations of Pius XI and Pius XII and even of Paul VI and the Sacred Congregation for the Doctrine of the Faith. One is not necessarily tampering with the substance of that teaching. The distinction between substance and formulation is not only present in Vatican II explicitly. It is clear in St. Thomas, specifically in the I-II, g. 100, a. 8, where he discusses the dispensability of the precepts of the Decalogue. There he discusses the possible difference between the original or intended senses and the formulated letter, thus laying the basis for *mutatio materiae* (as it was later known) due to circumstances.

What is the substance of the classical moral position? Distin-

[7] "Déclaration des évêques belges sur l'avortement," *Documentation catholique*, 70 (1973), 434.

guishing the abiding substance from its enveloping and changeable formulation is a tricky and difficult business—even, it would seem, an arrogant one. At a certain point one has to assume the posture of a person standing over history and filtering out the limitations of others when one is at least knee-deep in historical limitations oneself.

With that caution, I would like to repeat and expand in three statements the substance of the classical Christian moral position in our time.

1. Human life as a basic gift and good, the foundation for the enjoyment of all other goods, may be taken only when doing so is the only life-saving and life-serving alternative, or only when doing so is, all things considered (not just numbers), the lesser evil. I have said here "human life," not the "human person," for the word "person," as I suggested, only muddies the moral discussion. "Person," as Albert Outler of Emory University, Atlanta, notes, is a code word for a self-transcending, transempirical reality. Self-transcendence is not, contrary to the notions or wishes of so many, a part of the organism. It is the organism as oriented to its self-transcending matrix. I have said "life-saving and life-serving" for two reasons. First, not every life-saving action is life-serving. (For example, some actions could, while saving numerical lives, actually and simultaneously undermine other basic goods in a way that would be a disservice to life itself by attacking an associated value; for the further explanation of the notion of associated values, consult the Appendix.) Second, it seems to me that the exceptions historically tolerated (for example, ectopic pregnancies) fit this general category.

2. By "human life" I mean human life from fertilization or at least from the time at or after which it is settled whether there will be one or two distinct human beings (the phrase is Ramsey's). There are phenomena in the preimplantation period that generate evaluative doubts about the claims the fetus at this stage makes, at least in some cases. I refer to twinning, the number of spontaneous abortions, the possibility of recombination of two fertilized ova into one (chimeras), the time of the appearance of the primary organizer. These phenomena create problems—doubts only. After all, one could and should counter, the only thing that stands between an eight-cell embryo in a petri dish and Louise

Brown is a uterine home for 266 days. I find it remarkable—to wit, worth remarking—that Louise Brown is referred to as the "test-tube *baby*." The answer to the question, Where did Louise Brown begin? is clearly: In the petri dish, if "baby" means anything. We do not say "test-tube tissue." In doubt one generally favors life— but I think not always.

3. For an act to be life-saving and life-serving, to be the lesser evil (all things considered), there must be at stake human life or its moral equivalent, a good or a value comparable to life itself. This is not what the traditional formulations say, but it is where the corpus of teachings on life-taking lead (for example, just war, capital punishment). For instance, if human beings may go to war and take human life to defend their freedom (political autonomy) against an enemy who would strip them of it, something is being said about human freedom compared with life. I realize that life and liberty cannot be compared, as apples and oranges cannot. But in daily life we somehow manage to parse this incommensurability in many areas. We choose to smoke or to drink or to eat creamy butter for enjoyment's sake at risk of a shorter life in which to enjoy anything. We elect a heart bypass operation to relieve oppressive and continuous chest pains, although we know the operation is still being investigated and itself may kill us. We choose a contemplative or a more active career for ourselves.

In all these instances it is not inaccurate to say that we somehow manage to weigh incommensurables, to overcome indeterminacy. As philosopher Donald Evans has been known to say: Such compromises are a part of everyday morality, but they raise serious problems for ethical theory, for their logic and rationale are obscure. So we may grant with philosopher W. D. Ross that we are faced with great difficulties when we try to commeasure good things of very different types. But I would suggest that the difficulties are not insuperable. I make this very slight opening in fear and trembling because it is made in a world and at a time where it can be terribly misused and misunderstood. If that is a serious danger, I withdraw it—and here and now. But I have known cases where failure to terminate a pregnancy has resulted in complete and permanent loss of freedom for the mother (insanity). We die for our freedom, do we not? "Give me liberty or give me death" resonates with all of us, though there are still some who would rather be "red than dead"—but, I suspect, because they think they will really have their liberty after all.

I have presented at least, and perhaps at best, a defensible account of the substance of the Catholic community's evaluation of nascent life over the centuries. It is an evaluation I share. I want to make three points about the notion of evaluation. First, evaluation is a complex concept, involving many dimensions of human insight and judgment. It cannot be reduced simply to rational arguments or religious dogma. Persons with profound religious faith often make judgments that coincide with those of a genuine humanism. Having said that, I would add, however, that the best way to state why I share the traditional evaluation is that I can think of no persuasive arguments that limit the sanctity of human life to extrauterine life. In other words, arguments that justify abortion seem to me equally to justify infanticide—and more.

Second, by saying I share the evaluation, I do not mean to suggest that all problems are solved. They are not. For instance, the moral relevance of the distinction between direct and indirect abortion (really direct/indirect anything) remains a theoretical problem of the first magnitude. I am inclined to agree with John Noonan, Bruno Schüller, Denis O'Callaghan, and, most recently, Susan Teft Nicholson that the distinction is not of crucial moral significance. For instance, O'Callaghan wrote: "If it was honest with itself, it [scholastic tradition] would have admitted that it made exceptions where these depended on chance occurrence of circumstances rather than on free human choice. In other words, an exception was admitted when it would not open the door to more and more exceptions, precisely because the occurrence of the exception was determined by factors of chance outside of human control."[8] He gives intervention into ectopic pregnancy as an example. The casuistic tradition, he believes, accepted what is in principle an abortion because it posed no threat to the general position, though this tradition felt obliged to rationalize this by use of the double effect. Tubal pregnancy, as a relatively rare occurrence and one independent of human choice, does not lay the way open to abuse.

The Belgian hierarchy, perhaps unwittingly, seems to agree. Of

[8] Denis O'Callaghan, "Moral Principle and Exception," *Furrow*, 22 (1971), 686–96.

those very rare and desperate conflict instances (where both mother and child will die if abortion is not performed) they note: "The moral principle which ought to govern the intervention can be formulated as follows: Since two lives are at stake, one will, while doing everything possible to save both, attempt to save one rather than to allow two to perish."[9]

Similarly, in her recent study *Abortion and the Roman Catholic Church*, Susan Nicholson has suggested that abortion might be reconceptualized. If it is viewed dominantly as a killing intervention, we might come out one way. If it is conceptualized above all as withdrawal of maternal assistance, different questions arise— and possibly different answers. Thus this question comes up: Is a woman bound (heroically) to provide assistance (nourishment, etc.) when the pregnancy is the result of rape?[10] I shall not dialogue with Nicholson here except to say that she raises legitimate questions.

The third point to be made about this evaluation is its historicotheological rootage. Albert Outler puts it well: "One of Christianity's oldest traditions is the sacredness of human life as an implication of the Christian convictions about God and the good life. If all persons are equally the creatures of the one God, then none of these creatures is authorized to play God toward any other. And if all persons are cherished by God, regardless of merit, we ought also to cherish each other in the same spirit. This was the ground on which the early Christians rejected the prevalent Graeco-Roman codes of sexuality in which abortion and infanticide were commonplace. Christian moralists found them profoundly irreligious and proposed instead an ethic of compassion (adopted from their Jewish matrix) that proscribed abortion and encouraged 'adoption.' "[11] Thus the value of human life leading to the traditional evaluation was seen in God's special and costing love for each individual—for fetal life, infant life, senescent life, disabled life, captive life, enslaved life, yes, and most of all, unwanted life. These evaluations can be and have been shared

[9] "Déclaration des évêques belges sur l'avortement," 434.
[10] Susan Teft Nicholson, *Abortion and the Roman Catholic Church* (Knoxville, Tenn.: Religious Ethics, 1979).
[11] Albert C. Outler, "The Beginnings of Personhood: Theological Considerations," *Perkins Journal*, 27 (1973), 28–34.

by others than Christians, of course. But Christians have particular warrants for resisting any cultural callousing of them.

I now want to turn to public policy. What makes this so enormously difficult is that public policy is precisely that—public. It cannot exist successfully if there is not some ground of agreement to support it and the principles on which it stands. And at some point that agreement must be on evaluation of fetal life. There is no such agreement. Indeed, there is virulent disagreement, as the recent and unfortunate manifesto *Call to Concern* (issued by a group of over two hundred largely Protestant and Jewish scholars) indicated once again.[12] Furthermore, there is already a public policy in place—the *Wade* and *Bolton* decisions—but one I regard as bad law and bad morality.

In the face of such difficulties all one can do is say what one thinks the law ought to be and why. Let me do this in three steps: procedures, principles, and applications.

Procedures. We should accept that, in a pluralistic society, legal positions tracing back to almost any moral position (whether it be that of Vatican Council II or that of the U. S. Supreme Court) are going to be experienced as an imposition of one view on another group. Thus many view the *Wade* and *Bolton* decisions as an imposition, the introduction of legalized killing into their world. Such a matter should be decided in the Congress, not by nine men in a use of "raw judicial power." Congress is the place where all of us, through our representatives, have a chance to share in the democratic process. This process, as I noted earlier, is often halting, messy, and frustrating, but have we not learned that it is the most adequate way to live with our differences? Furthermore, it gives a reasonable chance from year to year to tighten and purify the policies that have emerged from compromise. Certainly it is a way more adequate than that of a decision framed and finalized by a Court that imposes its own poorly researched and shabbily reasoned moral values as the bases for the law of the land. There are reasons to believe that if this matter were returned to the electorate through its representatives, the nation would have a remarkably different policy. At least there is the chance

[12] "A Call to Concern," *Christianity and Crisis,* 37 (1977), 222–24.

that the gap between the good and the feasible would be narrowed.

Principles. I believe three general guidelines are called for as bases for specific policy if one accepts the traditional Christian (and my) evaluation of fetal life and competing interests. First, there should be a strong presumption in law for the legal protection of fetal life. Second, exceptions should be as clearly and precisely delineated as possible, and such exceptions should contain their own substantive and procedural controls. This statement is but an entailment of the strong presumption favoring fetal life and coincides with the sound policy advocated by the Catholic-Evangelical episcopates of the Federal Republic of Germany. Without both substantive and procedural controls, there is simply no strong presumption in law for protection. Thus to leave the abortion decision simply to the woman ("prochoice") is legal forfeiture of any presumptive claims by the fetus. In bioethics two questions are often distinguished: What is the right decision? Who decides? (At some point a loose answer to the second question destroys in principle the possibility of a disciplined answer to the first.) Third, the policy should be under constant review. The values at stake are fundamental to the continuance of civilized society. That being the case, not only legal protection of nascent life is required, but also social protection—getting at the causes of abortion. Abortion exists because of a cluster of factors that make up the quality of a society. It will disappear only when that quality is changed. Optimistically I contend that the quality can be altered and that therefore the legal provisions must be under constant review lest they themselves become factors corrosive of this quality.

Applications. When I try to fit the Christian evaluation of fetal life into the contemporary American scene and to develop a feasible protective law, I believe it is realistic (feasible) to say that many people would agree that abortion is legally acceptable if the alternative is tragedy, but unacceptable if the alternative is mere inconvenience. Furthermore, I believe that Americans are capable of distinguishing the two in policy—certainly not in a way that will satisfy everyone, but in a way that at least very many can live with. In other words, I do not believe the distinction can or ought to be left entirely to individuals. Such a policy would prohibit

abortion unless the life of the mother is at stake; there is a serious
threat to her physical health and to the length of her life; the
pregnancy is due to rape or incest; fetal deformity is of such magnitude that life-supporting efforts would not be considered obligatory after birth. (I hesitate to list this last exception because it is
accordionlike and easily abused. Furthermore, it is problematic because the very situation of life supports for disabled neonates is itself problematical.)

This list is for all practical purposes and with a few changes the
American Law Institute's proposals in the Model Penal Code. I do
not list these indications because I judge them to be exceptions
that are morally right. I do so only because at the present time
many people believe that continuing the pregnancy in such circumstances is heroic and should not be mandated by law. I list
them also because among the evils associated with any law, these
seem to represent the lesser evil. I am confident that such a policy
will completely satisfy no one—including me. Certainly it will not
satisfy the prolife advocates, and certainly it will not satisfy the
advocates of prochoice. It ought to be more acceptable to those
morally opposed to abortion than to others. But again this acceptance is rooted solidly in one's assessment of fetal life.

Several more issues in regard to this policy require attention.
First, is it a realistically possible policy now? Probably not, unless
some of the cultural changes I will cite occur. Second, does not
this policy force some women to bear pregnancies that they do
not want or that they find terribly onerous? Yes, and I think it
should do so. If it does not do this, if it leaves this decision simply
in the hands of the individual, the law has forfeited all sanctity of
fetal life to personal value judgments. The law does this in no
other area where human life is at stake. Third, would a great number of people suffer under such a policy? Yes, they would. But a
great number of people are suffering under the present policy. It is
a question of measuring suffering and choosing the lesser. In such
a measuring one returns to evaluation of fetal life.

In connection with suffering the picture is incomplete without
taking seriously—personally and at the level of social policy—genuine alternatives to abortion. There are such and there ought to be
more. We have some experiences of this at Georgetown; and we
know that when genuine, supportive alternatives are provided, the

felt need and the actual experiences of abortion are remarkably
lower. Any policy on abortion ought to live in an atmosphere
where alternatives exist. The policy I have proposed can only be
evaluated if such an atmosphere is assumed to be present. I know
it is not present in some places—perhaps not in many. But that
does not attack the policy; it says only that more work must be
done. And one reason such alternatives do not always exist is that
some do not see them as alternatives.

I want to raise a final point to anticipate an objection one frequently hears: How can you, a man—and a celibate priest to boot
—really know what it is to carry a pregnancy with your back
against the wall? It is women, and the individual woman, who
ought to make this decision, according to this objection. I want to
grant the element of truth in this way of thinking. The more one
knows experientially of a situation, the more it is one's own experience, the more sensitive one ought to be to the situation's many-
faceted circumstances, though I believe this is frequently not the
way things turn out. Self-involved agents are frequently self-in-
terested agents with a one-dimensional view of things obvious to
most reasonable and reflective people. Still, it remains true that if
I, as a moral theologian, am going to reflect on the moral problem
of terribly disabled neonates, I ought to learn all I can from
neonatal intensive-care units, from nurses, from experienced physicians, from parents.

After that element of truth has been granted, I must respond
that if the objection is pushed to the limit—as it often is by ex-
tremists—it does away with the possibility of generalization in
ethics—that is, with ethics or moral theology itself. Do I really
have to be a veteran of Vietnam to judge the disproportion of
that war? Do I have to be a politician to recognize obstruction of
justice in public office and judge it wrong? Do I have to be a male
to know that torture by castration is to be condemned? Hardly.
Those who assert that one must be a woman or a married person
to judge abortion a moral tragedy are saying, by implication, that
only the involved agent is capable of assessing the moral character
of his or her action. That is destructive of the entire ethical enterprise and, at the level of policy, leads to the total dissociation of
the moral and legal order.

Try an experiment in thinking about this question. If you were a fetus during the Great Depression, would you want your future to be in the hands of an individual undergoing economic hardship? I daresay you would not want that. Indeed, most of us would appreciate retrospectively the existence of controls (and their social supports) that allowed us to come to be. It is easy for adults undergoing hardship to forget this.

A constitutional amendment is needed to realize such a policy or any policy that legally protects fetuses. I wish to discuss that here only indirectly, to the extent that in order to get a constitutional amendment of any kind, more of a consensus on fetal evaluation must emerge than seems presently to exist, particularly on fetal evaluation with respect to competing claims of the woman (and family). In order to get closer to consensus, the climate of opinion that affects this evaluation must change. I want to list some of the factors that can easily (and corrosively) affect evaluation of nascent life. Attempts to alter policy that ignore and bypass these factors might easily prove shortsighted. Or, more positively, those who concern themselves (in thought and action) with these climatic factors are doing something very important to affect policy.

Human sexuality. What Americans as a culture think about sexuality and how they live it will have a strong influence on their evaluation of fetal life and abortion. One need be neither a eunuch nor a cassandra nor even a phallocrat to think that something has gone wrong in this area and that we must readjust our communal head on the matter. The latest right seems to be the right to sexual pleasure without incumbrance or consequence. Thus we have sex without marriage, sex outside of marriage, and a whole variety of couplings and noncouplings that increasingly separate sex and *eros* from covenanted *philia*—the one relationship that offers the best chance to retain quality in sexual expression. In other words, the culture has trivialized sexuality. Symbols of this trivialization are all about us, from "Charlie's Angels" and "Soap" to the teen-age illegitimacy rate. Not every loosening is a true liberation. Sexual trivialization means sexual irresponsibility, and that must deflate our esteem for the offspring of sexual activity. Unless a genuine cultural change occurs in regard to sexuality, I have little hope for a shift in fetal evaluation.

The concept of privacy. The assumption in American society that abortion is a private affair powerfully undergirds attitudes on the subject. The U. S. Supreme Court struck down all prohibitive state laws by appeal to the penumbral right of privacy. Basically the reasoning is that abortion is a private matter because the right to have a child is a private matter. But as John Noonan points out, it is not merely unpersuasive but also inaccurate to say that destruction of the unborn is private to the mother because it affects only her body. "It affects the child, the father, the grandparents, the physician, the nurse, and the hospital. It is not merely unrealistic but false to hold that a decision ending nascent life does not affect basic social attitudes about life, fidelity, and responsibility and does not touch the fabric of society."[13]

Abortion is not just a matter of the bedroom, as proponents sometimes argue. The right of privacy is increasingly confused with excessive individualism and autonomy—the "freedom to be let alone to do my own thing" syndrome. Many of the arguments surrounding the abortion debate reveal this lonely individualism. For instance, as was noted above, the New York *Times* welcomed the 1973 abortion decisions with this editorial statement: "Nothing in the Court's approach ought to give affront to persons who oppose all abortion for reasons of religion or individual conviction. They can stand as firmly as ever for those principles, provided they do not seek to impede the freedom of those with an opposite view."[14] This simply says: "Nobody requires you to kill. Just let others do it." That assumes that I am unrelated to, unaffected by, others' actions. It supposes that you and I are islands—individual and isolated from the society and atomized within it. From such beginnings comes the nonsense about abortion as an exercise of "privacy." The U. S. Supreme Court, in its 1976 abortion decision in *Planned Parenthood* v. *Danforth*, further intensified this individualism by declaring Missouri's requirement of spousal consent unconstitutional. This decision just atomizes individuals within the family. Unless the nation can somehow overcome this radical individualism, fetuses are at risk.

The interventionist mentality. As a highly technological and pragmatic people, Americans are possessed by the interventionist mentality. What Daniel Callahan calls the "power plasticity"

---

[13] John T. Noonan, Jr., "Abortion in the American Context" (manuscript).
[14] New York *Times* (Jan. 23, 1973).

model has shaped our imaginations and feelings.[15] The best solution to the problems of technology is more technology. We obliterate cities to liberate them. We segregate senior citizens in leisure worlds, and retarded "defective" children in institutions. What is efficient becomes the morally good and right. Technology creates its own morality. In this perspective we eliminate the maladapted condition rather than compassionately adjust the environment to it. We are moving toward what Paul Ramsey calls "administered death" much in the way that twenty years of liberated chat about sexuality has brought us "calisthenic sexuality." The society has the "fly now, pay later" attitude. Let me repeat here what I regard as a kind of ultimate in this interventionist mentality, the statement of Joseph Fletcher: "Man is a maker and a selector and a designer, and the more rationally contrived and deliberate anything is, the more *human* it is." He continues: "Laboratory reproduction is radically human compared to conception by ordinary heterosexual intercourse. It is willed, chosen, purposed, and controlled; and surely these are among the traits that distinguish *Homo sapiens* from others in the animal genus. . . . Coital reproduction is, therefore, less human than laboratory reproduction."[16] Welcome 1984! That something is wrong in this statement I have no doubt. Its surest symptom is that the fun has gone out of things. The "interventionist mentality" leads us to identify making a problem go away with a human solution. Unless we can somehow overcome this, fetuses are at risk.

Utilitarian attitudes. The prevalent popular morality, or structure of moral thinking, is utilitarian. By this I mean an attitude that measures rightness and wrongness in terms exclusively of "getting results," as Joseph Fletcher puts it. If the results seem urgent enough, then paying the price is morally justified regardless of who or what gets stepped on in the process. Not too thinly disguised in these attitudes is a highly functional concept of persons. This attitude is evident frequently in medical procedures involving experimentation, in military strategy, and in government decision-making. It emerged in the reaction of many people to *in vitro*

[15] Daniel Callahan, "Living with the New Biology," *Center Magazine,* 5 (1972), 4–12.
[16] Joseph Fletcher, "Ethical Aspects of Genetic Controls," *New England Journal of Medicine,* 285 (1971), 781.

fertilization with embryo transfer. Results are only one determinant of the moral quality of human conduct; and until this is realized, fetuses—and all of us are but grown-up fetuses—are in trouble.

The influence of the media. I do not wish to join the Agnews of this world in blackening a whole industry. Rather, I want to insist on the fact that via TV we are frequently and mediately exposed to the suffering and deprivation of others. Thus we experience media presentations of suffering and death in Lebanon, Biafra, Guatemala, El Salvador, Guyana, and a host of other places. (And here it should be added that the very prevalence of legal abortion is part of this picture. We are getting used to it. It is well known that wherever abortion laws have been made very permissive, thousands of women come forward feeling the need for abortion who did not feel it in a different climate. That they do this suggests the subtly coercive character of liberalized laws.) The "mediate" experience of suffering inevitably blunts our moral imaginations and sensitivities, and such blunting can chip away at our grasp on the uniqueness and equality of each of God's children, particularly the poorest of the poor and the weakest of the weak.

Attitudes toward childbearing and the family. A whole series of influences (divorce and instability of the nuclear family, population pressures, financial pressures, the emergence of a "comfort ethic" in a consumer society) has drastically modified the attitude toward childbearing. Many young couples now view children as nuisances, incursions on double careers, and so on. Sterilization has become the contraceptive method of choice. In some of the nation's hospitals obstetrics units are no longer active. I simply want to note this, not to analyze it.

Many will cheer this development as the American contribution to solving the "population problem." But before they do—thus adding to the antinatalist atmosphere—they would be well advised to take a long look at some statistics. For instance, the nation is now spending $112 billion (25 per cent of the federal budget) on Social Security for persons over 65. In 1977 the ratio of workers to dependents was 6 to 1. With present fertility rates, in the year 2025 the nation will be spending $635 billion (40 per cent of the federal budget) for those over 65. The ratio of workers to dependents will be 3 to 1. Therefore, a heavier burden will fall on fewer—the burden being 12 times what it is today. A narrow, unsophisticated attitude toward the "population problem" forms part of our evaluative preconditioning where fetal life is concerned. When some people see a pregnant woman in the supermarket, they groan about another polluter or another college education. Far too few of those who make such comments think of their own future Social Security checks and the people required to generate the funds for them. Until they do, fetuses will remain at risk.

The concepts of health and disease and the role of the medical profession. The concept of disease—and therefore of health—has gone through several stages. I noted this above when dealing with our moral responsibility for health. The upshot of this development was a gradual expansion of the notion of disease to include not only mathematical or predictive conditions (hyper, hypo), but also social functionality and sense of social well-being.

What is going on is the increasing desomatization of the notions of health and disease. That means that physicians are increasingly "treating" the desires of people in a move toward the discomfortless society. Columnist George Will mentions the woman who had a mastectomy because her left breast bothered her golf swing.[17] That this notion of medical service and of health and disease provides powerful support for an abortion ethic seems clear; for the fetus is a *soma*.

These are but a few of the cultural obstacles threatening the proper evaluation of nascent life. I am sure there are many more. In combination they suggest that our liberation from abortion as a "crime" has led many to reject any evaluation of abortion as a moral evil, a moral tragedy. Until we as a nation come seriously to grips with these cultural factors, I am afraid there is very little hope that we will move toward an abortion policy that is truly in our over-all best interests. We will continue to protect the redwood, the sperm whale, and the snaildarter more than we do nascent life—which is just plain sad.

17 Washington *Post* (June 25, 1978).

SECTION IV

CONTRACEPTIVE INTERVENTIONS

11. The Encyclical *Humanae Vitae*

[The encyclical *Humanae vitae* appeared at the end of July 1968. In July 1978 it had its tenth anniversary. The following two essays were composed on these two occasions, and represent the author's struggle to deal with these matters from within the Catholic context.]

The Magisterium and Contraception Before "Humanae Vitae"

In an earlier study of mine I concluded a discussion of Pope Paul VI's on the address of October 29, 1966, on birth control, as follows: "Only an authentic teaching statement is capable of dissipating a genuine doctrinal doubt. And that is why I would agree with the many theologians who contend that the matter of contraception is as of now, at least for situations of genuine conflict, just where it was before the papal address—in a state of practical doubt."[1] This conclusion was based on the opinion that the October 29 statement of Pope Paul was not an authentic teaching statement.

John C. Ford, S.J., and John J. Lynch, S.J., have challenged the conclusion that the teaching on contraception was practically doubtful (and subject to probabilism), and especially they have challenged it on the grounds on which I argued it.[2] The particular point at issue between us was the condition of certainty or doubt in the Church as this situation was affected by Vatican II and the papal address of October 29. An analysis of the situation in terms

---

[1] Richard A. McCormick, S.J., "Notes on Moral Theology," *Theological Studies*, 28 (1967), 799–800.

[2] John C. Ford, S.J., and John J. Lynch, S.J., "Contraception: A Matter of Practical Doubt?" *Homiletic and Pastoral Review*, 68 (1968), 563–74. That the article is a counterstatement to the conclusions I drew is made explicit in the July issue of *Homiletic and Pastoral Review*, 810.

of these two documents is no longer adequate since the issuance of *Humanae vitae*. However, the state of the Church from 1966 to 1968 is very helpful, perhaps even necessary, for an understanding of the over-all significance of *Humanae vitae*—that is, an understanding of *Humanae vitae* and the cognate problems it raises will depend to some extent on how one assesses the situation in the Church prior to the encyclical. Furthermore, because of the established competence and humaneness of the authors, and because the entire discussion touches sensitively on the matter of theological methodology, we stand to learn a great deal from a continuing exchange of views on this matter.

The Ford-Lynch argument was made in three steps: (1) the papal statement of June 23, 1964; (2) the doctrine of Vatican II; (3) the papal address of October 29, 1966. The thrust of their paper was that these three documents prevented the existence of a contrary practical probability. A word on each of these documents is called for here.

With regard to the first point, I am in full agreement with Ford and Lynch. The allocution of June 23, 1964, was an authentic noninfallible teaching statement. It was an authentic noninfallible assertion that the reasons adduced to that point were not sufficient to topple the norms of Pius XI and Pius XII. Those familiar with the articles published before that time would agree that they contained serious defects and inconsistencies, and that these shortcomings fully justified the judgment of Pope Paul.

As for Vatican II, Ford-Lynch state their conviction that the texts of the Council "deal with contraception and prohibit it." I have discussed this matter at length before and it is unlikely that further prolonged discussion of the matter could do more than deepen trenches already dug and occupied.[3] However, since the discussion concerned not only the document itself but also its relation to a practical doubt, several points bear repeating here.

First, it must be remembered that the Pope reserved the matter to himself. It is hardly likely, therefore, that the statement of Vatican II would be very definite or decisive. Indeed, those familiar with the *stylus curiae* recognize in the conciliar remarks a piece of masterful evasion. Hirschmann reminds us that the conciliar state-

[3] Richard A. McCormick, S.J., "Notes on Moral Theology," *Theological Studies*, 27 (1966), 651.

ment was very "cautious and open" and that the famous footnote 14 ends as follows: "With the doctrine of the magisterium in this state, this Holy Synod does not intend to propose immediately concrete solutions."[4] Such conciliar light-stepping is not to be wondered at when we read from a Council *peritus* and the editorial secretary of the subcommission that studied marriage questions: "The grave questions as to whether every act is subject to the end of procreation and whether an act of conjugal love in a generously lived marriage may not find more independent expression are left quite open. *The Council deliberately refrained from giving a decision in this theological dispute*" (emphasis added).[5]

Second, Ford-Lynch introduced two letters from H. J. Cardinal Cicognani to Alfredo Cardinal Ottaviani. One of their purposes in introducing these letters, the authors stated, was "to throw light on the meaning which Pope Paul himself attached to the conciliar text when he signed it." It can be argued that if such letters are needed to illumine the meaning a signatory attaches to a text, then the text hardly speaks too clearly and convincingly for itself. Furthermore, it must be said that the letters adduced throw light on the desires and intentions of Pope Paul, not precisely on the meaning he "himself attached to the conciliar text when he signed it," as the authors asserted.

Finally, if Vatican II spoke so clearly and decisively on contraception, one is puzzled by Pope Paul's later remarks about the conciliar statement: "The new pronouncement awaited from the Church on the problem of the regulation of births is not thereby [by the Council] given, because We ourselves, having promised and having reserved the matter to ourselves, wanted to consider carefully the doctrinal and pastoral applications which have arisen regarding this problem in recent years. . . ."[6]

[4] Johannes B. Hirschmann, "Eheliche Gewissenskonflikte und kirchliches Lehramt," *Geist und Leben*, 41 (1968), 143.

[5] Victor L. Heylen, "Fostering the Nobility of Marriage and the Family," in Group 2000 (ed.), *The Church Today* (Westminster: Newman, 1968), 117. This is also the conclusion of Michel Dayez: "*En effet, le Concile n'a pas voulu condamner les nouvelles tentatives de solution selon lesquelles on peut, pour des motifs objectifs . . . recourir à la contraception. Il a même explicitement rejeté plusiers amendments qui visaient à introduire dans le texte conciliarie lui-même des formulations favorissant la présentation classique de la doctrine*" (*Revue diocèsaine de Tournai*, 22 [1967], 520).

[6] *Acta Apostolicae Sedis*, 58 (1966), 1,169.

The Council, then, was hardly the place to turn for the type of statement that would unequivocally and authoritatively settle a matter that it knew the Pope had reserved to himself. I cannot but agree with Donald Campion, S.J., when he asserts that it seems generally agreed now that the Council did not alter "the state of debate on the matter that had existed since Pope Paul's own announcement of June 23, 1964, of his creation of a commission to study questions in dispute about marriage and birth control."[7]

This brings us to the papal allocution of October 29, 1966.[8] It was my contention that this allocution did not represent a genuine teaching statement dealing with the doubts that had arisen since 1964. Ford-Lynch disagree with this conclusion. Their reasons are two. First, they are "mystified when any theologian imagines that a Pope would attempt to deal with a problem like contraception by means of canonical legislation." I am too. But canonical legislation is not the only alternative to a teaching statement. It can be argued that the Pope was simply trying to calm the ruffled waters by suggesting an interim pastoral policy that would not make his genuine teaching more difficult than it should be. Still, a pastoral policy is not a teaching statement.[9]

Their second reason for regarding the allocution as a doctrinal statement is that "Paul himself explicitly declares in the document that the norm he is insisting on is one that is 'constituted best and most sacred for everybody by the authority of the law of God, rather than by Our authority.'" Here we must recall two facts. First, Pope Paul did not at this time make his decisive statement. Alluding to the enormous complications and tremendous gravity of the subject, he said: "This is the reason why our re-

[7] Donald R. Campion, S.J., and Gregory Baum, O.S.A., *Pastoral Constitution on the Church in the Modern World* (Westminster: Paulist Press, 1967), 43.

[8] AAS, 58 (1966), 1,166–70.

[9] F. Bersini asks the following question: May someone in the meantime freely follow the opinion he holds better, as in the situation of doubt? His answer is interesting because it casts serious doubt on the teaching character of the statement of Vatican II and Pope Paul (Oct. 29, 1966): *"La nostra risposta è negativa; perché, mentre la questione è posta allo studio dei competenti, il Concilio e il Summo Pontefice vogliono che nella practica pastorale si segua la dottrina tradizionale"* (Perfice munus, 43 [1968], 155–56 [emphasis added]).

sponse has been delayed and why it mus   ⸱ some
time yet." Second, in an earlier allocution   of the
Italian Feminine Center, Pope Paul, refe   ngoing
work of his special birth-control commission   magisterium of the Church cannot propose moral   is certain of interpreting the will of God. And to   ⸱tainty
the Church is not dispensed from research a⸱   ⸱ining
the many questions proposed for her consid⸢   every
part of the world. This is at times a long and n⸢   '⸴."10

These two statements must be weighed in ⸤   ith
each other. The following analysis is suggested. If   n
cannot propose (that is, teach) moral norms "u⸱   n
of interpreting the will of God," then the tradition⸱   ⸱s
reiterated by Pope Paul at that time must have rep⸱   ⸴-
tain teaching of the will of God. But if this was so, ⸝   ⸱
have delayed his decisive statement and done so pre   ⸱
grounds that time and research were needed to achie⸢   ?
The obvious conclusion would seem to be that the ⸱   n
was not *certain* that these norms represented God's wil⸱   ⸱n-
clusion is only reinforced when one recalls the conclu   ⸍ro-
posed by the majority of the papal study commission. If   ⸴ach
this certainty (*raggiungere questa certezza*) the Church ⸱s not
dispensed from research," then surely the conclusions of this research group must have some bearing on the achievement or
maintenance of certainty in this area. If it is argued that the papal
delay was to be attributed to problems of pastoral presentation
and not to uncertainty, we need only to return to Pope Paul's
statement (February 12, 1966) that the magisterium must be certain that it is proposing God's will when it proposes norms for
conduct and that to reach this certainty "is at times a long and
not an easy task."11

Summarily, then, if certainty is required to teach moral norms,
and if research is required to achieve this certainty, and if the
research sources produce anything but certainty, then the conclusion must be that the required certainty about these norms

---

10 *AAS*, 58 (1966), 219.

11 John Cardinal Heenan found the root of delay in the character of the devices that fall under the general term "contraception" ("The Authority of the Church," *Tablet*, 222 [1968], 489).

did not exist—hence that these norms could not be proposed (taught). And if this is so, how was the papal statement of October 29, 1966, a true teaching statement? This would not mean that the traditional norms were seen to be incorrect. It simply means that it is not clear how they could then be taught as certainly interpreting God's will.

Let us put it this way. Given the certainty necessary to teaching binding moral norms (a certainty asserted by the Pope himself), what was one to think of the Pope's assertion that "the thought and norm of the Church are not changed"? This might have meant two things. (1) The traditional thought and norm are *certainly* the will of God. The evidence seems heavily weighted against such a reading if Pope Paul's statement about certainty and its indispensable sources is given due consideration—that is, if in February 1966 the Pope needed the studies of the commission to achieve (*raggiungere*) the certainty necessary to propose moral norms, and if having received the majority report of the commission he achieved or maintained a certainty contrary to it, then perhaps we need a long, long discussion about the nature of the magisterium. We shall return to this point shortly. (2) The thought and norm just mentioned are not certainly the will of God, but they have not yet been formally admitted to be doubtful. The magisterium was not at that time prepared either to reverse these norms or to admit their doubtful character. In other words, the magisterium was certain only that it did not yet want formally and explicitly to modify or recall these norms. Such hesitation was, in my judgment, very understandable and very prudent. But certainty that the norms should not yet have been formally modified was not the same as certainty that they represented the will of God. The latter is a doctrinal certainty, the former is not necessarily such. Expression of the latter certainty is a doctrinal or teaching statement, whereas expression of the former is not necessarily such.

What then of the papal insistence that "they [traditional norms] demand faithful observance"? In 1966 this conclusion only raised the question: Why?[12] In other words, if the traditional

[12] By simply referring to the 1964 statement, the Pope does not thereby issue a similar statement in 1966; for the 1964 statement was a teaching statement on the reasons adduced to that time. If the 1966 statement were to have

norms were not clearly enough the will of God to allow a decisive statement to that effect, then the assertion that "the norms are still valid" simply had to rest on something other than the conviction that they were certainly the will of God. Consequently this assertion constituted something other than a doctrinal or genuine teaching statement. It was this line of reasoning that led me to the conclusion that the real doubts that had arisen since 1964 had not encountered a true teaching statement.[13] This in turn led to the assertion that contraception was in a state of practical doubt.[14] This still appears to me to have been a very defensible position.

We have dwelled at considerable length on this matter because of its importance to an understanding of the nature and function of the magisterium. In this perspective the discussion is far broader than the single issue that occasioned it. When weighty considerations are introduced against traditional norms of the natural law, and when a highly competent research group is assembled to sort out these problems, and when this group fails to uphold traditional norms, and when a subsequent episcopal com-

---

had a similar force, it would have to have passed authoritatively on the theological thought since then, and specifically on the report of the Commission. The Pope said of the Commission's conclusions only that "they cannot be considered definitive."

[13] Cardinal Heenan's remarks do not appear to be those of a man faced with a genuine teaching statement ("The Authority of the Church," 489).

[14] Dayez (see footnote 5) held explicitly the conclusion of practical doubt: "Given the state of doctrinal research, given the evolution which is developing, given the positive and reasonable doubt touching the statement that 'every contraceptive method is de se evil,' it appears to me that a confessor cannot *demand*, under pain of refusal of absolution, that the penitent renounce a contraceptive method motivated by grave reasons of conjugal life." Hirschmann gingerly avoided saying explicitly that probabilism was operative where contraception is concerned. But his whole treatment implied this conclusion. For example, he insisted that probabilism does not amount to minimalism or laxism. Furthermore, he suggested that clinging to a teaching which did not by any means clearly raise the claim of last authority can lead one to place himself in the path of a fuller appearance of the truth and thereby inhibit the final dynamic of the Spirit in the Church ("Ehelich Gewissenskonflikte und kirchliches Lehramt," 145). These conclusions, it must be noted, do not resemble those that drew from the French episcopal commission on the family the following castigation: "Even though the work and research of moral specialists are legitimate and necessary, still it is astonishing that some Catholic authors allow themselves to solve the question authoritatively in advance of papal teaching" (*Documentation catholique*, 65 [1968], 533).

mission produces the same results, then the contention that the norms are still certain (certainly the will of God) because the magisterium has not yet modified them would seem to be a contention that asks the magisterium to bear a burden it can hardly carry. Is it not asking it to be certain independently of the ordinary sources of clarity and certainty? At some point or other such a notion of the magisterium is all too easily a caricature of the teaching office of the Church.

Could we not put it this way? If a modification of traditional teaching is only plausible on the supposition that the inadequacy of traditional norms had already become clear *before the papal statement,* then it is not the official papal statement alone that gives this clarity. Norms are not certain up to the moment of modification, then suddenly uncertain or changed with the modifying statement. To say so is to adopt a theory of "magisterium by fiat."[15] Now, if the state of uncertainty is not produced by a papal statement of modification, but is the condition of its possibility, this means that the state of uncertainty is gathered from the best available evidence prior to such a statement. This in turn suggests that the state of certainty is gathered from the best available evidence, not from a papal assertion about the state of certainty.[16] To imply anything else is once again to adopt a theory of magisterium by decree and to deny the validity of Pope Paul's assertion that research is required to achieve certainty.

In summary, what very probably underlay the exchange be-

[15] Some of these same reflections can be urged against the guidelines produced in several American dioceses prior to the issuance of *Humanae vitae.* After calling attention to the direct and supreme jurisdiction of the Pope over all members of the Church, and referring to the Pope's insistence on the validity of then existing norms, the guidelines say: "In light of that statement it is clear that neither priest in the confessional, nor Catholic teachers in public or private instruction, may say or imply that the teaching of the Catholic Church either permits or condones the use of means of contraception, be they mechanical, chemical or simply behavioral." The guidelines mentioned greater understanding and compassion; "we repeat, however, that he [the confessor] may not permit or condone the contraceptive practices mentioned above" (*National Catholic Reporter* [July 3, 1968], p. 6). A somewhat different emphasis is found in the letter of Bishop Bernard Stein (Trier) to his priests (see *National Catholic Reporter* [May 22, 1968]) and in the remarks of Bishop Sergio Mendez Arceo of Cuernavaca (see Davenport *Messenger* [May 16, 1968]).

[16] The state of certainty, it would seem, is a fact, not precisely a doctrine about which the magisterium can teach.

tween Ford-Lynch and myself was the relationship of the magisterium to theological investigation. This relationship constitutes what surely is one of the most important theological problems of the day. In broader perspective, it is simply one aspect of a changing notion of the magisterium. The style and structure of authority in the Church (not excluding teaching authority) are undergoing development. Not all aspects of this development are clear, but at the root of it there seems to be a growing decentralization. It is possible, of course, to carry this too far; it is also possible not to allow it to occur at all. Somewhere in the middle lies the truth. But at a time of painful and groping transition it is hard to find this middle. It is quite possible that it was these larger issues that were operative in our disagreement. And that brings us to *Humanae vitae.*

The Encyclical "Humanae Vitae"

The problem prior to *Humanae vitae* was whether the positive doubts surrounding traditional teaching had encountered a true teaching statement. To view the problem in this way was, of course, to approach it from the restricted viewpoint of classical categories. Specifically, it was to imply that a true teaching statement would have destroyed, at least temporarily, any contrary practical probability. The focus of attention was on pastoral practice, once one had granted the existence of a genuine doctrinal doubt. It should not be forgotten that this discussion supposed the existence of a true doctrinal doubt. The problem after *Humanae vitae* is the extent to which this document, obviously a teaching statement, has truly solved the doubts.

Perhaps it were better to say that this is one of the problems occasioned by the encyclical; for if anything is clear, it is that *Humanae vitae* is inseparable from questions far more basic than the issue that occasioned it. These larger issues have been stated very clearly by a group of theologians at Marquette University in the following way:

> 1. In the areas of human understanding which are proper
> to human reasoning, such as natural law, what is the

function of the Church as the authoritative teacher of revelation?

2. What are the sources for the formulation of binding moral doctrine within the Christian community?

3. What is the precise role of the Pope as an authoritative teacher in these areas?

4. What is the role of the bishops, of the body of the faithful, and of the Church's theologians in formulating such moral teaching?

5. What qualifications may be attached to the individual Christian's assent to admittedly fallible statements of the merely authentic magisterium, especially when this involves practical judgments of grave consequence?[17]

These questions, touching as they do on the central nervous system of Catholic belief and life, explain why *Humanae vitae* caused such a profound reaction in the Catholic community.[18] Obviously, we cannot discuss these major theological themes here.[19] However, only their full discussion will position us to understand the phase of development we are presently experiencing. We can address ourselves only to the single assertion that is at the heart of the encyclical: Every contraceptive act is intrinsically evil. The following remarks may be gathered under three headings: (1) the analysis and argument of the encyclical; (2) the relation of theological analysis to a doctrinal conclusion; (3) some pastoral notes and conclusions.

After stating that each marriage act must remain open (*per se destinatus*) to the transmission of life, Pope Paul presents the following analysis.

---

[17] *Our Sunday Visitor* (Aug. 18, 1968).

[18] This reaction was not without its human inconsistencies. For example, one wonders whether the issue of collegiality would have been raised quite so sharply had the decision of Pope Paul been different. This issue should have been raised by theologians at a much earlier date. Similarly, in earlier days the celibacy of the theologian defending traditional teaching was underscored. This same celibacy seems a bit more tolerable where the theologian is presently a dissenter. Or again, the very ones who dissented most vigorously when *Mater et magistra* appeared are now the ones fervently urging that Rome speak.

[19] For example, the word *ecclesia* is used thirty-four times in the encyclical, according to my hasty count. It would be interesting to study the theological implications of its various uses.

That teaching, often set forth by the magisterium, is founded upon the inseparable connection, established by God and unable to be broken by man on his own initiative, between the unitive and procreative meanings, both of which are present in the conjugal act.

For by its intimate structure, the conjugal act, while most closely uniting husband and wife, also capacitates them (*eos idoneos etiam facit*) for the generation of new life, according to laws inscribed in the very being of man and woman. By safeguarding both of these essential aspects, the unitive and the procreative, the use of marriage preserves in its fullness the sense of true mutual love and its ordination to man's exalted calling to parenthood.[20]

The encyclical argues, therefore, that intercourse is a single act with two aspects or inner meanings, the unitive and procreative. It further argues that these two senses are by divine design inseparable, so that one who deliberately renders coitus sterile attacks its meaning as an expression of mutual self-giving. Thus we read later that contraceptive intercourse removes, "*licet solum ex parte, significationem et finem doni ipsius*" (n. 13). It seems that the whole weight of the encyclical's teaching that a contraceptive act is "*intrinsece inhonestum*" (n. 14) derives from this analysis. In fact, Pope Paul says just that. Because this is so, several remarks are in place.

First, the above analysis is not new. It will be recalled that *Casti connubii* approached the expression of marital love as a motive for sexual intercourse. In the years prior to the Second Vatican Council it became clear to theologians that this was an incomplete and imperfect analysis. They began to speak of the expression of marital love as one of the very inner senses (*finis operis*) of intercourse. Several allocutions of Pius XII adopted this point of view.[21] In recent years Joseph Fuchs, S.J., was more than anyone else associated with systematizing this notion. Speaking of

[20] *De propagatione humanae prolis recte ordinanda* (Rome: Typis Polyglottis Vaticanis [1968]), No. 12. This is a Latin version of *Humanae vitae*. Subsequent references will be to this text and by paragraph number.

[21] For example, *AAS*, 43 (1951), 850; *AAS*, 48 (1956), 470.

the relationship of the two meanings or aspects of coitus, Fuchs wrote in 1963:

> The Creator so arranged the sexual act that it is simultaneously both per se generative and per se expressive of intimate oblative love. He has so arranged it that procreation would take place from an act intimately expressive of conjugal love and that this act expressive of conjugal love would tend toward procreation. Therefore an act which *of itself* does not appear to be apt for procreation is by this very fact shown to be one which does not conform to the intentions of the Creator. The same thing should be said about an act which *of itself* is not apt for the expression of oblative love. Indeed, an act which is not apt for procreation is by this very fact shown to be one which is *of itself* not apt for the expression of conjugal love; for the sexual act is one.[22]

Many of us accepted this approach for a number of years and argued that contraceptive interference could not be viewed as a merely biological intervention.[23] Rather, we argued, it was one that affected the very foundation of the act as procreative and hence as unitive of persons; for by excluding the child as the permanent sign of the love to be expressed in coitus, one introduced a reservation into coitus and therefore robbed it of that which makes it objectively unitive.

This analysis, even though it represents a genuine advance, rests ultimately on the supposition that every act of coitus has and therefore must retain a per se aptitude for procreation.[24] This

22 Joseph Fuchs, S.J., *De castitate et ordine sexuali* (Rome: Gregorian University Press, 1963), 45. Speaking in another place (p. 80) of the separability of the two aspects of coitus asserted by some non-Catholics, Fuchs wrote: "They do not sufficiently grasp that the Creator *united* this double aspect. The sexual faculty has but *one* natural actuation in which the generative and oblative aspects specify each other." These same analyses are present in the earlier edition (1959, p. 61) of Fuchs' work.

23 See Richard A. McCormick, S.J., "Conjugal Love and Conjugal Morality," *America*, 110 (1964), 38–42; "Family Size, Rhythm, and the Pill," in *The Problem of Population* (Notre Dame: University of Notre Dame Press, 1964), 58–84.

24 For a refutation of the validity of the argument, see G. Grisez, *Contraception and the Natural Law* (Milwaukee, Wis.: Bruce, 1964), 34–35.

supposition is accepted and clearly stated in *Humanae vitae*. The encyclical's formulation and repetition of traditional teaching speaks of the necessity that each marital act *"ad vitam humanam procreandam per se destinatus permaneat"* (n. 11).[25] Furthermore, the encyclical speaks of the restriction of man's dominion over the genital powers "because of their intrinsic ordination toward raising up life, of which God is the principle" (n. 13). Also, of coitus we read that "by its intimate structure coitus . . . capacitates them for the generation of new life . . ." (n. 12). Now, the immediate and often-stated difficulty with such a contention is that, starting with an obsolete biology, it attributes a meaning to all coitus on the basis of what happens with relative rarity.

Unless I am mistaken, *Humanae vitae* reflects the strength of this difficulty in what appears to be almost a contradiction within the encyclical. Speaking of coital acts during infertile periods, the encyclical says that they are legitimate *"cum non cesset eorum destinatio ad conjugum conjunctionem significandam roborandamque"* (because their ordination toward the expressing and strengthening of conjugal relations does not cease) (n. 11). The rather clear implication here is that any *destinatio ad procreationem* ceases. Otherwise why did the encyclical not say, *"cum non cesset eorum per se destinatio ad procreationem"*? Why did the document use the phrase *"non cesset"* of a single aspect of coitus, thereby implying that the other of the two ordinations or aspects did indeed cease? The unstated but obvious reason is that any *destinatio ad procreationem* is absent in infertile acts. And if it is absent, it is clearly separable from them. In these infertile acts the unitive and procreative aspects are separable. This means that at one point the encyclical seems unwittingly to imply a factual separation of the unitive and procreative aspects of individual coital acts during the infertile period. At another (n. 12) the doctrine that each act must remain open to new life is said to rest on the inseparable connection between the procreative and unitive meanings *"quae ambae in actu conjugali insunt."*

A second point must be noted here. Theologians have found

---

[25] This wording seems to represent a great broadening of the notion of a forbidden contraceptive act. In *Casti connubii* those interventions were condemned in which the act was deprived of its natural power to procreate (*AAS*, 22 [1930], 560).

the per se aptitude for procreation of each act of coitus an extremely difficult analysis to sustain, because it seems to imply and
demand an unacceptable criterion for the assessment of the meaning of human actions. The criterion apparently inseparable from
this analysis is an approach that measures the meaning of an act
by examining its physiological structure. In any number of places
in the encyclical biological structure and the processes of nature
are accepted as the determinants of meaning.[26] They are said to
represent God's plan and therefore to be morally normative.

Contemporary theological thought insists that the basic criterion for the meaning of human actions is the person, not some isolated aspect of the person. Vatican II, while speaking of marriage
and responsible parenthood, pointed out that the moral character
of any procedure must be determined by objective standards "ex
personae ejusdemque actuum natura desumptis."[27] It is interesting
to note the shift in emphasis found in Humanae vitae. There the
criterion is "ipsa matrimonii ejusque actuum natura" (n. 10).

It is important to understand what it means to say that the person is the criterion of the meaning of actions. Authors have always
admitted that the total object (or significance) of an action cannot be identified merely with the physical object. Physical objects
as such have no relation to the moral order. Thus "taking another's property" is only a physical act; it is not yet a moral object.
Similarly "uttering an untruth" is only a physical act or object.
The Majority Report points this out in the case of arms whose use
is good when in self-defense, but evil when turned to unjust killing.[28] The materiality of the act is not the same as its meaning.

If, however, "taking another's property" contains an attack on
persons or a person, it contains the malice of theft (and is an

---

[26] "Deus enim naturales leges ac tempora fecunditatis ita sapienter dis-
posuit . . ." (No. 11); "humana ratio . . . biologicas deprehendit leges, quae
ad humanam personam pertinent . . ." (No. 10); "actum amoris mutui, qui
facultati vitam propagandi detrimento sit, quam Deus omnium Creator secun-
dum peculiares leges in ea insculpsit . . ." (No. 13); ". . . leges conservans
generationis . . ." (No. 13); ". . . conjuges legitime facultate utuntur, sibi a
natura data; in altera vero, iidem impediunt, quominus generationis ordo suos
habeat naturae processus . . ." (No. 16); "Qui limites non aliam ob causam
statuuntur, quam ob reverentiam, quae toti humano corpori ejusque naturalibus
muneribus debetur . . ." (No. 17).
[27] AAS, 58 (1966), 1,072.
[28] "The Birth Control Report," Tablet, 221 (1967), 512.

unloving act). If "uttering an untruth" jeopardizes man's life in community, it contains the malice of a lie. After examination of the goals and conditions of the human person (his potentialities and relationships as known from all sources—above all, revelation), we have concluded to the meaning of material goods and man's relation to them. The basic common destiny of material goods allows us to conclude to the inherent limitations on property rights. Only those actions that violate genuine property rights constitute an attack on persons and merit the name of theft. We say genuine property rights—that is, rights as defined and delimited within the whole hierarchy of personal value. This relationship to the hierarchy of personal value we have encapsulated in the phrase "against his reasonable will." Therefore only those acts that take another's property against his reasonable will constitute the category of theft, and represent an attack on the person through those things that are necessary to personal growth and good. It is the total good of the person that has determined which physical acts are theft, which not. The same might be said of speech.

Clearly, then, significance does not refer to mere physical acts; rather it is an assessment of an action's relation to the order of persons, to the hierarchy of personal value.[29] This same methodology must also apply in the area of sexual ethics. The significance (the total moral object) must be determined, as in other instances, by relating the physical act to the order of persons and by seeing it as an intersubjective reality.

Of course, sexuality is founded in biological realities, and just as obviously sexual intercourse, materially considered, has some orientation toward fecundation. We are not calling these "thresholds of objectivity" into question here. We are only suggesting that the meaning of sexual activity cannot be derived narrowly from biological materialities; for this does not take account of the full range and meaning of human sexuality. It is not the sexual organs that are the source of life, but the person. As the Majority Report noted, "the biological process in man is not some separated part (animality) but is integrated into the total personality of

[29] W. van der Marck, O.P., refers to this personal aspect of the act as "intersubjectivity" in *Toward a Christian Ethic* (Westminster: Newman, 1967), 48–59.

man."[30] Thus the material fecundity in this process gets its moral meaning from its finalization toward the goods that define marriage. This is what it means, one would think, to draw objective standards *ex personae ejusdemque actuum natura*. Just as we refuse to identify "taking another's property" with theft, so we must refuse to identify the physiological components with the full meaning of sexual actions.

The third point to be made about the argument of the encyclical is its handling of the analysis made by the now famous Majority Report. This report had suggested that infecund acts (even those deliberately made such) are incomplete, and derive one aspect of their moral quality from their relationship to the fertile acts already placed or to be placed. This analysis is rejected by the encyclical on the grounds that an act deprived of its procreative power is intrinsically evil. But this is precisely the point to be shown. In my judgment the encyclical does not succeed in doing this.

If the analysis and argument used in an authoritative moral teaching on natural law do not support the conclusions, what is one to think of these conclusions? Concretely, *Humanae vitae* taught the intrinsic immorality of every contraceptive act. At least very many theologians will agree that there are serious methodological problems, even deficiencies, in the analysis used to support this conclusion. What is one to say of the conclusion in these circumstances?

The encyclical itself, after exhorting priests to be examples of loyal internal and external *obsequium*,[31] stated: "That *obsequium*, as you know well, obliges not only because of the reasons adduced, but rather (*potius*) because of the light of the Holy Spirit, which is given in a particular way to the pastors of the Church in order that they may illustrate the truth" (n. 28). This statement summarizes the accepted notion of the authoritative but noninfallible moral magisterium. It says in effect that the authoritative character of the teaching is not identified with the reasons adduced for it. On the other hand, it clearly implies that

---

[30] "The Birth Control Report," 512.

[31] I have left the word *obsequium* untranslated because a satisfactory English equivalent is lacking. Several Latin scholars have suggested that "obedience" is too strong.

the certainty of the teaching cannot prescind from the adequacy of the analyses given. Establishing the proper balance is the problem we face.

It might be helpful to point out the extremes to be avoided where authoritative noninfallible teaching is concerned. One extreme is that the teaching is as good as the argument. This makes the Pope just another theologian and destroys the genuinely authoritative character of the papal charism. It also implies a one-sidedly rationalistic epistemology of moral cognition. The other extreme is that the teaching is totally independent of the argument. This makes the Pope an arbitrary issuer of decrees and edicts. It dispenses completely with the need of theological reflection and ends up ultimately as an attack on the *teaching* prerogatives of the Holy Father.

It is important to stress this point. If a teaching is considered valid independently of the reasons and arguments, then the possibility of objectively founded dissent is eliminated on principle—that is, if noninfallible teaching must be accepted independently of the reasons supporting it (understanding "reasons" in a broad, not excessively rationalistic, sense), on what grounds is dissent still possible? And if dissent is impossible, in what sense is the teaching noninfallible? At this point the truth of the teaching is simply identified with the authority proposing it. And who has greater moral authority than the Sovereign Pontiff? Many of us will find it uncomfortable to live with a notion of noninfallible teaching that demands that it be treated as practically infallible. Somewhere between these two extremes lies the truth.

The middle ground between these extremes has traditionally been formulated in terms of a presumption to be granted to authentic noninfallible statements. This is a presumption that they are correct.[32] The strength of this presumption will vary in individual instances according to many circumstances too numerous to detail or discuss here. We have already suggested that the response generated by this presumption is religious docility of mind and will. Furthermore, it was suggested that this docility would

[32] Here some further precisions are probably in place. When the word "correct" is applied to moral teaching, it could mean "speculatively true," "a valid value judgment," "a justifiable jurisdictional act in protection of moral values," etc.

concretize itself in several ways. These ways include a readiness to reassess one's own position in light of the teaching and an attempt to discover whether the conclusion taught might be established on grounds other than those adopted by the magisterium. Finally, it was stated that such steps will generally lead to full and grateful acceptance of the teaching. And this acceptance will manifest itself in one's decisions.

But precisely because we are dealing with noninfallible teaching, the steps that express one's radical docility and submission could end somewhat differently. This will not happen often, otherwise the magisterium would cease to be truly authoritative.[33] But if the very possibility is excluded on principle, then are we really dealing with noninfallible teaching? Now, if the steps stimulated by docility are carefully and conscientiously taken, and one still finds it personally impossible to justify the doctrinal conclusion, it seems to me that the presumption supporting the doctrine prevails until a sufficient number of mature and well-informed members of the community share this same difficulty. Until this stage is reached, our difficulties will suggest to us our own limitations, if we are honest and realistic. But once it becomes clear that a large number of loyal, docile, and expert Catholics share this same difficulty, then it would seem that the presumption supporting the certain correctness of the teaching would be weakened, at least to the extent that the doctrine could be said to be doubtful. If the presumption would not be weakened in the instance just described, when would it ever be? At this point one would wonder whether such a doctrine could give rise to a certain obligation in conscience.

How does all of this apply to the doctrine of *Humanae vitae* that a contraceptive act is "instrinsically evil" (n. 14) and "always illicit" (n. 16)? By way of preface it must be said that a theologian's answer to this question is only his own honest, conscientious, but very fallible opinion. He submits it to his colleagues for appraisal and correction, and then to the bishops for their prayerful consideration. It seems necessary to make this point because in recent years theological opinions, including some of my own, have occasionally been used as if they enjoyed doctrinal sta-

---

[33] G. Baum, O.S.A., "The Right to Dissent," *Commonweal*, 88 (1968), 553–54.

tus. This being said, we may attempt an answer to the question raised by proceeding in stages.

First, in the past years a good number of theologians, after literally thousands of hours of diligent study and discussion, had concluded that the traditional norms as proposed by Pius XI and Pius XII were genuinely doubtful—that is, there were serious and positive reasons against them. I am convinced that for many of us the word "doubt" meant just that.[34] It did not mean certainty one way or the other, though increasingly many of us viewed the analysis presented in the Majority Report as by far the more probable and persuasive view. Hence, when *Humanae vitae* appeared, we read it eagerly looking for the new evidence or the more adequate analyses that led Paul VI to his reaffirmation of traditional norms.

Second, a rather well-educated guess would say that the vast majority of theologians will conclude that the analyses of *Humanae vitae* build upon an unacceptable identification of natural law with natural processes—that is, they will assert that the argument does not justify the conclusion.

Third, at this point the theologian's docility will stimulate him to ask: Can the intrinsic immorality of contraception be established in some more acceptable way, and on other grounds? Possibly. But in the past six or seven years of intense discussion we have experienced little success, and not for lack of trying, to be sure. It is not that the arguments do not conclude with the force of mathematical demonstration. Few ethical arguments do, even the most suasive. It is rather that there seems to be no argument capable of sustaining the intrinsic malice of contraceptive acts, and a good deal of evidence that denies this thesis. Indeed, past attempts to establish the doctrine have imprisoned us, step by inexorable step, in totally unacceptable presuppositions.

This is not to say that a strong indictment of contraception is out of place. Quite the contrary. For very many people, contraception could easily represent a way of life springing from and reflecting the materialism and secularism of Western man. We live in a contraceptive world where the pill (etc.) has assumed the character of a human panacea. Contraception cannot be viewed in

---

[34] We say "many" here because there are certainly some, perhaps quite a few, theologians who are convinced of the complete moral integrity of contraception, at least in certain circumstances.

isolation from basic attitudes toward life and sexuality. There is
mounting evidence that in contemporary culture contraception is
part and parcel of an attitudinal package that includes sterilization
(even coerced), abortion, artificial insemination, and ultimately
euthanasia. Furthermore, contraception might be associated with
a certain amount of marital selfishness, marital infidelity, and pre-
marital irresponsibility, though we must be careful here to document any generalizations we would make.

Perhaps it was a cultural criticism such as this that Paul Ricoeur had in mind when he wrote:

> What gives force to the anticontraceptive position are
> not, in my opinion, the arguments based on the meaning
> of "natural" and "unnatural," but an argument which is
> rarely made use of: the knowledge that contraception
> risks destroying the quality of the sexual act by making it
> facile and ultimately insignificant. I would develop the
> implicit argument of those who oppose contraception in
> these terms: Of course, birth control is necessary, but
> there is the danger that the meaning and value of sexual-
> ity will disappear. Today we are perhaps more worried
> about overcoming the fatality of reproduction. The price
> of this victory—a price costly from the point of view of
> psychology and spirituality—will inevitably become ap-
> parent. It may be that tomorrow's greatest problem will
> be to preserve the expressive and meaningful value of
> sexuality. But if this is tomorrow's problem, is it not al-
> ready today's? Must we not, come what may, retain the
> distinction between natural and unnatural, not because
> this distinction is of value in itself, but because nature it-
> self proposes an exterior limit to man's demands on sex,
> and also maintains the sole objective bulwark capable of
> sustaining the quality of the sexual act?[35]

Ricoeur then added that

> the partisans of birth control should be aware that con-
> traception, considered as a simple technique in general,

[35] Cross Currents, 14 (1964), 246–47.

> helps to precipitate sexuality into meaninglessness; it is
> probable that a rational use of contraception can only
> succeed where men are spiritually aroused to the need
> for maintaining the quality of the sexual language.[36]

Clearly Ricoeur himself believes that contraception can be put
at the disposal of a responsible conjugal ethics and that it can be
in the service of rational fertility rather than sterility. I am not arguing here that this approach to the question is persuasive or that
it will lead to the conclusions of *Humanae vitae*. I am only
suggesting that it seems to represent the only kind of approach
left toward those conclusions. One might argue that we live in a
culture where very many are not spiritually aroused to the need
for maintaining the quality of sexual language. Sexual expression
is more facile and insignificant than ever. Its increasing mechanization poses a serious threat to its viability as a human experience.

If we approach the question of contraception from this point of
view, could we arrive at the conclusion that it is intrinsically evil?
I doubt it. We would conclude only that it is dangerous and that
the duty of the individual couple is subject to their ability to de-
tach the practice from these poisonous concomitants. However,
the dangers might be so considerable that ecclesiastical authority
would wish to impose a norm of conduct in virtue of its jurisdictional authority. There is some indication in the documents of
the magisterium that propositions about natural-law matters do at
times conform more to jurisdictional precepts than to teaching.[37]
If this were the case, it would seem that the teaching would be, to
use Daniel Maguire's phrase, "open to the soothing influence of
epikeia."[38] In any event, these reflections do not lead to the conclusion of the intrinsic immorality or absolute illicitness of contraceptive acts.

[36] Ibid., 247.

[37] For example, Pope John XXIII wrote in *Mater et magistra:* "It is clear,
however, that when the hierarchy has issued a *precept or decision* on a point
at issue, Catholics are bound to obey their directives. The reason is that the
Church has the right and obligation, not merely to guard the purity of ethical
and religious principles, but also to intervene authoritatively when there is
question of judging the application of these principles to concrete cases" (*AAS*,
53 [1961], 457).

[38] Daniel Maguire, "Morality and the Magisterium," *Cross Currents*, 18
(Winter 1968), 57.

If theologians have not been able to sustain the conclusion of intrinsic malice, and if increasingly they have found sound theological reasons to justify contraception at least in some instances (compare the Majority Report), on what grounds did the Pope reaffirm traditional teaching? It is not from arrogance that one seeks to discover how Pope Paul VI arrived at the conviction that he must reaffirm traditional norms. Only when one knows what factors were operative in this decision is he positioned to appropriate the decision as fully as a docile and intelligent Catholic would desire. We are dealing here, after all, with the natural law, as the encyclical states. This means that the exclusion of contraception is a demand based on the person's being as person. Now, the demands of natural law are determined by evidence gathered from many competences and evidence available to all of us. This evidence either yields a reasonably convincing case or it does not.

If it does, should this not recommend itself to the reflections of at least very many devoted and reflective Christians, and manifest itself in the convictions of a majority of expert theologians and episcopal advisers, even though our formulations of this may be awkward?[39] It did not. How, then, are we to explain the reaffirmation? Pope Paul VI gives some hint of an explanation when he refers in *Humanae vitae* to the work of the Birth Control Commission. He states that its conclusions could not be considered definitive and gives as the special reason for this (*praesertim*) "because certain criteria of solutions had emerged which departed from the moral teaching authority of the Church" (n. 6). There are many other indications in the encyclical that the Holy Father felt keenly the weight of tradition.[40] Ultimately, however, one

---

[39] Here it must be noted that many reactions to *Humanae vitae* were couched in terms of support or nonsupport for the Pope, of acceptance or rejection of his authority. Hence they cannot be reckoned a truly accurate guide of Catholic conviction on the issue at stake.

[40] For instance: ". . . *ut saepenumero Decessores Nostri pronuntia-verunt* . . ." (No. 4); ". . . *Ecclesia congrua dedit documenta* . . ." (No. 4); ". . . *hinc constans Ecclesiae doctrina declarat* . . ." (No. 10); ". . . *quam constanti sua doctrina interpretatur* . . ." (No. 11); "*huiusmodi doctrina, quae ab Ecclesiae Magisterio saepe exposita est* . . ." (No. 12); ". . . *sicut Ecclesiae Magisterium pluries docuit* . . ." (No. 14); "*Ecclesia sibi suaeque doctrinae constat* . . ." (No. 16); "*Cum Ecclesia utramque hanc legem non condiderit, ejusdem non arbitra, sed tantummodo custos atque interpres* . . ." (No. 18).

must conclude that the constant proposal of a teaching by the Church guarantees not its absolute correctness (unless it is infallibly proposed) but only its longevity.

At this point perhaps the theologian ought to ask himself whether he has read the encyclical properly. Certainly, before anyone concludes that the teaching of *Humanae vitae* is gravely doubtful or even in error, he must determine what that teaching is. To do that, he must have some hermeneutic for papal documents. We are familiar with the contention of theologians that earlier authoritative condemnations must be understood as condemnations of a teaching or tenet as it was then understood (for example, religious liberty). Pius XII's elaboration of the principle of totality had to be read, theologians argued, in light of the totalitarian abuses of which he was so acutely aware and that he wished to counteract. And so on.

A concrete application of this method to *Humanae vitae* might suggest the following approach. Beneath the explicit and dated language of faculties and processes, of intrinsic evil and per se ordinations, there is a message that carries beyond these categories. Perhaps the document should be read as one that points in a general direction and prophetically defends the great values of life and marital love. In other words, perhaps it can be read as delineating an ideal toward which we must work. Just as marriage is growth in unity, so the expression of marriage (marital intimacy) is an activity whose purity and perfection we have not reached, but for which we must constantly struggle. It is quite possible that we are collectively insensitive to this ideal.

However, if this is the basic message of the encyclical, if it is outlining a horizon toward which we must move rather than a casuistry to which we must conform, then the integrity of marital relations would be determined by the couple's acceptance or rejection of this ideal in their present situation. If contraceptive acts were performed without a resolve or desire to grow toward this ideal, then they would be immoral. But as long as the couple resolves to do what they can to bring their marriage (and societal conditions) to the point where the fullness of the sexual act is possible, their practice of contraception would not represent moral failure.

I am not suggesting here that the encyclical can or should be read in this manner. I doubt that it can. I am only attempting to illustrate how the theologian will exhaust every reasonable means to understand and defend authoritative teaching before he ultimately questions its validity. In this instance one feels particularly reluctant to develop a hermeneutic in the face of the practical statements of *Humanae vitae* precisely because such attempts will almost certainly provoke immediate howls that they are devious and ignominious attempts to water down the clear teaching of the encyclical. And up to a point this reaction is justified. But those who insist on reading the encyclical with theological literalism must live with the presuppositions of theological literalism. And in this instance that would be a hard life.

In the light of these reflections it is my opinion that the intrinsic immorality of every contraceptive act remains a teaching subject to solid and positive doubt. This is not to say that this teaching of *Humanae vitae* is certainly erroneous.[41] It is only to say that there are very strong objections that can be urged against it and very little evidence that will sustain it. One draws this conclusion reluctantly and with no small measure of personal anguish. With proper allowance made for one's own shortcomings, pride, and resistance, what more can a theologian say? He can say, of course, that the teaching is clear and certain simply because the papal magisterium has said so. But ultimately such an assertion must rest on the supposition that the clarity and certainty of a conclusion of natural-law morality are independent of objective evidence. In the discussion that has followed *Humanae vitae*, those who have supported the conclusions of the encyclical have argued in just this way. I believe this is theologically unacceptable.

If other theologians, after meticulous research and sober reflection, share this opinion in sufficient numbers, if bishops and competent married couples would arrive at the same conclusion, it is difficult to see how the teaching would not lose the presumption of certainty ordinarily enjoyed by authoritative utterances. How-

[41] That is why I stated in the *National Catholic Reporter*: "I am not prepared to say that it is the only way traditional norms could be established and that therefore this teaching is *clearly inadequate*. More time and study are required to reach such a conclusion" (Aug. 7, 1968, p. 9). "Gravely doubtful" is not the same as "clearly inadequate." This latter suggests reasonable certainty of error. There are other theologians whose position would be far stronger than this.

ever, the ecclesial value of dissenting judgments in the present circumstances remains a problem in its own right.

Because of the proximity of the encyclical and some unfortunate reactions associated with its issuance (unfortunate because agreement was allowed to be equated with loyalty, disagreement with disloyalty), one's honest expression of this theological opinion risks appearing as a kind of private magisterium that has entered into conflict with the authoritative papal magisterium. John Reed, S.J., was assuredly correct when he noted that "whatever the limits on one's obligation to accept the judgment of the latter [magisterium of the Church], one is certainly not entitled, either singly or in company with other theologians, to enter into conflict with it."[42] It is very difficult in the present circumstances to question the papal magisterium in one form or another without seeming to be in conflict with it. But the two notions (dissent from, in conflict with) are radically different. The theologian who conscientiously questions a particular teaching of the magisterium is deeply convinced that he is actually supporting and contributing to the magisterium. Indeed, the continuing health of the magisterium depends on his ability to do just this.

But he will be disinclined to discharge his duty of personal reflection if the results of his study are viewed as a private and defiant magisterium. The only ones capable of preventing this are the bishops. They are the magisterium in a way no theologian can claim to be. They must be in close contact with theologians (and the sources theologians draw upon), so that the best and most responsible Catholic thought will feed into the magisterium and shape its authoritative directives. If a much closer working relationship between the episcopal and the theological communities fails to mature, the theologian will be faced with only two alternatives, both of which are disastrous for himself and the Church: to abandon his honesty and integrity of thought, or to keep it and to become a private magisterium distinct from and sometimes in conflict with the genuine magisterium of the Church.

We are too close to the neurological issue and too far from the solution to the great theological problems inseparable from the encyclical to lay down pastoral directives with any degree of

[42] John J. Reed, S.J., "Natural Law, Theology and the Church," *Theological Studies*, 26 (1965), 59.

confidence. Furthermore, such a task is properly that of the bishops. However, certain avenues of approach may be suggested here with the hope that they will stimulate others to make them more precise. We may touch on three points: bishops, bishops and priests, priests and the married.

Bishops. It is a mistake for an individual bishop or the conference of bishops to accept this, or any noninfallible teaching, without serious personal reflection and consultation. The teaching charism of bishops demands of them a truly personal reflection. The Dutch bishops gave us an example of this. They stated: "It is obvious, therefore, that your bishops will be able to give the guidance you so badly need only after consultation with theologians and other experts. This guidance will undoubtedly be given, but cannot be given until after some lapse of time."[43] It would seem that decisions to "support the Pope" without a true personal reflection are policy decisions. Such decisions can all too easily deprive the Pope and the faithful of the wisdom they have a right to expect from their bishops. They also fail to tell us whether the bishops are truly accepting and teaching a doctrine rather than just enforcing it. In this connection it must be said in all candor that the statements of several American bishops fail to distinguish "accepting the authority of the Pope" from "accepting what is authoritatively taught."

Bishops and priests. Given the fact that the teaching is noninfallible and error is possible (though one does not start with this emphasis in his own reflections), it is a mistake for bishops to insist on assent from their priests. We shall only grow in knowledge and understanding in the Catholic community if acceptance of this or any teaching is completely uncoerced, and if it represents, as far as possible, a truly personal assimilation, even though this assimilation may be somewhat delayed.

It would seem more appropriate that bishops, in dealing with their priests, should insist on a basic Christian and religious docility and the need for arduous reflection, study, and consultation. Bishops should do everything possible to encourage and facilitate a personal assimilation of authoritative teaching on the part of their priests. Second, bishops should insist on responsible conduct,

[43] *National Catholic Reporter* (Aug. 14, 1968), p. 5.

whether one's study has issued in acceptance or dissent. Responsible conduct would include the following: respect for the Pope and his office; respect for the fact that he has a personal charism authoritatively to teach and lead the faithful. In other words, a priest's conduct will reflect a realization that the virtue of faith may not be weakened 'in the process of discussing one teaching that does not pertain to the faith.

Priest and faithful. It seems to me that the priest's first task is to distinguish for his faithful between his own personal opinion and authoritative teaching. The Church needs the reflections and opinions of all of us. But our assimilation of any teaching is subject to our own imperfections and shortcomings. Concretely, if a priest in his professional capacity (confessor, preacher, counselor) asserts that "it is legitimate to practice contraception in certain circumstances," this is his opinion. If he presents it as any more than this, is he not equivalently setting himself up as a teacher in conflict with a far more authoritative teacher? It is precisely the impossibility of doing this that constitutes the problem we are now facing.

The priest's second task is to aid the faithful toward a personal reflection and assimilation of the encyclical. Just as growth in understanding in the Church depends on a careful reflection by the authentic teachers in the Church (the bishops), so their reflections remain incomplete if they are not informed by the uncoerced reflections of those most vitally concerned and most directly involved in the question—the married. Therefore anything a priest says must represent an aid to the faithful in forming their consciences. He should not attempt to form their conscience for them. This would represent a form of paternalism detrimental to personal and corporate growth.

Third, we come inevitably to what in the past we have referred to as "confessional practice" or its equivalent. Perhaps the matter could be approached in the following way, pending further developments.

1. When asked, we must unambiguously state that the present but noninfallible teaching of the papal magisterium is that every contraceptive act is immoral. This conclusion should, of course, be stated within the context of a rounded assertion of the positive values contained in *Humanae vitae*.

2. The dissent of reflective and competent married people should be respected and the teaching on contraception should not be made a matter of denial of absolution.

3. The truly anguishing aspect of the problem has been put well by the National Association of Laymen Executive Board. They state: "We are, therefore, not concerned for ourselves but for the millions of silent Catholics on whom this decision will fall as an unnecessary and harsh burden. They will obey because this is the main thrust of their religious training—to obey. They have not been allowed to reach spiritual adulthood, so they have no way to make independent judgment. For them to disobey or ignore this edict would destroy the very root of their religious belief."[44] There is no genuinely satisfactory solution for these people in terms of a practical conclusion. Indeed, if there were such a solution, the problem would not exist in its present poignancy. But here we may propose two suggestions that may help priests structure their pastoral practice.

First, in the present circumstances (widespread public confusion, episcopal and theological dissent, difficulty of the doctrine, frequent good faith, unclarity of related theological questions, etc.) this teaching should not be allowed to become an issue of refusal of absolution. When the problem arises in the confessional situation, the faithful should be encouraged, and they should be urged to exercise Christian patience and confidence as the unanswered questions and difficulties connected with this problem work themselves out.

Second, if a couple are trying to live responsibly their married life as defined by the values stated in *Humanae vitae*, a strong case can be made for saying that their individual acts of contraception should not be viewed by them or judged by the confessor to be subjectively serious sin.[45] Furthermore, the statement just

---

[44] *National Catholic Reporter* (Sept. 14, 1968), p. 2.

[45] Three considerations suggest this conclusion. (1) *The difficulty of the faithful in understanding the doctrine.* Consider the following factors: confusion from priestly and theological discussions; a sensate, pansexualized culture; hardness of the doctrine; discussion before *Humanae vitae* and the expectations associated with it; subtlety of the argument; *"asperas vitae conditiones"* of families and nations (No. 19); *"sine dubio multis talis videbitur, ut nonnisi difficulter, immo etiam nullo modo servari possit"* (No. 20). (2) *The difficulty in practicing the doctrine.* Note: *"multosque labores postulat"* (No. 20);

made suggests to theologians the need to determine more precisely and satisfactorily what constitutes serious matter where the practice of contraception is concerned. I realize that these pastoral notes do not solve the basic underlying problems of the encyclical and its application to daily Catholic practice. But they do not intend to do this. They intend only to formulate possible approaches—tentative and imperfect—during difficult, transitional, and therefore challenging times.

"asceseos sit opus" (No. 21); the grave difficulties of married life (No. 25); the fact that married people tend to judge the importance of an act by its relation to the goals and values of married life, not by a physiological openness, etc. (3) *The compassion and understanding urged by the encyclical.* "In their difficulties may married couples always find in the words and the heart of a priest the echo of the voice and the love of the Redeemer" (No. 29). Similarly, "if sin should still keep its hold over them, let them not be discouraged, but rather have recourse with humble perseverance to the mercy of God" (No. 25). The Belgian hierarchy, after referring to attempts of Catholics in difficult circumstances to adapt their behavior to the norms of *Humanae vitae,* stated that "if they do not succeed immediately, they should not, however, believe they are separated from God's love" (*Catholic Chronicle* [Sept. 6, 1968]). In this connection see the interesting remarks of John Dedek, *"Humanae vitae* and the Confessor," *Chicago Studies,* 7 (1968), 221–24. Dedek believes that true evaluative cognition would be lacking in very many instances in the present circumstances.

12. On the Tenth Anniversary of *Humanae Vitae*

In the tenth-anniversary year of the issuance of *Humanae vitae* it was to be expected that we would see a good number of statements and studies on that controversial document. That expectation has not been disappointed. Public reactions differ from Andrew Greeley's ("a dead letter")[1] to John Cardinal Carberry's statement of gratitude to the Holy Father for these "courageous conclusions."[2] The late Pope Paul VI touched briefly on the matter in his address to the College of Cardinals (June 23, 1978). He said that this document "caused us anguish, not only because the issue treated was serious and delicate but also—and perhaps especially—because among Catholics and public opinion in general there was a certain climate of expectancy that concessions, relaxations, or liberalization of the Church's moral doctrine and teaching on marriage would be made."[3] He referred somewhat puzzlingly to "confirmations which have come from the more scientific studies."[4] He concluded his reference to the encyclical by repeating "the principle of respect for the natural laws, which—as Dante said—'takes its course from divine intelligence and from its art,' the principle of aware and ethically responsible parenthood."

One might ask whether the late Pontiff thought he was referring to one principle or to two principles here. In other words, did he mean to identify "respect for the natural laws" with "the principle of . . . ethically responsible parenthood"? Or are they dis-

[1] *Catholic Chronicle* (Oct. 20, 1978).
[2] "U.S. Bishops at the Vatican," *Origins*, 8 (1978), 91 (text of an address by John Cardinal Carberry to Pope Paul VI [June 15, 1978]).
[3] "Paul VI Comments on Today's Church," *Origins*, 8 (1978), 108–10.
[4] "Puzzlingly" because it is not clear what he means. Does he refer to the medical dangers associated with the pill? Or that there is now a better scientific foundation for periodic continence?

tinct principles, one (respect) in service of the other (responsible parenthood)? Whatever the case, it is clear that Paul VI provided no reasons to think he had changed his mind on the question. And it is clear that the association of "natural laws" with "divine intelligence" tends to yield intangibility.[5]

In his address at the opening of the spring meeting of the National Conference of Catholic Bishops (May 2, 1978), Archbishop John R. Quinn sensibly urged that the encyclical be read in a broader context—the integration of sexuality with the sacrificially selfless love that is the soul of the Christian life.[6] Quinn suggests that the tensions of "discussion, and sometimes painful and strident controversy" would be reduced in this way. I agree with Archbishop Quinn's concern to provide a broader context for any ethic of sexuality. But at some point, the question returns: Can *Humanae vitae* be read as saying *only* this?

Cardinal Jean Villot wrote a letter in the name of Paul VI to participants in a natural family planning symposium (New York, May 23–24, 1978).[7] The letter emphasizes areas of papal concern: continued research; promotion of natural family planning ("in which the dignity of the human person is fostered"); personal commitment of husband and wife and pastoral support for their efforts to lead a holy, conjugal life.

The bishops of India issued a declaration (January 17, 1978) commemorating the tenth anniversary of *Humanae vitae*. They note that the specific doctrines of the encyclical (on contraception, sterilization, and abortion) are "integrated into a comprehensive vision of man, evangelical love, and responsible parenthood." After affirming their unqualified acceptance of *Humanae vitae*, they state that they have seen the fears of the Holy Father (about the powers that governments would have if contraception were approved) realized and his views vindicated "at least in some

[5] In his homily of June 29, 1978, Pope Paul VI singled out *Humanae vitae* as a document that defends life, especially against the twin evils of divorce and abortion. "This document," he said, "has become of new and more urgent actuality. . . ." (*Civiltà cattolica*, 129 [1978], 181).

[6] "A Broader Perspective on '*Humanae vitae*,' " *Origins*, 8 (1978), 10–12.

[7] Jean Cardinal Villot, "La planification naturelle de la famille," *Documentation catholique*, 75 (1978), 555–56. A similar letter was sent by Cardinal Villot to a conference in Melbourne on family planning (*Documentation catholique*, 75 [1978], 257–58) and to the University of San Francisco (*L'Osservatore romano* [Aug. 3, 1977]).

degree." They urge their priests to show great compassion but "from now on, they must avoid spreading any personal views which may be opposed to the teaching of the Church. This teaching is clear and admits of no ambiguity."[8]

Archbishop Matagrin, the archbishop of Grenoble and vice president of the French Episcopal Conference, wrote in an article in *Le Progrès* that *Humanae vitae* had stirred up controversy. Matagrin admits that the language used was, in the eyes of many, obsolete, but he underlines the validity of the profound intuition. Just as populations ought not to be manipulated, so procreation itself ought not to be ruled by physical and chemical means. In a time of ecological awareness we ought to be sensitive to the concerns of Paul VI for "the quality of life, the biological rhythms not simply of the universe but of man himself."[9]

An anonymous moral theologian ("he will be risking his chair if his name is published, so it is withheld at his request and the shame of all of us")[10] from a "prestigious ecclesiastical establishment" summarizes the situation for the *Tablet*. One of the results to settle in over the past ten years is the loss of confidence in Roman pronouncements on moral questions. This "special correspondent" believes that the *sensus fidelium* must be taken more into account in the formulation of doctrinal and moral teaching. He regards the early liberal dissent as counterproductive because it hardened the traditionalism of some theologians and bishops.[11] It would have been better to interpret *Humanae vitae* very flexibly—a thing that the Vatican would live with provided the document is accepted in principle. As for the future: "The time is not yet ripe for the theoretic formulation of an ecclesial consensus on all the complex moral aspects of human procreativity in the present-day world, simply because as yet there is no ecclesial consensus about them."

Dr. Denis Cashman, an English physician and former medical adviser to the Catholic Marriage Advisory Council, takes issue

---

[8] *"Humanae vitae* Ten Years Later," *The Pope Speaks,* 23 (1978), 183–87.

[9] Monsignor Matagrin, "Le pape d'*Humanae vitae,*" *Documentation catholique,* 75 (1978), 752.

[10] "After *Humanae vitae,*" *Tablet,* 232 (1978), 852.

[11] On this see Brigitte Andre, "*Humanae vitae:* rigeur et compassion," *Informations catholique internationales,* 530 (Sept. 1978), 28–29. Andre mistakenly refers to "l'Université pontificale de Georgetown."

with *Humanae vitae* on some very practical issues.[12] Contraception, he believes, does not lead to loss of respect for women. The discipline involved in periodic abstinence is often a source of harm to marriages. He argues that the "observance of natural rhythms" will never be more than "marginally satisfactory."

This is certainly not the prevailing view. Arthur McCormack reports on a tenth-anniversary congress (its theme: "Love, Fruitful and Responsible") held in Milan, June 21–25, 1978.[13] It is of particular interest because two of its major presenters were Gustave Martelet, S.J. (widely considered one of the major influences on *Humanae vitae*), and Cardinal Karol Wojtyla.[14] Two points became clear in the discussions about natural family planning: (1) Natural methods have been very much improved. (2) Many more Catholic doctors and counselors are involved in teaching such methods.[15]

One of the more interesting points is McCormack's report of Martelet. It reads:

> He said that paragraph 14 of the encyclical (which includes the ban on contraception) was only meant to clarify the position of the Church because of the "redoubtable volume of opinion in favor of contraception" which had developed in the sixties: It was not meant to harass individual Catholics who found themselves in the dilemma of having to limit their families but were unable

[12] Denis Cashman, "Letter to Editor," *Tablet*, 232 (1978), 852.

[13] Arthur McCormack, "*Humanae vitae* Today," *Tablet*, 232 (1978), 674–76.

[14] One of Italy's most respected newspapers, Milan's *Corriere della sera*, carried an article (Oct. 18, 1978) entitled "The Thought of the Pope on Love and the Pill." According to many interpreters of John Paul II (as reported in *Corriere*), in the Pope's thought "a natural law that imposes itself as an absolute is unacceptable." Furthermore, it continues: "It is the phenomenological philosophical formation of Wojtyla that led him to this conclusion: That which counts most is the intention inspiring the acts of husband and wife. Simply put: The differences between the use of the pill and other contraceptive methods is secondary if, beneath all, there is always a loving act." Finally, the author, Dario Fertilio, states that many believe it to be the papal view that contraception is "*sempre un 'male,' ma un male a volte comprensibile*" (always an evil but at times an understandable one). I tend to think this is idle speculation.

[15] See Rhaban Haacke, "Zur Frage der Zeitwahlmethode," *Münchner theologische Zeitschrift*, 29 (1978), 64–70.

to use methods allowed by the Church. He called their use of contraceptives a "disorder" which was not sinful if they acted in good conscience and had tried their best to obey the encyclical in the circumstances of their life.[16]

Similarly Diogini Tettamanzi, professor of moral theology at the Seminary of Milan, is reported to have "confirmed the possibility of the use of methods other than natural ones on the service of this love when a couple decided in sincere conscience that this was necessary in their concrete circumstances." Moreover, three or four Italian moralists argued that the use of contraceptives by couples who felt that they must was not a question of choosing the lesser evil, but rather "of making a choice within a hierarchy of values: the preservation of married love, of life together, of the welfare of the family being a greater good than the methods used to achieve it."

This is all quite puzzling, for of this conference McCormack notes that "no dissenters were invited." As I read this report, the conference was fairly crawling with dissenters,[17] for *Humanae vitae* presented the contraceptive act as a *moral* evil, not just a "disorder."[18] If it can be read to have said that it was a disorder (disvalue, nonmoral evil, ontic evil, etc.), many problems would vanish. Indeed, this is precisely the analysis that some prominent dissenters (Janssens, Fuchs, Schüller) have made. Furthermore, I

[16] McCormack, "Humanae vitae Today," 676.

[17] This conference is also reported by Lino Ciccone, "Congresso internazionale sul tema 'amore fecondo responsabile a dieci anni dall' *Humanae vitae*,'" *Divus Thomas*, 81 (1978), 177–87. He is very critical of McCormack.

[18] This point is clear from many sources, most recently the Irish bishops. Of contraception they say: "*L'enseignement de l'église est clair: Elle est moralement mauvaise*" (*Documentation catholique*, 75 [1978], 424–25). Furthermore, reporting favorably on a new moral textbook by Dom Anselm Günthör, Luigi Ciappi, O.P., states: "He accepts the pastoral provisions of the encyclical, without mentioning 'conflict of duties' or 'hierarchy of values' in married life. He shows in this way that he does not consider worthy of acceptance those interpretations given by some pastoral conferences, which had not offered a correct and acceptable interpretation of the document of the Sovereign Pontiff" (*L'Osservatore romano* [English edition], No. 43 [Oct. 26, 1978], 11). One could, of course, draw a different conclusion from that of Cardinal Ciappi. For instance: "Günthör shows that he does not even consider the conflict character of reality" or "that he has absolutized the physical integrity of sexual intercourse."

am puzzled by the contrast stated between "making a choice within a hierarchy" and "choosing the lesser of two evils." These are simply various ways of wording the same thing, although one *sounds* better (to wit, more positive).

Charles Curran rejects this approach. He does not think that contraception violates an ideal or involves premoral or ontic evil. "In my judgment both of these approaches still give too much importance to the physical aspect of the act and see the physical as normative."[19] He sees these approaches as attempts to preserve greater unity in the Church. By contrast, Curran argues that the matter must be faced from the more radical perspective of papal error. "The condemnation of artificial contraception found in *Humanae vitae* is wrong." The remainder of Curran's study takes up the possibility and implications of dissent in the Church, and on a wide variety of topics. Curran grants that this means greater pluralism and that his model will somewhat reduce the prophetic role of the Church. He thinks the present situation where official teaching is one thing and accepted practice another is intolerable. It is clear where Curran thinks change is indicated. "If the hierarchical Church refuses to change here, there will probably be no change on other issues."

A different point of view is taken by Lawrence B. Porter, O.P. He has written a perceptive study comparing Martelet's work with *Humanae vitae*, particularly with regard to the underlying anthropology.[20] The study produces good internal evidence for saying that the "Pope's response to the birth-control controversy is indeed conceived in terms of Martelet's own thought." Rather than Curran's "physicalism," Martelet asserts in his study *Amour conjugal et renouveau conciliare* (1967) that the "Church has never seen in nature, or its functions a purely biological reality, but a living index of the demands of God and the spiritual being of man."[21] Martelet conceives the birth-control issue as a confrontation between technological domination on the one hand and human dominion on the other.

[19] Charles E. Curran, "Ten Years Later: Reflections on 'Humanae vitae,'" *Commonweal*, 105 (1978), 425–30; and "After *Humanae vitae*: A Decade of Lively Debate," *Hospital Progress*, 59 (July 1978), 84–89.

[20] Lawrence B. Porter, O.P., "'Humanae vitae' a Decade Later: The Theologian behind the Encyclical," *Thomist*, 42 (1978), 464–509.

[21] See Martelet 43, as cited by Porter.

This is a careful study,[22] and I have a great deal of sympathy for the broad anthropological perspectives Porter lifts out of Martelet. Technology *can* be inhumane and manipulative. The body does condition human love, and to avoid this does carry certain risks. But what that leads to is not clear. Martelet himself seems to have been aware of this, for he stated in *L'existence humaine et l'amour* that "an encyclical is nothing other than a means by which the Pope makes everyone and primarily Christians stop and think about something important. . . ."[23] Furthermore, Martelet concedes the inadequacy of expression in *Humanae vitae*:

> It is a fact, however, that this vocabulary of "intrinsically evil" used by both encyclicals to denounce in contraception something truly wrong, sadly allows one to believe that this always represents in itself the most grave failure of love. This is one of the *lacunae* of both *Casti connubii* and *Humanae vitae*, that neither one nor the other sufficiently protects its readers from the awful errors of such a misunderstanding.[24]

A word here about Curran's rejection of the notion of contraception as a nonmoral evil. This is technical terminology and it can strike people as "too strong," "misleading." What some contemporary authors are trying to do is discover a language that will recognize certain effects as deprivations or disvalues without calling them *moral* evils. For instance, when in the course of a just national self-defense certain enemy soldiers are wounded or killed, what are we to call those killings? They are certainly not the results of *morally* wrongful acts, for the defense is *ex hypothesi* just. Nor are they neutral happenings.

In this light we once again encounter the assertion that the basic message of *Humanae vitae* is (= ought to be) to caution couples who use contraception because they feel they must, against the danger of confusing responsible parenthood with an

[22] At one point Porter is less than cautious. He writes: "As a dogmatist, and more than any moral theologian, Martelet was aware of the importance of . . . the comprehensive Christian anthropology that underlies *Gaudium et spes'* teaching" (483). That sweeping statement would be difficult to establish.

[23] Porter, " '*Humanae vitae*' a Decade Later," 508.

[24] Ibid.

un-Christian hedonism or selfishness. In other words, it is a reminder that we are dealing with a disvalue—though not necessarily a terribly great one.

In light of this, I have recently worded the matter as follows:

> This, I believe, is very important. Some reactions to *Humanae vitae* framed the matter as follows: "Contraception is wrong vs. contraception is right," this latter being the case since the argument for the former was seen as illegitimate. This is terribly misleading and, in my judgment, erroneous. It leaves the impression that contraception and sterilization are right, that nothing is wrong with them, and eventually, that they are values in themselves. When compared abstractly to their alternatives, contraception and sterilization are nonmoral evils, what I call disvalues. To forget this is to lose the thrust away from their necessity. To say that something is a disvalue or nonmoral evil is to imply thereby the need to be moving constantly and steadily to the point where the causing of such disvalues is no longer required. To forget that something is a nonmoral evil is to settle for it, to embrace it into one's world.[25]

An analogy may help here. While speaking before the United Nations, Pope Paul VI prophetically and powerfully urged "no more war, never." This plea, however, would be misread if it were taken as an invalidation of the just-war theory, as a condemnation of a forceful national self-defense as intrinsically evil. It was rather a very useful cry by a highly respected spiritual leader about the disvalue (nonmoral evil) that is war.[26] Something similar is in place where contraception and sterilization are concerned —to wit, constant reminders that they are disvalues, yet allowance

[25] Richard A. McCormick, S.J., "Moral Norms and Their Meaning," *Lectureship* (St. Benedict, Ore.: Mount Angel Seminary, 1978), 45.

[26] James F. Childress has written a fine essay on just war, using the categories "*prima facie* wrongfulness" and "actual wrongfulness." He notes that this language is similar to the language of proportionate cause. See James F. Childress, "Just War Theories: The Bases, Interrelations, Priorities, and Functions of Their Criteria," *Theological Studies*, 39 (1978), 427–45.

for the fact that there is, in a world of conflict, still place for a "theory of just sterilization."

In other and technical language, the issue is not "contraception is wrong vs. contraception is right"; it is rather "contraception is intrinsically evil vs. contraception is not intrinsically evil." This point is clear in the writings of Schüller, Janssens, Fuchs, and others.

I suspect that Curran still will want to reject this analysis. But that only raises this question: Has his language of "physicalism" not possibly carried him too far? Has it possibly led him to deny *any* significance to the bodily involvement of our beings in these instances? After all, no one gets sterilized for the fun of it, but only for the purpose of it. Sterilization and (to a lesser degree) contraception remain nondesirable interferences. People would welcome the chance to limit their families without them.[27] This suggests that sterilization is not merely a neutral technique. It is something people want to avoid if possible. Curran's admirable resistance to the idea of describing certain physical actions as morally evil prior to their contextualization and his term "physicalism" to convey this may have led him to deny any meaning to such interventions.[28] At least the question deserves continued discussion.

One of the more interesting recent studies is that of Joseph A. Selling.[29] Of the phrase *"intrinsece inhonestum"* (*Hv*, n. 14), Selling correctly remarks that "the text clearly shows that what the encyclical was speaking of was moral evil and not, as some commentators would have it, some category which would allow

[27] This is increasingly clear in the medical literature in its description of the ideal contraceptive. It must be simple, easily reversible, cheap, medically safe, etc., all of which point to the disvalues involved when such qualities are absent.

[28] There is some indication of an overreaction in Curran's statement (footnote 19, "After *Humanae vitae*") that he holds "artificial insemination with donor semen (AID) is not always wrong." Furthermore, in holding that contraception and sterilization are not disvalues, he reveals an inconsistency, for he says: "If contraception is morally acceptable, so is sterilization, although a *more* serious reason is required if the sterilization is permanent." If a "more" serious reason is required where permanent sterilization is involved, then clearly some reason is required even when it is not permanent—that is, it is not simply a neutral thing but also has the elements of a disvalue.

[29] Joseph A. Selling, "Moral Teaching, Traditional Teaching and 'Humanae vitae,'" *Louvain Studies*, 7 (1978), 24–44.

for choosing the lesser of two evils. The introduction of this reasoning runs directly counter to what *Humanae vitae* was saying. . . ." Thus some of the following categories used to mitigate
its conclusions are at variance with the language of the encyclical:
conflict of duties, lesser of two evils, *Humanae vitae* as an ideal,
redefinition of totality, and "probably most important, the distinction between moral and premoral evil." I agree with Selling
here.

Selling then provides a brief but accurate history of moral tradition in this area. It is summarized in three expressions: *actus naturae, natura actus,* and *actus personae*—that is, the earlier tradition involving Augustine and Aquinas viewed sexual intercourse as
an *actus naturae* (with procreation as its biological finality). Over
a period of time nonprocreative purposes were introduced and tolerated as long as the nature of the act was respected (*natura
actus*). Finally, in *Gaudium et spes,* the analysis became that of
actus personae. This brief outline cannot do justice to the persuasiveness of Selling's account.

It is his contention that while the basic values of marriage
remain constant, the way in which they are protected and explained has gone through a real evolution. In essence "the realization of the procreative end had become totally detached from the
individual act of intercourse. Sexual relations were licit on the
basis of their connection with expressing conjugal love alone.
Consequently, a new set of norms was necessary to evaluate those
relations." Yet *Humanae vitae* represents a continuation of the
notion of *actus naturae* and "represents a regression in the evolution of concrete norms which had been elaborated in Vatican II."
Selling, therefore, feels that the document was dated at the time
it was promulgated because it repeated a "physicalistic interpretation of natural law."

He concludes by asking why Paul VI did this. It is Selling's
opinion that he did so because he feared that any sanctioning of
contraception would be interpreted as license for any form of sexual behavior. To change norms in one area inevitably would have
repercussions in all other areas. Thus Selling believes that Pope
Paul never "intended to condemn every form of artificial birth

control for the mature, responsible, loving married couple."
Rather he feared the floodgates and took a "safe" position.
The broad lines of Selling's analysis have been drawn by
others.[30] Hence no comment is called for except to say that his
study will probably be greeted with hails or harpoons. Neither is
appropriate; just calm study.

Two of the most serious studies on contraception appeared in
Theological Studies. John C. Ford, S.J., and Germain Grisez, in a
long and careful study, argue that the Church's condemnation of
contraception (what they call the "received Catholic teaching")
has been infallibly proposed by the ordinary magisterium.[31] "We
think that the facts show as clearly as anyone could reasonably
demand that the conditions articulated by Vatican II for infallibility in the exercise of the ordinary magisterium of the bishops
dispersed throughout the world have been met in the case of the
Catholic Church's teaching on contraception." The long Ford-
Grisez study explains that conclusion by examining the conditions
articulated in Vatican II for infallible teaching, the statements of
the papal and episcopal magisterium, and objections against this
position.

In the same issue of *Theological Studies* Joseph Komonchak
reached a different conclusion.[32] He argues that three conditions
must be fulfilled before a teaching is infallibly taught by the ordinary universal magisterium: (1) It must be divinely revealed or be
necessary to defend or explain what is revealed. (2) It must be
proposed by a moral unanimity of the body of bishops in com-
munion with one another and the Pope. (3) It must be proposed
by them as having to be held definitively. Komonchak discusses
these conditions at length and concludes: "I do not see, then,
how one can reply to the question of the infallibility of the magisterial condemnation of artificial contraception with anything but
a *non constat.*"

It is noteworthy that these two studies are basically essays in

30 Louis Janssens, *Mariage et fécondité* (Paris: Duculot, 1967).

31 John Ford, S.J., and Germain Grisez, "Contraception and Infallibility,"
Theological Studies, 39 (1978), 258–312. A popular summary of this is found
in Russell Shaw, "Contraception, Infallibility and the Ordinary Magisterium,"
Homiletic and Pastoral Review, 78 (July 1978), 9–19.

32 Joseph A. Komonchak, "*Humanae vitae* and Its Reception: Ecclesiological
Reflections," *Theological Studies,* 39 (1978), 221–57.

ecclesiology.[33] It would be immodest for a moral theologian to attempt to referee such a dispute, though it is clear that many theologians (what Komonchak calls "something like a *consensus theologorum*") would favor the Komonchak thesis. There is one point I would like to raise here for reflection. In an essay on the changeable and unchangeable in the Church, Karl Rahner highlights the distinction between a "truth in itself and in its abiding validity" and its "particular historical formulation."[34] By this he means that dogmas are always presented in context and by means of conceptual models that are subject to change. He uses transubstantiation and original sin as examples. For this latter, for example, those who accept polygenism must rethink what is meant by saying that Adam is the originator and cause of original sin.

Rahner then applies this to ethics. He states:

> Apart from wholly universal moral norms of an abstract kind, and apart from a radical orientation of human life toward God as the outcome of a supernatural and grace-given self-commitment, there are hardly any particular or individual norms of Christian morality which could be proclaimed by the ordinary or extraordinary teaching authorities of the Church in such a way that they could be unequivocally and certainly declared to have the force of dogmas.[35]

This does not mean, Rahner states, that certain concrete actions cannot be prescribed or proscribed authoritatively. They can, as demanded by the times. But they pertain to man's *concrete nature* at a given point in history. And this concrete nature is subject to change. Rahner's analysis would deny the very possibility of infallible teaching where contraceptive acts are concerned. It would further invite us to discover—not a simple task—the abiding and

[33] Komonchak does, however, address the argument of *Humanae vitae*. Particularly enlightening are his reflections on pp. 253–56, where the *ordo generationis* is explained as a "total complex," not simply as individual acts.

[34] Karl Rahner, "Basic Observations on the Subject of Changeable and Unchangeable Factors in the Church," *Theological Investigations*, 14 (1976), 3–23.

[35] Ibid., 14.

unchangeable concern of the Church encapsulated in this vehicle (condemnation of contraception).

Several impressions are generated by this literature. First, there is praise for the "over-all vision" of Paul VI, though that phrase is often left very general and unspecified. And there are invitations to read *Humanae vitae* within a broader context. Second, there is criticism of the language of the encyclical (*intrinsece inhonestum* —intrinsically evil) as if the Pope did not find the proper vehicle for his message. Third, there is increasingly the suggestion that there is a middle position between *Humanae vitae* and some of its critics, one that would see a value in naturalness without canonizing it, that would see a relative disvalue in artificial interventions without condemning them as intrinsically evil. Equivalently, this view agrees that technology can be of great assistance to us, but should not be allowed to dominate us. Finally—and this is but a personal reflection—there is need for a profounder analysis of sexuality in our time, a broad and deep systematic synthesis that can control and direct our reflections on family planning. When that is present we may be able with greater assurance and fairness to retain what is of abiding importance in *Humanae vitae*, and reformulate what is defective.

Nearly everyone who comments on the tenth anniversary of the 1968 encyclical calls attention to the fact that the past ten years have led to a reconsideration of authority in the Church, and particularly the nature of the magisterium. This traces, of course, to the fact that there was so much dissent associated with *Humanae vitae*. A few entries here will have to suffice.

Richard M. Gula, S.S., reviews the teaching of the manualists on dissent.[36] They do not see dissent as undermining the teaching of the ordinary magisterium, and at least one (Lercher) recognizes that suspending assent may be one way of protecting the Church from error.[37] Furthermore, Gula correctly notes that the responses to the *modi* on *Lumen gentium* (n. 25) state the very same thing.

[36] Richard M. Gula, S.S., "The Right to Private and Public Dissent from Specific Pronouncements of the Ordinary Magisterium," *Église et théologie*, 9 (1978), 319–43.

[37] "It is not absolutely out of the question that error might be excluded by the Holy Spirit in this way, namely, by the subjects of the decree detecting its error and ceasing to give it their internal assent" (L. Lercher, *Institutiones theologiae dogmaticae*, 4 [Barcelona: Herder, 1945], I, 297).

The charismatic structure of the Church further supports this notion. Gula argues that we must develop an approach to public dissent that is more realistic and adequate to our time.

One of the more interesting statements on the meaning of dissent from authentic teaching of the magisterium was made by Bishop Juan Arzube at the Catholic Press Association convention Mass.[38] He notes that, in contrast to infallible teaching, ordinary teaching has sometimes to "undergo correction and change." As example Arzube offers *Dignitatis humanae* and the teaching of previous popes on religious liberty. Such development could not have occurred "unless theologians and bishops had been free to be critical of papal teaching, to express views at variance with it. . . ." Our faculty of judgment cannot give assent to a proposition that it judges to be inaccurate or untrue. After detailing the conditions for legitimate dissent (competence, sincere effort to assent, convincing contrary reasons), Arzube argues that dissent must be viewed "as something positive and constructive" in the life of the Church.

Arzube's statement strikes this reviewer as being realistic, calm, and theologically correct. It is particularly encouraging because it comes from a bishop. Theologians also received very warmly the remarks of Archbishop John Roach at the opening of the Catholic Theological Society of America meeting. Roach touched enlighteningly on the publics he felt obliged as bishop to listen to carefully, even if at times critically.[39]

An entire issue of *Chicago Studies* is devoted to the theme "The Magisterium, the Theologian, and the Educator."[40] It is one of the finest issues of that seventeen-year-old journal that we have had. Here only a few highlights can be reported.

After Archbishop Joseph Bernardin's introductory essay, there follow useful "setting the stage" articles by Carl Peter and John F. Meyers. Eugene A. LaVerdiere, S.S.S., has a fine treatment of

[38] Juan Arzube, "When Is Dissent Legitimate?" *Catholic Journalist* (June 1978), 5.

[39] John Roach, "On Hearing the Voices That Echo God," *Origins*, 8 (1978), 81–86.

[40] *Chicago Studies*, 17 (1978), 149–307. The issue includes articles by Joseph L. Bernardin, Carl J. Peter, John F. Meyers, Eugene LaVerdiere, S.S.S., John E. Lynch, C.S.P., Yves Congar, O.P., Michael D. Place, T. Howland Sanks, S.J., Avery Dulles, S.J., Timothy O'Connell, and Raymond E. Brown, S.S.

teaching authority in the New Testament period. This is followed by John Lynch's detailed study of the magisterium and theologians from the Apostolic Fathers to the Gregorian Reform. During this period it was the councils that promulgated creeds and dogmatic definitions but "it was the theological teachers who carried on the vital interpretative task." Indeed, with the exception of Tertullian, Origen, and Jerome, one cannot speak of a differentiation of the magisterial and theological functions. That came with the rise of the universities.

Yves Congar covers the following period up to Trent. It was in this period that a new form of teaching developed, "the 'magisterium' of the theologians, the schools, and the universities." This reflects what Congar calls "two different modes of teaching." Thus the University of Paris considered itself and was generally thought of as exercising an authentic theological authority in Christianity. As a result properly theological terms were employed by the councils to express the data of the faith (*transubstantiatio* [transubstantiation], *anima forma corporis* [soul as the form of body]). Trent achieved a balance between *inquisitio* (inquiry) and *auctoritas* (authority), but a balance conditioned by four centuries of scholastic theology. The result: "The teaching of the magisterium has been woven with 'theology' which has gone far beyond the pure witness of the Word of God and apostolic tradition." Congar concludes that the distinction of charisms must be preserved but within a necessary and felicitous collaboration.

Michael Place traces developments in the relationship between scholars and what he calls "the authoritative hierarchical solicitude" (for the faith) from Trent to Vatican I. The upshot of these developments was a growing isolation of the papal and episcopal competency from the rest of the Church. Place outlines the political and theological threads that led to an increasingly powerful papacy. For instance, in the late eighteenth century the key category by which papal action in matters of faith was understood was that of jurisdiction—the concern of one who was not first a teacher but was to provide for unity. As Place puts it: "The theologian is the teacher. The papacy is the ruler that provides for the right ordering necessary to preserve ecclesial unity." However, early in the nineteenth century, categories from Germany (teach, rule, sanctify) were introduced rather than the powers of orders and jurisdiction. With this came also the usage "magisterium" around 1830 and it was "situated in a cultural milieu where the papacy is understood as having absolute spiritual sovereignty. . . ." In this new context the function of theologians is differently understood. He is now related not to the "governor of ecclesial unity" but to a supreme teacher. In such a context his role changes. It is Place's thesis that the relationship of magisterium to theologians is determined by the manner in which the Church perceives herself at a given time in history.

T. Howland Sanks, S.J., treats the relationship of theologians and the magisterium from Vatican I to 1978. He argues (rightly, I think) that the conflicts that existed—and still exist—are between various forms of theology, various theological paradigms, not precisely or first of all between theologians and the magisterium. During this period (up to Vatican II) the ahistorical, neoscholastic theology of the Roman school achieved an ascendancy. It got enshrined in official statements. It is present in Vatican I (*Dei filius, Pastor aeternus*) and continued to be the official theology used by the magisterium in its dealings with the historically conscious leanings of Loisy, Tyrell, and Pierre Rousselot. Furthermore, it was responsible for the suppression of Teilhard and John Courtney Murray (as well as de Lubac, Bouillard, and their colleagues at Fourvière). In *Humani generis* (August 12, 1950) this ahistorical approach peaked. Vatican II constituted a definitive break with such an approach but Sanks believes the problem is far from gone because this theology has "formed the thinking and attitudes of many of the hierarchy."

Avery Dulles provides a theological reflection on the magisterium in history. His over-all conclusion is that "the structures commonly regarded as Catholic today are relatively new and thus do not reflect God's unalterable design for his Church." Dulles passes in review the salient features of the models of the Church in various periods and uses these features to raise questions for our time. For instance, in the patristic period, what Dulles calls a "representational model" prevailed. The Catholic faith is identified with the unanimous belief of all the churches—and the bishops were the responsible heads of such local churches. The bishops were seen as teaching with full authority when they gather in councils representing the churches of the entire Christian world. On the basis of this model (not without imperfections) Dulles asks: Can we reactivate the idea of a unity achieved "from below" through consensus? Furthermore, instead of thinking of the bishop as the representative of the Holy See, should we not see him more as the local community's representative? Or again, Dulles wonders whether we can credibly view the bishop as the "chief teacher" in our time. This notion fits more easily the fourth and fifth centuries, when prominent theologians were bishops.

When he discusses the medieval model characterized by the rise of the universities, Dulles asks: "Could theologians, individually or at least corporately, be acknowledged as possessing true doctrinal or magisterial authority?" The notion is well founded in tradition, he insists. Dulles criticizes the excessive privatizing of theology as if theologians "indulge in nothing other than airy speculations." He suggests that statements would occasionally be issued jointly by bishops and nonbishops, by the Pope with the International Theological Commission. This would reduce the cleavage between the pastoral magisterium and theology.

The neoscholastic period (nineteenth and twentieth centuries) saw the magisterium as a power distinct from orders and government. Thus this period regarded the hierarchy not simply as judges, but also as true teachers, whereas in the eighteenth century teaching was viewed as a command or along more disciplinary lines. Under this neoscholastic model the Holy See exercised a vigorous doctrinal leadership. But because papal teaching was drawn up by theologians of the Roman school, they "gave official status to their own opinions." Vatican II changed many of the perspectives associated with the neoscholastic approach, especially the identification between magisterium and jurisdiction. It neither affirmed nor denied a complementary magisterium of theologians. However, it is clear that Dulles (along with Congar) believes such a notion is valid. "The concept of a distinct magisterium of theologians, as we have seen, is not simply a medieval theory; it is accepted in neoscholastic manuals of the twentieth century."

These papers were discussed at a seminar of the Catholic Theological Society of America (June 1978) in Milwaukee. Timothy O'Connell reports the results of those discussions in this issue of *Chicago Studies*. The key issue in relating theology to the magisterium was seen to be doctrinal development. Specifically, the seminarists asked: How do we account for the various changes in teaching that have occurred in the past? Can we develop a theology of Church teaching that accommodates without embarrassment the twin phenomena of divided opinion and ignorance?

The issue concludes with the address of Raymond Brown, S.S., to the National Catholic Education Association (March 29, 1978).[41] The prestigious exegete argues that the dispute among theologians and bishops has been "greatly exaggerated." He identifies four fictions that surround the dispute: belief that the main opponents in matters of doctrine are the magisterium and theologians; that their prevailing relationship is one of disagreement; that theologians and magisterium can be spoken of as if they were monolithic groups; and that they conflict because even centrist Catholic theologians deny many matters of Church doctrine. Brown argues, persuasively in my judgment, that third parties such as the secular media and the ultraconservative Catholic press are more damaging than any polarization of bishops and theologians. Furthermore, though there has been dissent (especially in matters of sexual morality), Brown asserts that this has been seriously exaggerated. With regard to centrist theologians denying many matters of Church doctrine, Brown insists that we must not inflate (as many do) what constitutes Catholic doctrine and we must realize that doctrines change. In his words, "Seeking a new formulation to meet a new problem" is hardly a denial of a teaching.

Though his paper was delivered to religious educators, both theologians and bishops could read it with profit. Brown approaches delicate problems with a combination of precision, wisdom, and pastoral sensitivity that is admirable. Neither those on the extreme right or the extreme left will be happy with his reflections. But that suggests more about the geography of their position than about the accuracy of Brown's analysis. One point that might deserve more emphasis than Brown's irenic analysis suggests: The differences on a single issue such as *Humanae vitae* have enormous implications with regard to moral theological method, no-

---

[41] See also Raymond E. Brown, S.S., "Bishops and Theologians: 'Dispute' Surrounded by Fiction," *Origins*, 7 (1968), 673–82.

tions of pluralism and authority, notions of the Church. Increasingly it is these issues that come to the fore in moral discussions and that perhaps accounts for the impression of polarization between some bishops and some theologians.

In another symposium (held in Philadelphia, January 6–8, 1978), William May discusses the moral magisterium.[42] He insists, quite rightly, that the Church expects that the faithful "will, in faith, make their own through acts of faithful understanding" the teachings of the Church. However, dissent remains possible. But this does not mean that there is a "double truth." He takes issue with Congar, Dulles, and myself who "speak of two magisteria within the Church." The unity of the Church demands one magisterium, and the scholar must be willing to allow his or her positions to be judged by this one magisterium.

Any differences between May and myself on this subject appear to be nonsubstantial and a matter of emphasis. But two comments might be in place. First, while May admits the possibility of dissent, he does not carry this far enough—that is, he does not relate it to the development of doctrine. It remains privatized. Concretely, if dissent on a particular point is widespread, does this not suggest to us that perhaps the official formulation is in need of improvement? To say otherwise is to say that scholarly (and other) reflection has no relation to the Church's ongoing search for truth and application of her message. As Bishop Arzube notes, we would never have gotten to *Dignitatis humanae* if the reflections of John Courtney Murray had been merely tolerated and not taken as new sources of evidence.

This leads to the second point: May's rejection of two magisteria in the Church. It is easy to understand how this can be a confusing verbal vehicle and I, for one, am not wedded to it. Raymond Brown notes: "Magisterium is a fighting word. I think the attempt to reclaim it for theologians will not succeed; and I personally do not think the battle worth fighting so long as, under any other name, the legitimate role of theologians in shaping the teaching of the Church is respected."[43] I agree with that statement of things and with Brown's subsequent addition: "All that I

[42] William E. May, "The Magisterium and Moral Theology," in John J. O'Rourke and Thomas Greenburg (eds.), *Symposium on the Magisterium: A Positive Statement* (Boston: Daughters of St. Paul, 1978), 71–94.
[43] Brown, "Bishops and Theologians," 675.

want is that scholarly evidence be taken into account in the formulation and reformulation of Catholic doctrine."

What is important, then, is not the word; it is the idea beneath it—that is, the Church in her teaching makes use of (and probably must) theologies and philosophical concepts, as Congar repeatedly reminds us. In moral theology, an example would be *direct* killing, *direct* sterilization. These formulations are only more or less adequate and may even be wrong at times. It is one of theology's (and philosophy's) tasks to make that determination, not precisely the magisterium's.

Here an example is in place. Masturbation for infertility testing has been condemned officially (the Holy Office, Pius XII). Yet very few theologians of my acquaintance see this procedure as having the malice of masturbation. When theologians say this, they are stating (at least they think they are) a truth, and in this sense teaching. Or must one wait until something is officially modified to recognize that it is true or false? Personally, I would have no hesitation in saying to an individual that that condemnation is obsolete even if it has not been modified by the Church's more official teaching organs.

What theologians (and other scholars) have been searching for is a formula that would admit two things: (1) the practical admission of an independent competence for theology and other disciplines; (2) the admission of the indispensability of this competence for the formation, defense, and critique of magisterial statements. They are not interested in arrogating the kerygmatic function of the Holy Father and the bishops.[44] By "independent"

[44] William Cardinal Baum has a thoughtful paper on the episcopal magisterium. He suggests that the theology of this magisterium must be based on the evangelical notion of the proclamation of the kerygma and on the sacramental nature of the episcopal order. "The episcopal magisterium is thus not above, below, or alongside the role of theologians and others. It is a reality of a different order. It pertains to the sacramental transmission of the divine realities. . . ." See "Magisterium and the Life of Faith," *Origins*, 8 (1978), 76–80. A similar analysis was made by the then Archbishop Karol Wojtyla. He emphasizes the magisterium of bishops as proclamation, leading people to Christ. Bishops are first of all *fidei praecones* and only secondly *doctores*. The faithful defense of the *depositum* and its proclamation "entails its growing understanding, in tune with the demands of every age and responding to them according to the progress of theology and human science." He argues that the magisterium "as systematic and doctrinal teaching should be put at the service of the announcement of the gospel." See "Bishops as Servants of the Faith," *Irish Theological Quarterly*, 43 (1976), 260–73.

I do not mean "in isolation from" the body of believers or the hierarchy. Theologians are first and foremost believers, members of the faithful. By "independent" competence is meant one with its own proper purpose, tools, and training. The word "practical" is used because most people would admit this in theory.

However, in practice this is not always the case. And this practical problem can manifest itself in three ways. First, theologians are selected according to a predetermined position to be proposed, what Sanks calls "co-optation." Second, moral positions are formulated against a significant theological opinion or consensus in the Church. Such opinion should lead us to conclude that the matter has not matured sufficiently to be stated by the authentic magisterium. Third, when theologians sometimes critique official formulations, that is viewed as out of order, arrogating the teaching role of the hierarchy, disloyalty, etc. Actually, it is performing one of theology's tasks. All three of these manifestations are practical denials of the independent competence of theology.

As for the third manifestation mentioned above, it ought to be said that when a particular critique becomes one shared by many competent and demonstrably loyal scholars, it is part of the public opinion in the Church, a source of new knowledge and reflection. And certainly this source of new knowledge and reflection cannot be excluded from those sources we draw upon to enlighten and form our consciences. For conscience is formed *within the Church*.[45]

An unsolicited suggestion might not be totally irrelevant here. Bishops should be conservative, in the best sense of that word. They should not endorse every fad, or even every theological theory. They should "conserve," but to do so in a way that fosters faith, they must be vulnerably open and deeply involved in a process of creative and critical absorption. In some, perhaps increasingly many instances, they must take risks, the risks of being tentative or even quite uncertain and above all reliant on others in a complex world. Such a process of clarification and settling takes

---

[45] In "The 'New Morality' v. Objective Morality," *Homiletic and Pastoral Review*, 79 (1978), 27–31, Joseph Farraher, S.J., states: "Most present-day liberals in both dogmatic and moral theology . . . treat his [the Pope's] statement with no more acceptance than they would the statements of any individual theologian who disagrees with them." That statement is, I believe, simply false.

time, patience, and courage. Its greatest enemy is ideology, the comfort of being clear, and above all the posture of pure defense of received formulations.

In all fairness, at this point something should be added about theologians. Amid the variation of their modest function in the Church, they must never lose the courage to be led. "Courage" seems appropriate because being led in our times means sharing the burdens of the leader—and that can be passingly painful. They should speak their mind knowing that there are other and certainly more significant minds. In other words, they must not lose the nerve to make and admit an honest mistake. They should trust their intuitions and their hearts, but always within a sharp remembrance that the announcement of the faith and its implications in our times must come from the melding of many hearts and minds. The Church needs a thinking arm, so to speak; but that arm is dead if it is detached.

13. Sterilization and Theological Method

Recently two documents on sterilization have come to public attention. One is a response of the Sacred Congregation for the Doctrine of the Faith, the other a letter of the American hierarchy communicating the substance of the Congregation's response.[1] The background for the Congregation's document consisted of doubts about, and inconsistencies in applying, Directives 18 and 20 of the Ethical and Religious Directives for Catholic Hospitals. These directives read as follows:

18. Sterilization, whether permanent or temporary for men or for women, may not be used as a means for contraception.

20. Procedures that induce sterility, whether permanent or temporary, are permitted when (a) they are immediately directed to the cure, diminution, or prevention of a serious pathological condition and are not directly contraceptive (that is, contraception is not the purpose); and (b) a simpler treatment is not reasonably available. Hence, for example, oöphorectomy [removal of ovaries] or irradiation of the ovaries may be allowed in treating carcinoma of the breast and metastasis therefrom; and orchidectomy

---

[1] The first is entitled *Documentum circa sterilizationem in nosocomiis catholicis* (Responsa ad quaesita Conferentiae episcopalis Americae septentrionalis [Prot. 2,027/69]). It was issued March 13, 1975, is published in English translation in *Origins*, 6 (1976), 33 and 35, and is cited extensively by Kevin O'Rourke, O.P., in an article on sterilization, "An Analysis of the Church's Teaching on Sterilization," *Hospital Progress*, 57 (May 1976), 68–75. Archbishop Joseph L. Bernardin's letter of April 14, 1975, communicating this to the American bishops, is given in full in *Linacre Quarterly*, 42 (Nov. 1975), 220.

[excision of testicles] is permitted in the treatment
of carcinoma of the prostate.[2]

There can be no doubt that this represents the traditional formulation of the matter, a formulation officially stated and repeated by Pius XII and recently by Paul VI (*Humanae vitae*).
Several factors have conspired to make implementation of these
directives in at least some Catholic health facilities a source of
problems. Among these I would highlight the following: the increasing resort to sterilization as a method of birth regulation in
America; the division in the Church on the formulations of *Humanae vitae* on contraception and sterilization; the pluralistic
makeup of Catholic hospital personnel (staff, patients) and the
increasingly public character of these institutions; doubts surrounding the understanding and morally decisive character of the
notions of directness and indirectness where sterilization is concerned. In combination, these and other influences were responsible for a pluralism of practice in Catholic hospitals, with some
of the practices clearly incompatible with the directives and the
official formulations that stand behind and support them.

It was to this situation that the Congregation spoke. What did
the Congregation say? After defining direct sterilization in the traditional way,[3] the document continues: "Therefore, notwithstanding any subjectively right intention of those whose actions
are prompted by the cure or prevention of physical or mental illness which is foreseen or feared as a result of pregnancy, such sterilization remains absolutely forbidden according to the doctrine of
the Church." Following this general statement, the Congregation
makes two points.[4] Since they have very important theological im-

---

[2] *Ethical and Religious Directives for Catholic Health Facilities* (St. Louis:
Catholic Hospital Association, 1975), 10–11.

[3] "*Quaecumque sterilizatio quae ex seipsa, seu ex natura et conditione
propria, immediate hoc solummodo efficit ut facultas generativa incapax red-
datur ad consequendam procreationem, habenda est pro sterilizatione directa,
prout haec intelligitur in declarationibus Magisterii Pontificii, speciatim Pii XII.*"

[4] The document concludes with an application of the standard principles of
formal and material cooperation to the hospital situation. Since I do not wish
to discuss these here, I refer the reader to the careful study of O'Rourke (see
footnote 1).

plications and since I wish to comment on these implications in this chapter, I cite the document in full on these points:

1. And indeed the sterilization of the faculty itself is forbidden for an even graver reason than the sterilization of individual acts, since it induces a state of sterility in the person which is almost always irreversible. Neither can any mandate of public authority, which would seek to impose direct sterilization as necessary for the common good, be invoked; for such sterilization damages the dignity and inviolability of the human person.[5] Likewise, neither can one invoke the principle of totality in this case, in virtue of which interference with organs is justified for the greater good of the person; sterility intended in itself is not directed to the integral good of the person properly understood (*recte intentum*), "the proper order of good being preserved,"[6] inasmuch as it damages the ethical good (*bono ethico*) of the person, which is the highest good, since it deliberately deprives foreseen and freely chosen sexual activity of an essential element. Thus Article 20 of the directives promulgated by the Conference in 1971 faithfully reflects the doctrine which is to be held, and its observance should be urged.

The Congregation then makes the second point of theological importance. It continues:

2. The Congregation, while it confirms this traditional doctrine of the Church, is not unaware of the dissent against this teaching from many theologians. The Congregation, however, denies that doctrinal significance can be attributed to this fact as such, so as to constitute a "theological source" which the faithful might invoke in order that, having abandoned the authentic magisterium, they might follow the opin-

5 The document refers here to Pius XI, *Casti connubii* (*Acta Apostolicae Sedis*, 22 [1930], 565). Hereinafter cited as *AAS*.
6 Reference is made here to Paul VI, *Humanae vitae* (*AAS*, 60 [1968], 487).

ions of private theologians dissenting from the magisterium.

After recalling the legitimacy and applicability of the traditional doctrine on formal and material cooperation, the document concludes as follows: "This Sacred Congregation hopes that the criteria recalled in this letter will satisfy the expectations of the episcopate, in order that, with the uncertainties of the faithful removed, the bishops might more easily respond to their pastoral duty."

The two points I wish to discuss here are (1) the argument used by the Congregation and (2) the Congregation's assessment of the significance of theological dissent.

The Congregation says of direct sterilization that it is absolutely forbidden (*absolute interdicta*). By this the Congregation almost certainly means that direct sterilization is intrinsically evil, for it speaks not only of official *approbation* of direct sterilization as intrinsically evil, it also adds immediately "a fortiori, its management and execution in accord with hospital regulations is a matter which, in the objective order, is by its very nature (or intrinsically) evil." Any doubt on this point is removed by the argument used against direct sterilization. The Congregation argues that the principle of totality may not be invoked, because sterility intended as such (*in se*) is not directed to the integral good of the person because it is an assault on (*nocet*) the ethical good (*bono ethico*) of the person. Now clearly, anything that harms the ethical good of the person is impossible to justify. Indeed, by its very definition (analytically), it is intrinsically wrong; for the human person, in Catholic thought, finds his or her *raison d'être* in the moral order—the order of relationship to the "ground of being," the Creator, the God of Salvation. This is where the person begins and ends. Or, as the document notes of the good in question, *quod est supremum* (a good which is the highest). Clearly, to compromise this good for whatever other conceivable benefit is incoherent; for it harms the supreme good of the person, and indeed on the grounds that this is good for the person. That violates not only the well-known Kantian moral maxim (a person must always be treated as an end also, and never merely as a means) but also the whole Christian notion of human person as we gather this from the sources of revelation.

Why does direct sterilization attack (*nocet*) the ethical good of the person, according to the Congregation? Because it deliberately (*ex proposito*) deprives "foreseen and freely chosen sexual activity of an essential element." That essential element is, of course, the potential to procreate.

In summary, then, the Congregation argues that deliberately to deprive freely chosen sexual relations[7] of the potential to procreate deprives those relations of an "essential element." But to do so is to harm the moral good (*bono ethico*) of the person. But since this good is the highest good (*quod est supremum*), an intervention that harms it (*nocet*) clearly cannot be justified by the principle of totality—a principle that justifies interventions precisely on the grounds that they are required by the over-all good of the person. In still other words, an intervention that harms the moral good of the person is intrinsically evil. But direct sterilization does this.

What is to be said of this analysis? I believe that it rests on a *petitio principii*. No one would quibble with the assertion that an intervention that harms the *moral* good of the person cannot be justified by the principle of totality. That is clear from the very meaning of that principle. What is not clear, however, is that the power to procreate is an element so essential to sexual intimacy that to deprive freely chosen intimacy of this power is in every instance to assault the ethical or moral good of the person. That is precisely the point to be proved. If it were clear, we would not have had the birth-control controversy of the past ten or twelve years. So, to draw the conclusion it does (*absolute interdicta* [absolutely forbidden], *intrinsece mala* [intrinsically evil]), the Congregation must assume what is to be established—that to deprive freely chosen sexual intimacy of the power to procreate always harms the ethical or moral good of the person. Until this is illumined, the analysis of the Congregation is less an analysis than a reassertion. One cannot fault the Congregation for saying that

---

[7] The wording here is very careful. By saying "freely chosen" the document rather clearly excludes sterilizing interventions (whether temporary or permanent) that are carried out as protection against sexual activity that is not freely chosen (for example, rape).

this reassertion is official Catholic teaching. It can be faulted, however, for failing to illumine this teaching.

Here two additional points are in order. First, the moral issue is not precisely the understanding and reach of the principle of totality. This "principle" is, under analysis, nothing more than a way of formulating the reasonableness or unreasonableness of medical interventions. In other words, whether earlier theologians and Pius XII understood the principle of totality as covering goods beyond the integrity of the organism (goods such as relationship to family and others) is not the issue. Clearly Pius XII did not view totality in this comprehensive way. The issue is rather the reasonableness or unreasonableness—all things considered—of certain surgical or medical interventions that have as their purpose the *over-all* good of the person, "the dignity and well-being of man as a person in all his essential relationships to God, to his fellow men, and to the world around him," as Bernard Häring words it.[8] Whether one calls this the "principle of totality" or not is quite secondary. Human and Christian reasonableness is the issue, a point suggested by the Church's long support of the notion communicated by the term "natural law." In the following chapter I shall suggest that it is indeed at times humanly and Christianly reasonable.

Second, my suggestion that the Congregation's analysis involves a *petitio principii* should not and may not be taken as a promotion of direct sterilization. The point I am making is methodological. The first thing that is to be said about direct sterilization is that it is an evil to be avoided insofar as possible—but an evil that, until it has been properly placed in the context of its circumstances, remains nonmoral in character (Louis Janssens would say an "ontic evil," Joseph Fuchs a "premoral evil," philosopher W. D. Ross would term its avoidance a "prima-facie obligation"), much as killing is a nonmoral evil until more of its circumstances have been revealed. Indeed, by putting the matter in this way, one implies that we must individually and corporately thrust toward a world where the values preserved or achieved by direct sterilization can be achieved without such an intervention. In other words, the issue is not "sterilization is an evil v. sterilization is a

[8] Bernard Häring, *Medical Ethics* (Notre Dame: Fides, 1973), 62.

good"; it is rather "direct sterilization is intrinsically evil v. direct sterilization is not intrinsically evil." If it is not intrinsically evil, many theologians argue, there remain instances of values in conflict where it cannot be shown to be morally wrong.[9]

Now to the second point: the Congregation's assessment of theological dissent. The document admits the existence of dissent on the part of many (*plurium*) theologians. But it denies that such dissent has doctrinal significance as such (*ut tali*), so as to constitute a theological source (*locum theologicum*) that the faithful might invoke in the formation of their consciences. It is absolutely correct to say that dissent has no doctrinal significance "as such." But I do not believe that anyone ever made that claim. No mere ("as such") aggregation of dissenters constitutes a *locus theologicus*. That would be to "Gallupize" moral issues.

Any doctrinal significance attributable to dissent comes from the *reasons* for the dissent. Thus, in the traditional understanding of probabilism, the opinions of four or five reputable theologians had significance because, being reputable, such external authority created the presumption of internal evidence or reasonableness. But it is this latter (internal evidence or reasonableness) that has doctrinal significance and becomes a *locus theologicus*. To deny this is to imply that a moral conclusion has little or no relation to the reasons and analyses available to support it or weaken it.[10] Such an implication would depart from the Catholic tradition of a natural moral law based on right reasoning and would juridicize the search for truth by pitting theologians against official statements, as if the ultimate reasonableness of a formulation depended above all on the ecclesiastical position of those proposing it.

On this matter the document of the Congregation seems strangely to be of two incompatible minds. First, by saying accu-

---

[9] I am not including in this statement coercive policies of sterilization, since these involve other considerations.

[10] The letter communicating the response of the Congregation to the American bishops is quite sweeping. It states: "I am writing to give assurance that the 1971 guideline stands as written, and that direct sterilization is not to be considered as justified by the common good, the principle of totality, the existence of contrary opinion, *or any other argument*" (emphasis added). If taken at face value (and I am not sure it should be), this last phrase puts moral reasoning out of order in the area of sterilization.

rately that the dissent of many theologians has no doctrinal significance "as such," the Congregation must clearly imply that it is the reasons or internal evidence that provide doctrinal significance. That is the force of the words "as such." If the Congregation would not admit this, then moral theology as a discipline would simply cease to exist. It would be unnecessary because moral positions would be conclusions unrelated to human analytic efforts and legitimated by the official position of those who issued them. If, contrarily, the Congregation would admit (as it seems to imply in the use *ut tali*) that reasons and analyses do have doctrinal significance, then it is these that must be weighed to determine whether dissent constitutes a *locus theologicus* that may rightly influence the formation of conscience.

Second, however, while seeming to imply this, the document does not examine the reasons and analyses of those who have dissented.[11] Rather, it offers its own argument (one that involves a *petitio principii*) and concludes that direct sterilization is absolutely forbidden and suggests that this should remove all doubts of the faithful (*incertitudinibus fidelium sublatis*). This too easily suggests that uncertainties and doubts are removed not by persuasive reasons but by official statements.[12]

I raise these points not because I wish to suggest any particular institutional policy on sterilization or a change in policy on sterilization for Catholic hospitals. There are many reasons why Catholic health-care facilities should be extremely cautious about sterilization.[13] I do so for methodological reasons. The Congre-

[11] I do not discuss these analyses here because my emphasis is above all on methodology.

[12] The statement that this document should remove the uncertainties of the faithful—including theologians—raises several serious theological questions. For instance, what is it about the document that removes doubts and uncertainties? What is the doctrinal significance of a statement of a Roman congregation responding on its own (to wit, without claiming to be an act of the Holy Father) and one destined only for a particular episcopate? Is it properly a document of the magisterium and one that carries doctrinal weight even in other countries? If so, what is this weight and how is it to be explained? A decade or two ago the answers to these questions seemed relatively simple and clear. But it can be doubted that such clarity is present in the contemporary Church.

[13] For instance, the fact that direct sterilization is a nonmoral evil almost always irreversible, the fact that today's exceptions become tomorrow's rules or habitual practices, the fact that in a technologically oriented and comfort-

gation, in facing the institutional-policy issue, has gotten deeply involved in theological presuppositions. These must be lifted out and examined, not only because of the importance of the specific question under discussion, but above all because these presuppositions will be operative in other, and even more important, matters.

Some may view pointing out the questionable theological implications in statements of a Roman congregation as defiance and disloyalty. Quite the contrary is the case. As Avery Dulles, S.J., pointed out in his excellent presidential address to the Catholic Theological Society of America (June 1976), "Recognizing the stern demands of intellectual integrity, theology must pursue truth for its own sake no matter who may be inconvenienced by the discovery. Unless we are true to this vocation, we shall not help the Church to live up to its calling to become, more than ever before, a zone of truth."[14] When the theologian follows Dulles' advice with honesty, courtesy, and a realistic awareness of his own limitations, the only threat is to an excessively juridical notion of magisterium.

---

conditioned culture many will seek sterilization where it is objectively unjustifiable, the fact that some countries may be weighing coercive sterilization policies, the fact that a prohibitory policy may be justified symbolically (even if the action is not inherently wrong)—these and other considerations could provide most Catholic health facilities with a defensible basis for a very stringent policy against sterilization. However, I do not wish to argue this at length here.

[14] Avery Dulles, S.J., "The Theologian and the Magisterium," *Proceedings of the Catholic Theological Society of America*, 31 (1976), 246.

14. Sterilization as a Catholic Institutional Problem

My title is important because it suggests the limited scope of the problem I wish to discuss. The limits are the following. First, I do not discuss vasectomy *explicitly* (though a thorough moral analysis will touch it at least implicitly) because this is an office procedure—and thus not a "Catholic institutional problem." Therefore, the restriction of the discussion is to tubal ligation. Second, I do not discuss the participation of Catholics in sterilizations done in non-Catholic hospitals—even though an adequate moral analysis would have something to say relevant to this too. Finally, for purposes of completeness, I do not discuss the sterilization of minors or incompetents, since these raise problems beyond the moral character of sterilization of requesting and consenting adults. In summary, then, my remarks are explicitly addressed to the *policy* problem of *tubal ligation* within a Catholic hospital.

Before approaching the problem, it would be well to review the factual situation in Catholic hospitals throughout the country as this emerges from conversations, letters, and a dossier of responses. Some administrators state simply: "There is no problem; we do not do tubal ligations." Generally there is no problem, I take it, because other facilities are available in the area. Hence there are relatively few requests. Yet, in my judgment, this may disguise a real problem. Even though the requests and pressures are not there *now*, we must ask if the current policy is *inherently* justifiable. Factual situations can and do change, and it would be administratively shortsighted to fail to grapple with a moral problem simply because there are no present pressures to do so. This is especially the case within a context of growing medical and theological conviction that some sterilizations are medically and morally sound procedures.

Others feel the pressures and are wondering what to do. This is especially—though not exclusively—true of the Catholic hospital that is the sole facility available to a physician and patient personnel often heavily non-Catholic. There are several possibilities here for policy and I shall list them briefly.

1. *Do no sterilizations and suffer the consequences.* The rationale for this policy is twofold. First, direct sterilization is always wrong (as several popes have taught) and is explicitly forbidden by the *Ethical and Religious Directives for Catholic Health Facilities* (n. 20). Second, there is no reason for (material) cooperation in sterilization since it is better for a Catholic hospital to go under than to abandon the glorious witness value it exists to serve. I know of no one (not even the Sacred Congregation for the Doctrine of the Faith) who holds this *in theory*—since it is indefensible. No one would or could argue that any sterilization necessarily involves abandonment of witnessing to Catholic values. But *in practice* some bishops and administrators would certainly act this way. Indeed, a recent article in *Linacre Quarterly* by Vitale H. Paganelli attempted to give theoretical warrants for this attitude by erroneously interpreting the document of the Sacred Congregation for the Doctrine of Faith on sterilization.[1]

2. *Apply the doctrine of material cooperation.* Briefly stated, this means that a Catholic hospital could tolerate tubal ligation on an individual basis where, all things considered, greater harm than good would result from enforcement of policy. This is a quite traditional approach and was explicitly provided for by the Sacred Congregation for the Doctrine of the Faith. Some (for example, Thomas O'Donnell, S.J.) want to interpret this very strictly by saying that material cooperation ought to be an "isolated" and "extreme case" and is not to be admitted "as hospital policy."[2] Others would argue that what is policy depends on the factual situation. If local factual circumstances dictate that a policy is justified, then it is justified, for it is precisely circumstances that justify exceptions—whether isolated or more frequent. At any rate, underlying this second response (material cooperation) is

[1] Vitale H. Paganelli, "An Update on Sterilization," *Linacre Quarterly*, 44 (1977), 12–17.
[2] Thomas J. O'Donnell, S.J., "Letter to the Editor," *Linacre Quarterly*, 44 (1977), 9–10.

the assumption that direct sterilization is always morally wrong. Hence an institution may only materially cooperate with it.

3. *Sterilizations are permissible for serious medical reasons.* The rationale for this position is that when there are serious health problems that would be aggravated by pregnancy, the sterilization is indirect and not prohibited by the *Directives*. This is the interpretation in some places and by some ordinaries and by some theologians. It has the advantage of "getting the hospital off the hook." In my judgment, it is incompatible with the traditional understanding of the terms "direct" and "indirect" sterilization. By this I do not mean to suggest that such sterilizations are immoral; quite the contrary. I mean to suggest only that according to traditional theological literature, papal statements, and the *Directives*, these are direct sterilizations. For instance, if a woman suffers from cardiac decompensation or chronic kidney disease, and another pregnancy would endanger the life (or life-span) or health of the woman, then tubal ligation has as its immediate purpose the prevention of pregnancy. If that is the case, it is a direct sterilization. To say anything else would be to say that the sterilization is indirect *because it is justifiable.* That is a remarkable change in traditional language.

4. *Sterilizations are permissible for the over-all good of the person.* The rationale here (in contrast to n. 3) is that even though the sterilization is direct (to wit, it aims proximately—"as a means"—at sterilization), it is nonetheless justified. Various reasons can be given for such justification. Regardless of the name one gives such reasons, they are reducible to the claim that the moral justification for removing fertility is the total good of the person. Many call this the "principle of totality." The encyclical *Humanae vitae* and the document of the Sacred Congregation for the Doctrine of the Faith reject such a principle as applicable to direct sterilization. Hence those who appeal to this principle are in a position of dissent from those documents, in my judgment.

Having stated those *possible* policy responses, it is now necessary to turn to the morality of sterilization, for while policy need not be identical with morality, even in a Catholic hospital (for example, material cooperation), it is rooted in and based on morality.

What is the morality of sterilization—and by this term I mean

what we traditionally have called "direct sterilization" (since no
one questions the morality of sterility induced by treatment of or
removal of pathological reproductive organs themselves [for example, removal of cancerous ovaries])?

First, a brief look at the official (Pius XII, Paul VI, Sacred
Congregation for the Doctrine of the Faith) formulation of the
matter. In his "Address to the Midwives" (October 29, 1951),
Pius XII stated: "Direct sterilization—that is, the sterilization
which aims, either as a means or as an end in itself, to render
childbearing impossible—is a grave violation of the moral
law. . . ." Pius XII made it clear that this was simply an extension (a fortiori) of the rejection of a contraceptive act. Paul VI
repeated this teaching in Humanae vitae: "Equally to be excluded
. . . is direct sterilization, whether perpetual or temporary,
whether of the man or of the woman."[3] Pope Paul adverted to the
"so-called 'principle of totality'" but rejected its application to
contraception and direct sterilization.

The Sacred Congregation for the Doctrine of the Faith recently
put it as follows: "Any sterilization which of itself—that is, of its
own nature and condition—has the sole immediate effect of rendering the generative faculty incapable of procreation is to be considered direct sterilization, as the term is understood in the declaration of the pontifical magisterium, especially of Pius XII.
Therefore, notwithstanding any subjectively right intention of
those whose actions are prompted by the cure or prevention of
physical or mental illness which is foreseen or feared as a result of
pregnancy, such sterilization remains absolutely forbidden according to the doctrine of the Church."[4] The Sacred Congregation for
the Doctrine of the Faith explicitly rejected use of the "principle
of totality" to such cases.

Therefore, in the official teaching of the Church, two points are
utterly clear. First, direct sterilization is absolutely prohibited. Second, under the term "direct" must be included those sterilizations
"prompted by the cure or prevention of physical or mental illness
that is foreseen or feared *as a result of pregnancy*" (emphasis

[3] Paul VI, Humanae vitae as in Robert G. Hoyt (ed.), The Birth Control
Debate (Kansas City, Mo.: National Catholic Reporter, 1968), 124.
[4] Documentum circa sterilizationem in nosocomiis catholicis (Prot. 2,027/69).
An English version is available in Origins, 6 (1976), 33 and 35.

added)—to wit, "medically indicated sterilizations" that seek to prevent pregnancy.

The response of large segments of the Catholic community to this teaching is equally well known. It can be stated negatively and positively. Negatively, it is argued that it has not been persuasively established that direct sterilization is intrinsically evil. I shall not enter the niceties of the theological argument on this point except to point out that if the Church says that the direct taking of the full integrity of procreative capacity is intrinsically evil, she is asserting something about procreative capacity that she has refused to assert about life itself.

Positively, many theologians argue that procreative function or capacity is, like any other aspect of the human person, for the over-all good of the person. Being subordinated to the good of the person, this capacity may be negated when the good of the person so dictates. Whether one calls this the principle of totality or not is quite secondary. The main thrust of the assertion is that in some instances sterilization represents a reasonable disposition of the self, a reasonable act of stewardship. As Bernard Häring words it: "Whenever the direct preoccupation is responsible care for the health of persons or for saving a marriage (which also affects the total health of all persons involved), sterilization can then receive its justification from valid medical reasons. If, therefore, a competent physician can determine, in full agreement with his patient, that in this particular situation a new pregnancy must be excluded now and forever because it would be thoroughly irresponsible, and if from a medical point of view sterilization is the best possible situation, it cannot be against the principles of medical ethics, nor is it against 'natural law' (*recta ratio*)."[5] Many theologians would agree with this—and I include myself among them. The arguments *contra* are unpersuasive and, I believe, inconsistent with other modes of argument in our tradition. But there can be no doubt that this point of view is incompatible with official Church formulations.

It is at this point that the problem becomes critical and quite delicate. What is one to make of such disagreements in the Church? And more specifically, what is the Catholic hospital to

[5] Bernard Häring, *Medical Ethics* (Notre Dame, Ind.: Fides, 1973), 90.

do in light of such disagreements? The problem is basically one of moral epistemology and ecclesiology. *Epistemology* because it touches one's view of the relationship of analysis and recognized analyzers to a moral conclusion. Concretely, if there are very persuasive reasons for a conclusion and those reasons are held by very many reputable theologians (including bishops)—indeed, by most reputable theologians—can the opposite position be said to be clear and certain simply because it is proposed by official teachers? I think not. *Ecclesiology* because at stake is one's view of the magisterium—its nature and limits—and even more broadly of the Church itself.

When the epistemological and ecclesiological elements are shaken and mixed, two basic positions emerge. The first argues that in spite of dissenting views, the official position is correct and must be held. Direct sterilizations are intrinsically wrong. To say anything else is to be disobedient to authoritative teaching. Hence the only involvement of the Catholic hospital in such sterilization is by way of rare and isolated cases of material cooperation.

This view was recently expressed by Thomas O'Donnell, S.J., in the *Linacre Quarterly*. He wrote: "It is equally clear, however, that those in Catholic hospital work who are determined to ignore this directive of the Holy See and continue doing contraceptive sterilizations will have no trouble finding theologians who will be willing to 'waffle' on the matter and thereby seem to make the Catholic hospital's disobedience to the Holy See quite defensible and even virtuous."[6] I have profound disagreements with the ecclesiology underlying this statement—for example, an honest dissent is characterized as "waffling." That simply *supposes* the truth of the official position, and precisely because it is official.

The second view shakes and mixes its perspectives in a remarkably different way. It refuses to analyze the moral rightness or wrongness of sterilization dominantly in terms of *obedience* to the Holy See, for this subordinates the truth to a vehicle of the truth and supposes a highly juridical and neoscholastic notion of the Church, and of the Church as teacher (magisterium). Summarily, it puts truth in the service of official statements and positions. Rejecting this notion, the second view puts much more emphasis

6 O'Donnell, "Letter to the Editor."

on *analysis and reasons* for moral positions and argues therefore that official teachers must not simply command, but also persuade. This is particularly true of a moral tradition (the Catholic) that puts great emphasis on *recta ratio* or the natural law in moral matters. Within this perspective, it sees all of the reasons proposed to support the intrinsically evil character of any direct sterilization as unpersuasive—and indeed as various forms of the naturalistic fallacy, an error that attributes unalterable normative force to givenness or biological entities. Furthermore, it argues that when numerous moral authorities within the Church converge in their presentation of a point of view, this must be taken into account in determining what the *Church's* conviction on a moral matter is and ought to be at a certain time. Otherwise, this view contends, personal reflection has been ruled out of order in the teaching-learning process of the Church in a totally unacceptable way. Briefly, this view argues that it is fully Catholic to say (to wit, it is a tenable moral position) that not every direct sterilization is morally wrong. And since that is the case, the Catholic hospital ought not to adopt a policy that supposes that it is. Rather this policy should be one framed to assure, insofar as possible, that sterilizations are done with great caution and responsibility—namely, for serious indications.[7] This latter position is my own—but more importantly that of those I consider to be the most reputable and reliable theologians in the Church today.

Put differently, this position would argue that (1) sterilization cannot be shown to be inherently evil; (2) and therefore it is justifiable for a truly proportionate reason. This means that Directives 18 and 20 of the *Directives* are wrong. The reason is proportionate when continuing procreative function is, as far as humanly foreseeable, a threat to the over-all good of the person and no other reversible procedure is acceptable because it is (1) insufficiently effective (2) or incompatible with health (3) or inconsistent with respect for nascent life.

It is not the function of a moral theologian to list exhaustively

[7] I do not wish to imply that medical reasons are the only ones that justify sterilization. Rather, since the problem I address is one of hospital policy, I am concerned with hospital sterilization that should, generally speaking, be for medical reasons. However, I would argue that much greater caution is in place where an irreversible procedure is done for reversible indications—for example, socioeconomic ones.

those instances where procreative function is a threat to the over-all good of the person. Nor is it entirely a medical judgment; for what is to the over-all good of the person depends heavily on a patient's personal perspective, personal circumstances, personal biography. Thus it is one thing for a 20-year-old gravida 1, para 1 to undergo certain risks to have a child. It is quite a different thing for a 38-year-old gravida 7, para 7 to undergo the same risks. So the term "medically indicated" is not the same as "humanly indicated" or "morally indicated," for "medically indicated" is subordinate to the qualifier "depending on the patient's perspectives."

While it is not my function, then, to list exhaustively or even at length justifiable sterilizations, it is important to give an example simply to indicate that there are some. I have in mind the instances of severe renal disease and heart disease where further pregnancy would abbreviate the life-span. I have in mind women whose life-support medication is potentially incompatible with fetal health and well-being. I have in mind the woman who can never carry a pregnancy to the point of fetal survival. There are cases where it could be Christianly reasonable for this couple to conclude that they should never again conceive. Clearly, there would be many other less obvious instances. My only point here is to make it clear that there are medically related cases where the decision to undergo sterilization need not be unreasonable (contrary to *recta ratio*).

So these are the two basic general perspectives. In moral matters, when there is disagreement and controversy, one usually concludes that there is doubt. And when there is doubt, the usual principle is *in dubiis libertas* (in doubtful matters, there is freedom). But the matter is not that simple where policy for a Catholic hospital is concerned, for the two general perspectives I have outlined are shared by bishops. Concretely, some bishops follow Pope Paul VI and the *Directives*, regarding direct sterilization as inherently evil. Among these some allow for material cooperation; others (at least as they are interpreted) absolutely forbid it. Others apply the notion of *indirect* to medically justifiable sterilizations, thus quieting the problem but, in my opinion, doing so without realizing that they are going against Pius XII, Paul VI, the Sacred Congregation for the Doctrine of the Faith, and the

Directives. Still others, believing the matter is not sufficiently certain in the Church to justify absolute prohibition, allow hospitals to work out a policy of controlled selective sterilization. There is, in short, a regrettable cacophony of moral policies.

While I, as a moral theologian, am convinced with many other theologians that direct sterilization is objectively justifiable for the over-all good of the person, still the problem of policy must be faced. Specifically, what are hospitals to do when an individual bishop working with different epistemological and ecclesiological perspectives insists on following the *Directives,* a policy that at least very many physicians believe to be bad medicine and many theologians believe to be bad theology?

This is a political problem and because it is that I want to propose a political solution. It would be worded as follows: The policy of this Catholic hospital is, for many reasons (theological and institutional) not to intervene in individual cases where (1) sterilization is judged by patient *and* physician (or staff) to be essential to the over-all good of the patient, (2) and where more harm than good would result from intervention.

Like all political solutions, this is something of a compromise, but one I believe at least very many of us could live with. Let me point out some aspects of this approach that appear important.

1. The most important political aspect of this policy is that it can be understood as a classical statement of the principle of material cooperation. The policy speaks of "nonintervention" (or toleration) in situations where there is a proportionate reason ("more harm than good would result from intervention"). Because this is a statement of the traditional principle of cooperation, no one, including a bishop, is competent to deny such a principle. Indeed, its application is explicitly provided for in the recent document of the Sacred Congregation for the Doctrine of the Faith.

The only possible loophole is that an individual bishop might reserve to himself the judgment as to whether "more harm than good would result from intervention." I would hope, however, that the over-all position of the entire Church (not just official statements), the practice of other dioceses and national hierarchies, the principle of subsidiarity, and a host of other factors—not excluding the vulnerability of a bishop to the charge of "prac-

ticing medicine without a license"—would lead bishops to conclude that such assessments are best left to those on the scene.

2. The statement *need not* be interpreted as merely a statement
about material cooperation—and for that reason I could live with
it; for the thrust of the first condition ("essential to the over-all
good of the patient") is the inherent justifiability of the procedure
at times. If the policy is read that way, and it can be, then the
force of the second condition is cautionary—that is, the substance
of the statement is that direct sterilization is what we call a *prima
facie* evil (or an ontic evil), to be avoided insofar as compatibly
(with other conflicting values) possible. Furthermore, because at
least some individuals are likely to seek tubal ligation for less than
adequate reasons and because exceptions easily tend to become
rules, the second condition is a cautionary check, a kind of attempt to balance off this danger. Viewed in this way, the policy is
no longer one of material cooperation (*which supposes the objective evil of the procedure*), but one of cautious and controlled approval in individual instances. In this sense, it represents what I
regard as the best theological position—to wit, the best understanding of the meaning of concrete moral norms in this area.

Not all will be happy with this solution. It is, as I said, *political*
in character. But as I read my moral epistemology and ecclesiology, it is a justifiable policy. Other theologians and bishops
would agree that this is a defensible way, at the present time, of
facing a delicate situation in a Church somewhat divided on the
moral issue. What is above all necessary is that any policy avoid
leaving the impression that sterilization is a *simple, unqualified
good*, meriting *simple, unqualified approval*. It is an intervention
that needs justification—but one that can find it in individual
cases. That justification, if we are to be consistent with our statements and policies in other areas of moral concern, is the over-all
good of the patient.

SECTION V

REPRODUCTIVE TECHNOLOGICAL GENETICS

15. Genetic Medicine: Notes on the Moral Literature

The moral literature on genetic controls is enormous.[1] Furthermore, it touches on several different problems with ethical implications: eugenic engineering (both positive and negative), genetic counseling and screening, genetic abortion,[2] *in vitro* fertilization, cloning, etc. Much of the occasional writing is general in character.[3] The more systematic moral studies on genetics remind one of a masked ball: new disguises but behind them familiar faces. The familiar faces in this instance refer to the methodologies of well-known theologians on the (especially) American scene. Hence, even in the face of the exciting and/or frightening possibilities of contemporary biomedicine, there is a lingering sense of *déjà vu* in the moral literature. Briefly, since ultimate attitudes and judg-

---

[1] Literature of the 1960s can be found in Rosalind P. Petchesky's "Issues in Biological Engineering," *Institute for the Study of Science in Human Affairs Bulletin*, 7 (New York: Columbia University, 1969). See also *Theological Studies*, 30 (1969), 680–92, where I review the recent periodical literature. This literature will not be reviewed here. Another valuable bibliographical source is "In the Literature," which appears regularly in the *Hastings Center Report*.

[2] A conference at Airlie House, Virginia (Oct. 10–14, 1971) was devoted to "Ethical Issues in Genetic Counseling and the Use of Genetic Knowledge." It dealt heavily with counseling, screening, and abortion. The papers include thoughtful essays by Daniel Callahan, Paul Ramsey, James Gustafson, Leon Kass, and John Fletcher. For a brief report of this conference, see W. G. Peter, "Ethical Perspectives in the Use of Genetic Knowledge," *BioScience*, 21 (Nov. 15, 1971), 1,133–37.

[3] See, for example, Donald Huisingh, "Should Man Control His Genetic Future?" *Zygon*, 4 (1969), 188–99; S. E. Luria, "Modern Biology: A Terrifying Power," *Nation*, 209 (1969), 405 ff; Kenneth Vaux, "Cyborg, R. U. Human? Ethical Issues in Rebuilding Man," *Religion in Life*, 39 (1970), 187–92. Articles of this kind abound in the medical journals and in journals such as *Science* and *Science News*. See also New York *Times Magazine* (Mar. 5, 1972), pp. 10 ff.

ments vis-à-vis various genetic interventions depend heavily on
how the author builds his approach, the emphasis falls heavily on
methodology. Three approaches are discernible: a consequentialist
calculus, a more deontological attitude, and a "mediating" approach.[4]

Consequentialist Calculus

Joseph Fletcher, after reporting on some earlier writing on the
subject,[5] sees the whole difference of opinion in terms of
"apriorists" and "consequentialists."[6] This is, he says, "the rock-
bottom issue . . . the definitive question in the ethical analysis of
genetic control." The apriorists, relying on some kind of religious

[4] The very problems theologians decide to discuss are important, for a false
move here could bring theology and its important contributions to biomedical
decisions into disrepute with the scientific world. Furthermore, too great a
futurism would allow existing problems to get solved by default. The matter
is complicated by the fact that theologians are at the mercy of the scientific
world in deciding what problems are realistic, and this very world gives ambiguous answers. For instance, James D. Watson reports of Joshua Lederberg's
attitude toward cloning that "to him, serious talk about cloning is essentially
crying wolf when a tiger is already inside the walls" ("Moving Toward the
Clonal Man," *Atlantic* [May 1971], 52). Many authors view cloning as too
far into the future to merit serious discussion now. On the other hand, statements such as that of Bernard D. Davis, M.D., are not infrequent: "Cloning
is thus the aspect of genetic intervention that most requires public discussion
today" (*New England Journal of Medicine*, 285 [1971], 800).

[5] Inaccurately in at least several places. Speaking of "genetic engineering,"
Fletcher states that "Richard McCormick condemns it because, he believes,
only monogamously married heterosexual reproduction is morally licit." The
reference is to *Theological Studies* (see footnote 1), where a position on
"monogamously married heterosexual reproduction" is indeed endorsed; but
this endorsement is far from a condemnation of all "genetic engineering," as
even a quick reading will reveal. Similarly of Dr. André Hellegers, Fletcher
writes: "A Catholic obstetrician . . . has complained that it is 'arbitrary' to
start regarding a fetus as human at the twentieth week or at 'viability,' and
yet the physician himself insists on the even more arbitrary religious doctrine
that a fertilized ovum before implantation is human." Fletcher has misread
Hellegers' point (*Washington Post* [Jan. 9, 1971], Sec. A, p. 21). Hellegers
was simply challenging the *Post*'s concern over test-tube babies, since that paper
had for years supported the proposition that fetuses before the twentieth week
could be destroyed. If fetuses can be destroyed before this time, Hellegers rightly
wonders why it is improper for scientists to create such blobs of tissue. The
point is the *Post*'s consistency, nothing more.

[6] Joseph Fletcher, "Ethical Aspects of Genetic Controls," *New England
Journal of Medicine*, 285 (1971), 776–83.

or nonempirical cognition, "would say, therefore, that therapeutic goals are not enough to justify *in vitro* fertilization, positive eugenics, or designed eugenic changes, no matter how desirable they might be." In contrast to this is a pragmatic or consequentialist ethics, which Fletcher claims as his own. "We reason from the data of each actual case or problem and then choose the course that offers an optimum or maximum of desirable consequences." Or again, "results are what counts and results are good when they contribute to human well-being," a point to be situationally determined.

Fletcher then looks at a few cases and delivers his verdict. "I would vote for laboratory fertilization from donors to give a child to an infertile pair of spouses." As for cloning, Fletcher is a veritable cheerleader for the enthusiasts. "If the greatest good of the greatest number [that is, the social good] were served by it," he would "vote" both for specializing the capacities of people by cloning and bioengineering parahumans or modified men. There then follows one of the most remarkable sentences in the contemporary literature on genetics: "I suspect I would favor making and using man-machine hybrids rather than genetically designed people for dull, unrewarding or dangerous roles needed nonetheless for the community's welfare—perhaps the testing of suspected pollution areas or the investigation of threatening volcanoes or snowslides."[7]

Fletcher acknowledges several possible objections to all of this. First, it could be objected that since "fertilization or cloning result directly in human beings, or in creatures with nascent or protohuman status," the entailed practice of their sacrifice in the course of investigation is immoral. He dismisses this as "a priori metarational opinion," "belief in a faith assertion."

Having thus dismembered the first objection, he confronts the second—that is, that there might be something inhuman about the laboratory reproduction of human beings. If one has a sneaking suspicion that behind Fletcher's enthusiasm there lurks a concept of "the human," he is absolutely right. "Man is a maker and a selector and a designer, and the more rationally contrived and deliberate anything is, the more human it is." This opens on a

[7] Ibid., 779.

judgment that is at least competitive for "most remarkable statement of the year": "Laboratory reproduction is radically human compared to conception by ordinary heterosexual intercourse. It is willed, chosen, purposed and controlled, and surely these are among the traits that distinguish *Homo sapiens* from others in the animal genus, from the primates down. Coital reproduction is, therefore, less human than laboratory reproduction. . . ."[8]

To those who might object or hesitate, Fletcher has the reassuring word that "fear is at the bottom of this debate." But really we should fear not, for "to be men we must be in control. That is the first and last ethical word." Therefore, where cloning, donor insemination, etc., are concerned, "all this means that we are going to have to change or alter our old ideas about who or what a father is, or a mother, or a family."

Thus far Fletcher. I have cited him liberally because one has to, as it were, see it to believe it.

The time has come, I think, to blow the whistle on this type of thing. It is not a question of whether this genial Christian and gentlemanly ethician is right or wrong. We have all been a little bit of both, and much more of the latter. Rather, Fletcher continues to propose to do theology by setting up dubious polarities, promulgating unexamined premises, and flourishing rhetorical *non sequiturs*. The whole thing is then baptized into contemporary personalism with a now familiar ritualistic jargon: responsible, loving, pragmatic, personal. This is, of course, enormous fun; but it could be painfully expensive. If theologians are to retain any realistic hope of a dialogue with the scientific community, they must resolutely dissociate themselves from a type of discourse that too often dissolves into theology by anecdote.

First, the dubious polarities. An example is "apriorists v. consequentialists." The former are accused of "religious, metaphysical, nonempirical" thought. They "would say, therefore, that therapeutic or corrective goals are not enough to justify *in vitro* fertilization, positive eugenics or designed genetic changes no matter how desirable they might be. . . . Good consequences could not, to the a priori moralist, justify such acts or procedures since they are wrong as means. . . ." Here Fletcher's typologies, while re-

---

[8] Ibid., 781.

taining a certain pedagogical utility, simply ignore the possibility that it is precisely a form of consequentialism that could lead to a rejection of these things. In other words, what some theologians are saying is that the very desirability of therapeutic or corrective goals is not an isolated factor but must be weighed in light of the personal and social costs involved in moving toward such goals. They are saying that *in vitro* fertilization, cloning, etc., no matter what long-term pragmatic advantages and reliefs they would seem to provide, reveal the decisive disadvantage of containing an attack on the *humanum*, and for this reason (or consequence) are to be avoided. This is hardly metarational apriorism.

Second, the unexamined premises. At the very time Fletcher tells us that the notion of humanness "may well be the most searching and fundamental problem that faces not only ethicists but society as a whole," he announces that the search is really over: "The more rationally contrived and deliberate anything is, the more human it is." This is at best ambiguous and at worst a distortion of the human. Rational control, it is true, is a distinctive achievement of man. But he can use this rationality in inhuman ways. Deliberation and rationality tell us only that a human being is acting, not that he is acting humanly. One can, with utter control and deliberateness, do the most monstrously inhuman things. The Third Reich showed us how. Theology has always known that sin, by definition, is a deliberate, rational, controlled choice—but the most inhuman of acts. Rational control, therefore, is not the guarantor of humane choices but only the condition of their possibility. What happens to man in and as a result of his rationality and deliberate choices tells us whether these choices were more or less human, more or less desirable.

Similarly, Fletcher has argued that "if the greatest good of the greatest number . . . were served by it," he would approve cloning, bioengineering of parahumans, etc. This remains an "unexamined premise" in several senses. (1) Have we not repeatedly experienced the fact that the greatest good of the greatest number, unassailable as it might be as a theoretical criterion, is practically the warrant for present practices and policies that all but guarantee that this greatest good will not be served? (2) How is the social good to be spelled out even if we accept it as a goal? Who makes the determination? On what basis? (3) How would laboratory reproduction, cloning, etc., serve it? True, Fletcher has said "if," but his failure to confront the serious—indeed, decisive—problems buried in this "if" means that for him proportionate good too easily translates into "anything to get the job done." He seems not to suspect that it just might be more human to exist with volcanic threats or pollution than to create parahumans to help us overcome these things. It is possible, after all, that by engineering the engineer we would become very competent barbarians. Not to raise such an issue is, in a sense, to have solved it. The editorial page of a subsequent issue of the prestigious *New England Journal of Medicine* carried a (by and large favorable) commentary on Fletcher by Bernard D. Davis, M.D.[9] At one point Davis notes: "One therefore wishes that Dr. Fletcher had discussed the conflicting interests and values that lie at the heart of ethical problems." Exactly.

Finally, the rhetorical *non sequiturs*. Fletcher informs us that in view of the new biomedical achievements "we are going to have to change or alter our old ideas about who or what a father is, or a mother, or a family." Here it must be said that we *have to* change these notions only if what *can* be done biomedically *ought* to be done humanly. Fletcher has given us no persuasive reasons why these things ought to be done, because he has not seriously examined what would happen to the doers in the process. For this reason his "have to change" is an unwitting but two-handed surrender to the scientific imperative. The contention here, then, is not precisely that Fletcher is a consequentialist, but rather that he has provided us with no grounds for thinking that he is a good one.

Deontological Attitude

Paul Ramsey and Leon Kass can be taken as examples of the second approach. The writings of Princeton's Ramsey are about as contrary to Fletcher as it is possible to be. If there is a practical issue in moral theology, the chances are that Ramsey has been there digging, sorting, and giving forth with his version of Christian wisdom ahead of the pack. There is, it can be said, hardly

[9] See footnote 4 above. For other reactions to Fletcher's article, see *New England Journal of Medicine*, 286 (1972), 48–50.

anyone who has not learned a good deal from him. It must also be said that there is hardly anyone who has not snapped at Ramsey's pedagogical hand in the process, a point verified by the recent literature on biomedicine.

Ramsey's weighing of the issues raised by the new biology draws heavily on two basic principles.[10] First, there is the "nature of human parenthood." Human parenthood demands that the spheres of procreation and marital love not be separated. This means that we may not procreate apart from a context of responsibility for procreation. Repeatedly Ramsey asserts that the inseparability of these two spheres is human parenthood "as it came to us from the Creator,"[11] that we dare not put asunder "what God joined together in creation."[12] On this score alone he rejects AID (donor insemination), cloning, reproduction *in vitro*.[13]

His second basic principle concerns the difference between therapy and experimentation. It might be formulated as follows: We may never submit another human being to experimental procedures to which he cannot consent when these procedures have no relation to his own treatment. On this basis Ramsey believes that we could never *morally* get to know how to do certain things (for example, cloning) because the very first attempt would have the character of an experiment on the child to be. Thus he says:

> Because we ought not to choose for a child—whose procreation we are contemplating—the injury he may bear, there is no way by which we can *morally* get to know whether many things now planned are technically feasible or not. We need not ask whether we should clone a man or not, or what use is to be made of frozen semen

---

[10] Paul Ramsey, *Fabricated Man* (New Haven, Conn.: Yale University Press, 1970).

[11] Ibid., 124.

[12] Ibid., 38.

[13] Ramsey approves of AIH in a sterile marriage (p. 112). How this is consistent with his basic principle is somewhat hazy. He writes: "Their response to what God joined together . . . would be expressed by their resolve to hold *acts* of procreation . . . within the sphere of *acts* of conjugal love, within the covenant of marriage" (p. 36). AIH is certainly an act of procreation, and it is certainly within the covenant of marriage; but that it is "within the sphere of *acts* of conjugal love" is far from clear. Perhaps Ramsey stated his principle poorly here.

or ovum banks, or what sort of life we ought to create in hatcheries, etc., since we can *begin* to perfect these techniques in no other way than by subjecting another human being to risks to which he cannot consent as our coadventurer in promoting medical or scientific "progress."[14]

Similarly it is the distinction between therapy and experimentation that governs Ramsey's whole treatment of genetic surgery. Such treatment on an existing child, however drastic, is permissible if it does "not place the child at greater risk than now surrounds him as one of a specially endangered population." Here we are dealing with therapy. Where there is question, however, of an as yet unconceived child, Ramsey is rightly much more demanding. There would have to be *no discernible risks* in prospective genetic surgery before one could procreate a child likely to be burdened with Huntington's chorea, PKU, amaurotic idiocy, etc. Until such time as corrective genetic surgery is risk-free, the proper prevention of these diseases is "continence, not getting married to a particular person, not having any children, using three contraceptives at once, or sterilization." Any other procedure would be tantamount to illicit experimentation with human beings. Ramsey's study constantly returns to these two basic principles.

Ramsey's analysis is well informed, precise, and searching, even if frequently repetitious. Furthermore, one wishes that he were more successful in resisting the titillations of his own obiter dicta and neologisms. These more purple than persuasive asides simply blunt his theological punches. This being said, I would say that I find myself very close to nearly all of Ramsey's value judgments.[15] For this reason it is all the more important to raise several issues that seem to call for further attention.

[14] Ibid., 134.
[15] I say "nearly all" because I cannot agree with Ramsey that "we cannot rightfully *get to know* how to do this [use an artificial placenta] without conducting unethical experiments upon the unborn" (p. 113). If a pregnant woman with a nonviable fetus is dying and the only even remote hope of bringing her otherwise doomed child to term is an artificial placenta, I would think it legitimate—as therapy, not experimentation, or at least not exclusively experimentation.

First there is the manner of argument where Ramsey's two controlling principles are concerned. The first (the nature of parenthood as involving inseparability of the two spheres of love and procreation) he views as parenthood "as it comes to us from the Creator." He draws upon the Prologue of St. John and Ephesians 5 as loci where this divine plan is made clear.

> The Prologue of John's gospel (not Genesis) is the Christian story of creation which provides the source and standard for responsible procreation, even as Ephesians 5 contains the ultimate reference for the meaning and nature of conjugal love and the standard governing covenants of marriage. Since these two passages point to one and the same Lord—the Lord who presides over procreation as well as the Lord of all marital covenants—the two aspects of sexuality belong together.[16]

Ramsey contrasts this nature-of-parenthood perspective with a method that would weigh AID (etc.) in terms of consequences.

Perhaps Ramsey is right. But the question can be raised whether the two approaches are that different, a point suggested in the discussion of Fletcher's work. Ramsey is equivalently saying that there are some principles that hold no matter what the consequences. Others might argue that the principles have been arrived at and do indeed hold precisely because of the intolerable consequences. Specifically, Ramsey seems to say that the two spheres of sexuality are inseparable because God made them this way and told us so. Others would say that they are inseparable because to separate them would dehumanize us and *for this reason* we may say that God has joined them. It seems to me that Ramsey is not clear on how he derives this principle (and therefore, by implication, other principles). He seems to gather it from a reflective reading of Scripture and contrasts this with a consequentialist procedure. Yet over and over again he states it consequentially.

For instance, while discussing cloning Ramsey states: "The conquest of evolution by setting sexual love and procreation radically asunder entails depersonalization in the extreme. The entire ra-

16 Ibid., 37.

tionalization of procreation—its replacement by replication—can only mean the abolition of man's embodied personhood."[17] I agree, but is it not precisely because of these effects (alienation, depersonalization) that the statement is valid? We see more deeply into these things from John's Prologue and Ephesians 5, but the conclusion is not drawn independently of a consideration of effects or consequences, unless one has a very narrow notion of consequences.[18] Rather is it not precisely consequences that lead us to this conclusion? The dominating effect or consequence is the depersonalization of man, and this simply overrides any long-term eugenic goals. Therefore it is far from clear that Ramsey should speak of his principle as valid independently of consequences.

To say that a certain procedure is depersonalizing or dehumanizing demands, of course, both some notion of the *humanum* and the predictable effects on the *humanum* of prospective procedures. I shall return to this shortly.

Ramsey's second principle (the immorality of experimentation without consent) raises a somewhat similar problem. In *The Patient as Person* he has argued—dealing explicitly with infants—that the reason for this conclusion is that such experimental procedures make an "object" of an individual. In these cases, he contends, the parents cannot consent for the individual. Consent is the heart of the matter. If the parents could legitimately consent for the child, then presumably experimental procedures would not make an object of the infant and would be permissible. Therefore the basic question is: Why cannot the parents provide consent for the child? Why is their consent considered null here while it is accepted when procedures are therapeutic? To say that the child would be treated as an object does not answer this question; it presupposes the answer and announces it under this formulation.

As was noted earlier, adults may donate an organ to another

---

[17] Ibid., 89. Ramsey reveals a similar approach in many places. For instance, on cloning, he says it would not be right "because of its massive assaults upon human freedom and its grave violation of the respect due to men and women now alive and to human parenthood as such" (p. 61). Again, speaking of the separation of procreation and marital love, he notes: "Herein men usurp dominion over the human—the dominion they hold rightfully only over the animals. This is bound to pierce the heart of the *humanum* in sex, marriage and generation" (p. 88).

[18] By "consequences" I include two things: the immediate entailments or implications of an action, and the more mediate aftereffects.

(*inter vivos*) precisely because their personal good is not to be conceived individualistically, but socially—that is, there is a natural order to other human persons that is in the very notion of the human personality itself. The personal being and good of an individual do have a relationship to the being and good of others, difficult as it may be to keep this in a balanced perspective. For this reason, an individual can become (in carefully delimited circumstances) more fully a person by donation of an organ; for by communicating to another of his very being he has more fully integrated himself into the mysterious unity between person and person.

Must not something analogous be said of experimentation for the good of others? It can be an affirmation of one's solidarity and Christian concern for others (through the advancement of medicine), though it is easy to be naïve about the dangers and abuses of this idea. Becoming an experimental subject *can involve* any or all of three things: some degree of risk (at least of complications), pain, associated inconvenience (for example, prolonging the hospital stay, delaying recovery, etc.). To accept these for the good of others could be an act of charitable concern.

If these reflections are true of adults, must not the same be said of infants and children insofar as they are human persons? Therefore, precisely why is parental consent illegitimate in their case? Or perhaps more sharply, the parents' consent to therapy directed at the child's own good is both required and sufficient because it is the closest we can come to a *reasonable presumption of the child's wishes*. The fact that the therapy or surgery is for the child's good could be but a single example of a reasonable presumption of the child's wishes. Are there others? According to Ramsey, no. But I wonder. Above (pp. 51–71) I have stated a different approach, its rationale, and its ethical controls.

But we may not stop here. Since the individual has the right to make for himself decisions that involve risk, or pain, or notable inconvenience—a right that invalidates any presumption of his wishes—then he has a right to be protected against any possible violations of such a right, any dangers to it. It is here that one might argue the possible absoluteness of the personal-consent requirement—that is, our times are times of eager scientific research, enthusiastic eugenic ambitions, strong if subtle collectivistic tendencies, and growing impersonalization of health care. Thus it could be argued that we have a cultural situation with a built-in escalatory tendency to expose nonconsenting persons to violations of their rights. This means that there is a real danger of exceeding those limits to which the infant, for example, could be *reasonably* presumed to consent. He has a right to be protected against such a danger.

This danger is not sufficiently removed, it could be further argued, by the protections of parental consent, because this consent itself is in our day too often unstable and vulnerable to many noxious influences. Therefore, putting the nonconsenting person simply out of bounds where pure experimentation is concerned *might* be the only way to hold the delicate relation of individual to society in proper balance. I say "might" because if these dangers could be countered, then it would seem that some experimentation might be a reasonable presumption of the child's consent. If so, then this reasonableness would provide the basis for validating parental consent.

At this point it must be said parenthetically that in these matters it is always better to err, if err one must, on the side of conservatism. Hence if there is any doubt about the validity of these reflections, the personal-consent requirement should be viewed as a practical absolute. More specifically, whether there is any risk, pain, or inconvenience involved is a matter that cannot be left exclusively in the hands of medical researchers. The terrible examples in M. H. Pappworth's *Human Guinea Pigs* make this clear. Some of the researchers regard as "trivial" or "routine" procedures the ordinary patient would, with good reason, view as seriously bothersome and notably risky. Because a complication can be handled by subsequent therapy does not mean it is no longer a complication. Medical technology can dazzle us into distorted human judgments.

The approach proposed here moves away a bit from the absoluteness of Ramsey's analysis, though not necessarily from the absoluteness of his conclusions. Ramsey's analysis must conclude that *any* experimentation, even the most trifling and insignificant such as a buccal smear, on nonconsenting persons is beyond the reach of parental consent because it involves us in "treating another as an object." Perhaps. But this latter seems to be a rhetorical way of formulating a judgment concluded on other grounds.[19] I have suggested that we might approach the morality of risk-free, pain-free, inconvenience-free experimentation, rare as such experiments might be, through the notion of reasonable presumption of the child's wishes. In other words, is it not possible that the inviolability against all experimentation (if we ought to maintain such inviolability) of those incapable of consent is only a relatively necessary conclusion of human prudence rather than of intrinsic morality? At least I believe the question must be examined further.

The writings of Leon Kass reveal moral tendencies and judgments very close to those of Ramsey. For this reason Kass would probably fall into Fletcher's apriorist pigeonhole. In his major writings Kass realistically limits himself to the two questions that have some practicality in the future: *in vitro* fertilization (with eventual uterine implantation) and cloning.[20]

As for the first, its least controversial use will be the provision of their own child to a sterile couple. At first glance the intramarital use of artificial fertilization seems to resemble ethically AIH (artificial insemination by the husband). But Kass raises two moral objections. First, the implantation of the embryo fertilized *in vitro* involves the hazards of deformity and malformation. These hazards are being imposed nontherapeutically on a child-to-be without his consent. This, Kass argues, "provides a powerful moral objection sufficient to rebut the implantation experiments." Second, discarding unimplanted embryos raises another problem. Kass is undecided as to whether we are dealing with a protectable

[19] That Ramsey himself might agree with this and the underlying method is suggested by his attitude toward exceptional instances in situations of consent. He notes: "In the grave moral matters . . . a physician is more liable to make an error in moral judgment if he adopts a policy of holding himself open to the possibility that there may be significant, future permissions to ignore the principle of consent than he is if he holds this requirement of an informed consent always relevant and applicable" (*The Patient as Person* [New Haven, Conn.: Yale University Press, 1970], 9).

[20] Leon R. Kass, "Making Babies—the New Biology and the 'Old' Morality," *The Public Interest*, 26 (Winter 1972), 18–56. This long study is nearly identical with Kass's "New Beginnings in Life," an occasional paper privately published by the Hastings Center (Institute of Society, Ethics, and the Life Sciences), n.d. See also Leon R. Kass, "The New Biology: What Price Relieving Man's Estate?" *Science*, 174 (1971), 779–88, and his "What Price the Perfect Baby?" *Science*, 173 (1971), 103–4.

humanity at this (blastocyst) stage, but we certainly will be at a later state and therefore "had better force the question now and draw whatever lines need to be drawn." Apart from these objections, Kass finds no *intrinsic* reason to reject *in vitro* fertilization and implantation. But the argument must not stop here. A procedure possibly unobjectionable in itself makes possible other procedures. This is not an "argument from abuse." Rather he insists on

> the fact that one technical advance makes possible the next and in more than one respect. The first serves as a precedent for the second, the second for the third—not just technologically but also in moral arguments. At least one good humanitarian reason can be found to justify each step. Into the solemn and hallowed tent of human sexuality and procreation, the camel's nose has led the camel's neck and may someday soon, perhaps, even lead the camel's spermatozoa.[21]

I suspect Pius XII had something like this in mind when he condemned AIH.

As for cloning, Kass again raises the twin issues of production and disposition of defectives and contends with Ramsey that they "provide sufficient moral grounds for rebutting any first attempt to clone a man." He further urges the serious psychological problems of identity and individuality and finds them "sufficient to reject even the first attempts at human cloning."[22]

Kass eventually goes beyond this piece-by-piece approach and brings a broader cultural analysis to bear on the two questions. Here his writing is most powerful and persuasive. He argues that "increasing control over the product is purchased by the increasing depersonalization of the process" and that this depersonalization is dehumanizing. Against Fletcher's contentions he would insist that "human procreation is not simply an activity of our rational wills . . . it is more complete human activity precisely because it engages us bodily and spiritually, as well as rationally."[23]

---

21 "Making Babies," 38–39. The last sentence of the citation occurs only in the earlier ("New Beginnings in Life") version. Either his frivolity annoyed the editor of *Public Interest*, or Kass waxed formal when he went public.
22 Ibid., 45.
23 Ibid., 48–49.

The separation of reproduction from human sexuality Kass sees as a dehumanizing threat to the existence of marriage and the human family. "Transfer of procreation to the laboratory undermines the justification and support which biological parenthood gives to the monogamous (or even polygamous) marriage. Cloning adds an additional, more specific, and more fundamental threat: The technique renders males obsolete. All it requires are human eggs, nuclei, and (for the time being) uteri; all three can be supplied by women."[24]

Kass's concern for the family is not blind institutionalism. Rather he is concerned that "the family is rapidly becoming the only institution in an increasingly impersonal world where each person is loved not for what he does or makes, but simply because he is. The family is also the institution where most of us, both as children and as parents, acquire a sense of continuity with the past and a sense of commitment to the future."[25] For these and other reasons Kass urges that "when we lack sufficient wisdom to do, wisdom consists in not doing." He is sharply critical of theologians-turned-technocrats (for example, Karl Rahner[26]) whose no-

[24] Ibid., 50.

[25] Ibid., 51.

[26] The reference to Rahner is to "Experiment: Man," *Theology Digest*, 16 (1968), 57–69. (See "Experiment Mensch: Theologisches über die Selbstmanipulation des Menschen," *Schriften zur Theologie*, 8 [Einsiedeln: Benziger, 1967], 260–85.) Rahner's position is not accurately presented if it is drawn from "Experiment: Man" alone. His "Zum Problem der genetischen Manipulation," *Schriften zur Theologie*, 8, 286–321, must also be read. In this latter essay Rahner develops positions very close to those of Ramsey and Kass, and manifests a deep skepticism, even negativism, where eugenic genetic manipulation is concerned. He insists, for example, that not everything that can be done ought to be done (p. 318). In applying this to donor insemination, Rahner argues that personal sexual love has an essential relationship to the child; for the child is the expression and realization of the abiding unity of the spouses. But "genetic manipulation does two things. First it separates on principle the procreation of a new person (as the abiding expression of the love union of the spouses) from marital union. Second, it transfers procreation (sundered and separated from its human source) outside of the human sphere of intimacy" (p. 313). That Rahner would reject this is obvious. Furthermore, he speaks repeatedly of resisting "the temptation of the possible" and calls "immunity against the fascination of the newly possible" a virtue contemporary man must develop, and apply in the area of genetic manipulation. One of Rahner's major concerns is how his basic "no" to some of these possibilities can be made persuasive amid the existing moral pluralism. The Ramsey-Kass criticism of Rahner is, therefore, not only misleading in itself; it also *seems* to provide the support of a great theological name for utopian schemes and eugenic experiments that Rahner would resolutely disown.

tion of man as "freedom-event" provides no standards by which to measure whether self-modifying changes are in fact improvements. Those unfamiliar with Kass will find his writings both enlightening and entertaining. Charles H. Stinson of Dartmouth College demurs.[27] He takes a rather dim view of the attitudes and analyses of Ramsey-Kass. He sees both of them as biomedical pessimists. Behind Kass's pessimism he finds a body-soul dualism that contends: If mental-spiritual life is not a "separate entity" beyond genetic manipulation, it is somehow not as true as we had thought. Behind Ramsey's outlook Stinson sees a faulty theology of creation "which assumes that God *intended* certain aspects of natural structures and forces to remain *always* beyond the control of man's intelligence." Stinson then repeats in a variety of ways what he mistakenly takes to be a counterstatement to Ramsey-Kass: Increased empirical knowledge about the processes of life need not erode its divine meaningfulness. On the basis of such general assertions and the conviction that sooner or later we will be involved in "the socially regulated cloning of individuals," Stinson opts for the Rahnerian view that man's limitless power to experiment on himself is really a sign of the creaturely freedom given him by God.

Granted that the writings of both Ramsey and Kass do at times achieve liturgical fervor and leave them vulnerable to the accusation of both overstatement and pessimism, still Stinson's essay, interesting as it is, meets the serious issues they raise with little more than a gathering of evasions and begged questions.

Item: "No doubt, as Ramsey points out, accidental miscalculations and ignorance of variables will result in fetal monstrosities. Not a pretty picture to contemplate. Moreover, there will inevitably be abuses of power on the part of a small minority of insensitive or rash scientists and technicians. But are we to conclude that, because of its *risks* and possible abuses, all such work is intrinsically immoral?"[28] Since when is the certain ("no doubt") production of fetal monstrosities reducible to a mere risk? Ramsey may be wrong, but to talk of bench-made monstrosities as "risks" is hardly a persuasive way of showing it.

[27] Charles Stinson, "Theology and the Baron Frankenstein: Cloning and Beyond," *Christian Century*, 89 (1972), 60–63.
[28] Ibid., 60.

Item: "Ramsey's outlook is grounded . . . in a faulty theology of creation which assumes that God *intended* certain aspects of natural structures and forces to remain *always* beyond the control of man's intelligence."[29] Ramsey claims nothing of the kind. He does, indeed, argue (not "assume") that God intended certain aspects of natural structures as permanent, but he would insist that this is not to put them "beyond the control of man's intelligence"; it is only to say that certain controls may not be intelligent.

Item: "And why would a cloned human being not feel himself (or herself) to be a 'person' or 'embodied'? Possibly for a number of reasons, but Ramsey does not specify any."[30] To which two things must be said. First, when Ramsey refers to cloning as involving "the abolition of embodied personhood," he need not and does not refer primarily to the feelings of the cloned product, but to the parents and their concept of parenthood. Second, he does indeed with Kass specify reasons about the feelings of the cloned human being.[31]

Item: "Let me hazard a key theological concept for the future: It is the ongoing content of human life that is spiritually significant—not its origin whether natural or artificial."[32] Comment: It is precisely the Ramsey-Kass point that artificial origin will affect the "ongoing content of human life." One must wrestle with this contention if one is to meet Ramsey-Kass where they are.

Item: "This feat [the first cloning of a man] would certainly not invalidate Ramsey's ethical norms but it would make them irrelevant speculatively."[33] Does the first use of the atomic bomb make it speculatively irrelevant to urge this question: "Should we ever have done it?"? If such a question is utterly urgent—as it is— then the more urgent question is: "Should we do it?" Our mistakes of the past should teach us at least to take these earlier questions more seriously—unless one wants to hold the disastrous view that we can learn only from our mistakes.

[29] Ibid., 61.
[30] Ibid.
[31] Ramsey, *Fabricated Man*, 71–72.
[32] Stinson, "Theology and the Baron Frankenstein," 63.
[33] Ibid., 62.

Item: Of genetics a hundred years hence, Stinson notes: "And this will *no doubt* include the socially regulated cloning of individuals who are deemed to be especially valuable to the community."[34] Here, I believe, is the real and ultimate pessimism: Because we *can* do, we certainly *will* do. Is there a better way to render any present ethical reflection irrelevant than to think it really makes no difference anyway, and therefore to reduce the issue to: "What shall we do after we have cloned men?"?

Mediating Approach

James Gustafson and Charles Curran are examples of the third approach. A methodology midway between the rather structureless utilitarian calculus of Fletcher and the Ramsey-Kass insistence on the absolute immorality of some means is that of Gustafson. Under a nine-point division Gustafson lays out the many ethical issues in biomedicine.[35] Repeatedly he sets up groups of alternative approaches, states the warrants for them, unravels their latent presuppositions, and notes the questions they raise.

For instance, in perhaps the most substantive sections of his study, Gustafson approaches genetic medicine from the contrasting positions of inviolable individual rights and the benefits that might accrue to others and to society in general. He proposes three contrasting options: (1) The rights of individuals are sacred and primary and therefore under no circumstances are they to be violated in favor of benefits to others. (2) Anticipated consequences judged in terms of the "good" that will be achieved or the "evil" avoided ought to determine policy and action regardless of the restrictions on individual rights that this might require. (3) Both (1) and (2) are one-sided. Decisions require consideration both of individual rights and of benefits to others. One of the two will be the base line, the other will function as the principle justifying exceptions to the base line.

It is clear that Gustafson would opt for the third alternative, indeed for third alternatives in nearly every case where opposing methods or stances have been proposed. Thus, as between "re-

---

[34] Ibid.
[35] James M. Gustafson, "Basic Ethical Issues in the Biomedical Fields," *Soundings*, 53 (1970), 151–80.

stricting the kinds of experimentation that will be permitted through civil legislation . . . and clearly defined moral rules" and "ensuring the maximum possible freedom for research," Gustafson goes for a bit of both: maintaining maximum possible freedom but at the same time formulating principles and values that provide guidelines for procedures and for the uses of research. Similarly, he values summary rules but is uncomfortable with absolute rules. Or again, he argues that "the value of human physical life is primary" but this does not "entail that no other values or rights might override the right to bodily life." He wants societal benefits to count in genetic decisions, but not at all costs, just as he wants individual rights to be respected, but not at all costs. And so on.

What I believe Gustafson is doing is trying to hold in balance or bring to terms two intransigent elements of moral discourse: the complexity of reality, yet the abiding need to attempt to bring our decisions under objective rational scrutiny if our moral policies are to remain truly human. These two elements constantly surface as Gustafson's profound concerns. Equivalently he is suggesting that moral reasoning is neither as fixed and rational as Ramsey would sometimes lead us to believe, nor as shapeless and arbitrary as Fletcher's writing suggests.

Where does this leave Gustafson? With a goal and with a means to it. The goal is the counsel that for man the experimenter and intervener "the chief task is to develop with both sensitivity and clarity an understanding of the qualities or values of human life and a conception of the basic human rights that will provide the moral guidelines or touchstones for human development."[36] That is why Gustafson's recent work has been concerned with the "normatively human." The means: ongoing, rigorous conversation between those who best pose ethical questions and those who are shaping development in the biomedical field.

Gustafson's study—subtle, sensitive, sophisticated—resolutely avoids the blandishments of the shock statement and asks all the right questions. But there is one aspect of his approach that seems at least incomplete, even dissatisfying. For instance, he states that

[36] Ibid., 178.

while the right to physical life is primary, "this would not entail
that no other values or rights might ever override the rights to
bodily life. . . ." Thus he endorses an "ordering which gives *some*
guidance in particular decisions." Precisely at this point it is necessary to say what these other values and rights might be and why
they may be said to override the primary right.

Similarly, in dealing with biomedical procedures, Gustafson
says that both individual rights and societal benefits must be considered. One of the two is the base line, the other functions as a
principle justifying exceptions. Thus he says: "It might well be
that under certain circumstances it is morally responsible to make
the thrust of individual rights the base line, and under other circumstances the accounting of benefits." What are these circumstances? What is the criterion to make individual rights decisive in some instances, social benefits decisive in others? Until we
know this, Gustafson's middle position is incomplete and fails to
provide even "some guidance." It represents more a rejection of
the opposing alternatives than a satisfying synthesis of the two.

This point should be urged because of its further implications.
Let me put it this way. To say that there are overriding values
without stating what they might be, to state that there are circumstances in which the base-line priority shifts *without stating what
they might be,* is to do two things: (1) to empty the notions of
"primary" and "base line" of most of their significance for decision-making; (2) to suggest that these overriding values can be discovered only in individual decision. I do not think that these are
true. What Gustafson wants (and rightly) to say is that rational
moral discourse is limited, and that there comes a point when the
complexity of reality leads us beyond the formulations of traditional wisdom. That, I think, is true. And I believe that we have
always known it, even though we have not always admitted it. But
where that point is located is very important. Failure to specify at
least some of the values that can override a primary value or right
all too easily suggests that there is no point to which rational deliberation can lead us, that we cannot specify these values, and
that this can only be done in individual decisions. Does this not
remove moral discourse in principle from objective and rational
scrutiny? Gustafson does not want this, not at all. But how his ad-

mirable pastoral[37] sensitivities do not find their way to this theological cul-de-sac I fail to see.

I urge this point with a fear and trembling born of unqualified admiration for Gustafson's remarkable talents and work, of fear that the question may reflect my own overrationalization of the moral life, of the conviction that he as well as, and probably better than, any theological ethician on the American scene can bring light to those aspects of these remarks that hover in darkness.

Charles Curran states that moral theology, in facing biomedical problems, must proceed from a historical point of view, emphasize the societal aspects of the issues, and accept the self-creative power as a gift of equal importance with creatureliness.[38]

As for historical consciousness, we need a more "open" concept of man. For example, where Ramsey rejects Muller's eugenic proposals because they separate procreation and marital love, Curran agrees but believes that "the teaching Ramsey finds in Ephesians 5 might also be historically conditioned."

Similarly, in the past we were guilty of an individualist reading of the principle of totality. The task of contemporary moralists is to do justice to the social, cosmic aspects of man without falling into collectivism. Contemporary genetic possibilities force on us a realization of responsibilities beyond the individual.

Third, where the question of man's dominion is concerned, we must hold in tension man's greatness and creatureliness. Curran does not believe that Ramsey grants man enough dominion, just as he would believe that Fletcher uncritically grants him too much. Ramsey's one-sidedness Curran traces to an eschatology developed only in terms of apocalypse (discontinuity between this world and the next). Eschatology, Curran insists, must include three elements: the apocalyptical, the prophetic, and the teleological. After shaking and mixing these three ingredients, he ends with an eschatology where man's final stage is not totally con-

---

[37] I use the word "pastoral" because I wonder to what extent Gustafson is lifting the anguish of personal decision (to which, of course, it is all too easy to become insensitive) into a larger sphere of moral policy and general moral reasoning.

[38] Charles Curran, "Theology and Genetics: A Multifaceted Dialogue," *Journal of Ecumenical Studies*, 7 (1970), 61–89. (This also appeared as "Moral Theology and Genetics" in *Cross Currents*, 20 [1970], 64–82.)

tinuous with man's present existence (against the utopians) and
not totally discontinuous with it (against the apocalyptic likes of
Ramsey).

On the basis of these broad strokes Curran emerges with a position that states on the one hand that "there are importrant
human values which would stand in the way of the geneticist on
some occasions" (for example, adhering to the bond between procreation and marital union), and on the other that "one can en-
vision certain historical situations in which this bond *might be
sacrificed for greater values*" (emphasis added).[39]

The italicized words are interesting, for they indicate two
things: (1) Curran's basic position is very close to that of Ramsey
and Kass; (2) Curran's basic position is held on consequentialist
grounds. This latter seems clear even against Curran's explicit denial, because if a value is "sacrificed for greater values," clearly a
calculus model is operative. This leads one to force a question on
Curran that his essay does not satisfactorily answer: *Why* hold in
the first place that the spheres of procreation and marital love
must in our historical time be held together? Ramsey gets this
from a reflective reading of Scripture, the kind of argument Curran would reject as ahistorical and eventually deontological. Yet
he also rejects the more experiential (consequentialist) model.
What is left?

Curran's essay, like Gustafson's, is a helpful "both-and" balancing act, but at a different level—the level of broad cultural contrasts (for example, between the narrowly scientific and the fully
human, the utopian and the pessimistic, etc.). Ultimately, however, it finesses several of the hard questions and is less than complete in analyzing its own methodological presuppositions.

Thus far some recent moral literature; now to a concluding personal reflection. The two most commonly discussed issues seem to
be fertilization *in vitro* and cloning.[40] The first is upon us, and the

[39] Ibid., 83.
[40] Though with regard to *in vitro* fertilization several variations must be
weighed distinctly for their differences: (1) with husband's seed or donor's;
(2) with implantation in wife's uterus or someone else's; (3) with no implantation but use of artificial placenta, etc.—a development apparently rather
far off. For differing views on *in vitro* fertilization, see *Medical-Moral Newsletter*, 8 (Mar.–Apr. 1972), entire issue, and *Hastings Center Report*, 2 (Feb.
1972), 1–3.

second is possibly only decades away, though expert opinions differ about this. Furthermore, many of the moral issues in the more distant and exotic possibilities are essentially present in these problems. In both instances Ramsey and Kass have seen a serious issue in the production and destruction of embryos. I do too, though I am not certain of the exact way the issue should be formulated. But given the cultural attitudes now prevalent toward fetal life, I have little confidence that these points will be taken very seriously by most biotechnicians. In one sense, of course, this is all the more reason for raising them. However, because the discussion surrounding production and disposition of the "failures" to some extent suggests that in other respects we should go ahead and that "artificial children" are desirable if these objections can be met, the more basic moral issue strikes earlier. It is that of marriage and the family.

Briefly, I am in deep sympathy with the views of Ramsey-Kass and (less explicitly) Curran that these procedures are inimical to marriage and the family (Ramsey says the "nature of parenthood") and that therefore in terms of their immediate implications and foreseeable effects we should not take such steps (nor *allow* them to be taken, since a public good of the first order is involved) unless a value the equivalent of survival demands it.

If there is, among the eugenic dreams and apocalyptic fears surrounding biomedical technology, a single certainty, it is this: *In vitro* fertilization and cloning do factually debiologize marriage and the family. Ramsey and Kass have argued that this is depersonalizing and dehumanizing. I believe they are right, and for two reasons.

First, by removing the origin of the child from the sphere of specifically marital (bodily, sexual) love, that love itself is subtly redefined in a way that deflates the sexual and bodily and its pertinence to human love, and therefore to the human itself. The artificially produced child can obviously be the result of a loving decision, even a deeply loving one; just as obviously it can be loved, cared for, and protected within the family. And precisely for these reasons is it quite valid to say that this child is the "product of marital love." But at this point that term has undergone a change, a change that has to some extent debiologized and "debodified" the word "marital." The term has moved a step away from its full bodily and therefore *human* connotations. Man is everything we say of him: freedom, reason, body, emotions. He is the sum of his parts. To reduce his humanity to any one of these or, what is the same, to suppress any one of these from his humanity is dehumanizing. And that is what is happening here.[41]

Second, moving procreation into the laboratory "undermines the justification and support which biological parenthood gives to the monogamous marriage," as Kass puts it. In other words, the family as we know it is basically (not exclusively or eminently) a biological unit. To weaken the biological link is to untie the family at its root and therefore to undermine it. That this is dehumanizing and depersonalizing depends entirely on what one thinks of the family (or Kass's monogamous marriage).

The family, I would argue, embodies the ordinary conditions wherein we (parents, children, and others) learn to become persons. In the stable, permanent man-woman relationship we possess the chance to bring libido and eros to the maturity of *philia* (friendship). Through monogamous marriage we experience the basic (not the only) form of human love and caring, and learn thereby to take gradual possession of our own capacity to relate in love. That is why marriage is a sacrament: It is the human stuff eminently capable of mirroring God's own covenant-fidelity, His love. It is the ordinary societal condition of our coming to learn about responsibility, tenderness, fidelity, patience, the meaning of our own sexuality, etc. Without its nourishing presence in our midst, we gamble with our best hope for growth and dignity, our chances of learning what it means to love and be loved. For those created by and in the image of a loving God, and therefore destined to a consummation in this image, such a gamble is humanly suicidal. To undermine the family in any way would be to compromise the ordinary conditions of our own growth as persons, and that is dehumanizing.

Obviously marriages (and families) fail (as I noted in Chapter 2). And just as obviously the surrogate arrangements that pick up the pieces of our weakness, failure, and irresponsibility can and do succeed. Furthermore, it seems undeniable that the contemporary shape of family life cries out for restructuring if monogamous

---

[41] See Rahner, "Zum Problem der genetischen Manipulation," 313.

marriage is to survive, grow, and realize its true potential. But these facts do not negate the basic necessity of the monogamously structured family for human growth. They only say that it is worth criticizing vigorously because it is worth saving.

These reflections are not likely to be very persuasive to a culture that, it can be argued, is comfort-bent, goal-oriented, technologically sophisticated, sexually trivialized, and deeply secularized. But if they are true, they suggest that the moral theological analysis of the biomedical problems discussed in these pages must attend much more than it has to a Christian critique of the culture that not only generates such remarkable possibilities but above all shapes our reflection about them.

16. Ethics and Reproductive Interventions

In 1978, the world focused intense attention on Oldham, a town in northwestern England. At Oldham and District General Hospital on July 25, Lesley Brown gave birth to a baby girl fertilized *in vitro* with the sperm of her husband, Gilbert John Brown, through the efforts of Dr. Patrick Steptoe and physiologist Robert Edwards (Cambridge University). There is no doubt that this represents a stunning medical breakthrough. For until now the complicated process, especially of timing, of embryo transfer after laboratory culture has proved a stumbling block to physicians attempting to overcome the sterility associated with oviduct blockage.

But are such technological achievements necessarily steps forward? If there is a nagging uneasiness in the minds of many, what is its source? Or, more positively, if one responds to such brilliant technological feats with sheer exhilaration, is that perhaps premature? Perhaps uncritical? However one answers these questions, one thing is clear: The bottom line on *in vitro* fertilization is ethical, for the introduction of sophisticated technology into the fertilization-pregnancy process can touch sensitively on some basic human values: parenthood, the family, human sexuality. That being the case, it is a fairly safe bet that we shall see the resurrection of some quite weary arguments about tampering with nature or not tampering with it, about "playing God," about the "natural" and the "unnatural," about ends justifying means, about the purpose of faculties, and so on. Most such generalizations are tried and untrue, at least as they are so often used. They serve above all as slogan-summaries of one's value commitments. They do not argue and enlighten those commitments.

In this chapter I should like to detail some recent ethical reflection on the subject of *in vitro* fertilization and reproductive interventions in general.

The term "reproductive interventions" must be properly limited before its ethical dimensions are set forth. To be excluded under this title are abortion, contraception, delivery (including Caesarean sections, induced labor), amniocentesis, therapeutic interventions for mother or child (for example, ectopic pregnancies), and genetic counseling and screening. All of these legitimately qualify as "reproductive interventions" in the broadest sense of that term. Indeed, even the legal requirements of age and of registration for the mating couple, for a change in partners, or for the offspring can be called reproductive interventions.

The meaning of "reproductive interventions." The term "reproductive interventions" will be limited here to all procedures that replace, in part or totally, the natural (by sexual intercourse) process of conception and of *in utero* gestation. Practically this would include (1) artificial insemination (homologous when the insemination is from the husband's semen [AIH] and heterologous when the insemination is from a donor [AID]), (2) *in vitro* fertilization (with sperm of husband or donor, with ovum of wife or donor) with subsequent implantation (in wife or host womb) or without it (artificial placenta), and (3) cloning. Other interventions such as sperm banking, ovum banking, and zygote banking are generally ancillary and instrumental to those procedures. The ancillary procedures may raise specific ethical and policy problems rooted in effectiveness, danger, confidentiality, selection criteria, etc. On the other hand, they may raise very few problems. For instance, few would have any problem with totally artificial gestation (artificial placenta) if it were the only way of possibly saving an otherwise doomed fetus—that is, if the artificial placenta were therapeutic in purpose. However, the main ethical issues cluster around the three interventions noted.

Several things should be remarked about the three interventions. First, they progressively increase in the replacement of so-called natural processes. Just as artificial insemination replaces sexual intercourse, so *in vitro* fertilization does that and more. It replaces tubal fertilization and natural implantation, and could conceivably replace natural gestation. Second, many of the arguments used to justify or condemn one type of intervention reappear where another type is involved.

Motive for intervening. The reproductive interventions in question, or at least most of them, may be motivated by a variety of considerations:

1. They could be *individual* or *personal* in purpose, even though such purposes have social dimensions (marriage, parenthood). Thus AID could be and is employed to overcome the husbands' infertility secondary to oligospermia and azoospermia, or when fertilization by the husband is undesirable because of hereditary disease. Similarly, *in vitro* fertilization followed by artificial implantation could be used where the wife suffers from tubal blockage. Or again, embryonic transfer to a surrogate womb might be attempted where the wife is a habitual and intractable spontaneous aborter. Finally, under personal motivation would be included embryonic transfer to a host womb in situations where the only reason is convenience or dislike of pregnancy.

2. Reproductive interventions could be *eugenic* in purpose (planned breeding). Such eugenics are either positive or negative. Positive eugenics is "preferential breeding of so-called superior individuals in order to improve the genetic stock of the human race."[1] The best known of such eugenicists is Herman J. Muller, who proposed sperm banks from preferred donors to assure the continuance of desirable traits in the race. Negative eugenics is defined as "the discouragement or the legal prohibition of reproduction by individuals carrying genes leading to disease or disability."[2] This purpose can be implemented in a variety of ways (for example, genetic counseling, sterilization, and in its most intense form, abortion). These means have their own ethical aspects and problems.

The reproductive interventions discussed in this chapter would fall into the category of either personal interventions or interventions of positive eugenics. In other words, they are not by and large examples of negative eugenics.

The ethical discussion of such interventions could occur, then,

[1] Kurt Hirschhorn, "On Redoing Man," in Robert A. Paoletti (ed.), *Selected Readings: Genetic Engineering and Bioethics* (New York: MSS Information Corp., 1972), 63.
[2] Ibid.

at two distinguishable levels: the level of the personal and the level of positive eugenics. The types of ethical problems raised differ depending on the level of discussion. Furthermore, there are ethical assumptions hidden in the very level one chooses as the appropriate one to discuss the interventions. Thus one who derives the moral character of AID exclusively from the level of positive eugenics assumes that there is no objection to be made in terms of its possible violation of marital fidelity, the notion of parenthood, etc.

Interventions for Positive Eugenics

The ethical problems associated with any regime of positive eugenics, and therefore one that would use the reproductive interventions mentioned above, are enormous. In showing why both scientists and nonscientists have a powerful aversion to positive eugenics, R. A. Beatty has put the problems as clearly as possible.

First, wherever it has been attempted on a large scale it has been in the hands of evil men. Second, there is no proper measure of indefinable qualities such as nobility or courage; and if we cannot measure a character, we cannot select for it. Third, even if selection were effective, the results would not necessarily be something to look forward to with pleasure. The controllers of positive eugenics would probably be leaders of religious or political power groups. Desirable human qualities—those tending to perpetuate the power group—would no doubt include submissiveness to the power group and readiness to act rashly on its behalf. Undesirable qualities would probably include gentleness and the questioning of the power group's authority. With relief, one must conclude that mankind is simply not ready for positive eugenics.[3]

Similar objections to reproductive interventions as the tools of positive eugenics have come from others. Bentley Glass refers to

[3] R. A. Beatty, "The Future of Reproduction," in Robert A. Paoletti (ed.), *Selected Readings: Genetic Engineering and Bioethics* (New York: MSS Information Corp., 1972), 60.

"frightful dilemmas."[4] For example, how does one judge a "good" genotype when what is the optimum in one set of circumstances may be inferior in another? In selecting for certain characteristics, one sacrifices other desirable traits and compromises over-all adaptability. Who does the judging, and with what criteria? Is technical intelligence, even with reduced emotional and moral development, to be preferred to a less developed IQ in a person of profoundly human qualities (compassion, generosity, love)? Similar questions and objectives are registered by the community of ethicians.[5]

A further problem with approaching reproductive interventions as tools of positive eugenics is that positive eugenics is simply unworkable. Hirschhorn notes that "neither positive nor negative eugenics can ever significantly improve the gene pool of the population and simultaneously allow for adequate evolutionary improvement of the race."[6] Similarly, Peter Medawar argues that a regimen of selective inbreeding is not scientifically acceptable. The reason for this is that the end product of selective inbreeding (the supercattle, supermice, etc.) were expected to fulfill two functions. "The first function was to be end product itself, to be the usable, eatable, or marketable goal of the breeding procedure. The second function was to be the parents of the next generation of superanimals."[7] In order to fulfill the second function, the end product had to be homozygous or one that would breed true with regard to the desirable qualities that conditioned the selection process. Medawar argues that most geneticists think this view mistaken. On that basis he asserts that "it is *populations* that evolve, not the lineages and pedigrees of old-fashioned evolutionary 'family trees,' and the end product of an evolutionary episode is not a new genetic formula enjoyed by a group of similar individuals, but a new spectrum of genotypes, a new pattern of genetic inequality,

[4] Bentley Glass, "The Human Multitude: How Many Is Enough?" in Darrel S. English (ed.), *Genetic and Reproductive Engineering* (New York: MSS Information Corp., 1974), 119.
[5] Bernard Häring, *Ethics of Manipulation: Issues in Medicine, Behavior Control, and Genetics* (New York: Seabury Press, Crossroad Book, 1975), 170.
[6] Hirschhorn, "On Redoing Man," 67.
[7] Peter B. Medawar, *The Hope of Progress: A Scientist Looks at Problems in Philosophy, Literature, and Science* (Garden City, N.Y.: Anchor Press/Doubleday & Company, 1973), 75.

definable only in terms of the population as a whole."[8] Medawar concludes that the newer genetic conception (that it is *populations* that breed true, not its individual members) means that "the goal of positive genetics, in its older form, cannot be achieved, and I feel that eugenic policy must be confined . . . to *piecemeal genetic engineering* [emphasis in original]."[9] By that phrase Medawar means negative eugenics in the individual setting.

Because positive eugenics is scientifically problematic and because the ethical problems inseparable from it (were it workable) are enormous, the ethical discussion of reproductive interventions has generally taken a more modest path—the assessment of interventions as they relate to marriage, parenthood, sexual love, or the good of the child.

Interventions for Personal Purposes

Many in the scientific community—for example, Joshua Lederberg, R. G. Edwards, and R. Francoeur, along with such ethicists as Joseph Fletcher and Michael Hamilton—contend that the principal reproductive interventions already mentioned can be fully justified. Those writers share some definite presuppositions (to be examined at length later), three of which seem to be central to their arguments. First, they incline toward a consequentialistic or teleological normative position—that is, they hold that an act or practice is right and just if, on balance, it does more good than harm and helps to minimize human suffering. Second, they incline to the view that sharply distinguishes between sexual love and the generation of human life, seeing in them quite disparate activities. As Fletcher puts it, we have succeeded in separating completely "babymaking from lovemaking."[10] Third, they regard parenthood as a relationship essentially and primarily defined by acts of nurturing, not by acts of begetting.

Some members of the scientific community—for example, Leon Kass and the majority of religious ethicists—initially approach the

[8] Ibid., 90.
[9] Ibid.
[10] Joseph F. Fletcher, "Ethical Aspects of Genetic Controls: Designed Genetic Changes in Man," *New England Journal of Medicine*, 285 (1971), 781.

issues of reproductive interventions with a great deal more caution, principally because they share a different set of presuppositions. First, they are not pure teleologists in their moral thinking —that is, they argue that factors other than consequences need to be taken into account in offering a valid ethical evaluation of any human act, although many such writers do believe that a proportionately good enough end can justify the deliberate, direct intent to effect some kinds of disvalues or evils. Second, they maintain that a meaningful and reciprocal relationship between sexual love and the generation of human life exists and that it is no mere evolutionary accident that human beings come into existence through an act that is also capable of expressing love between a man and a woman. Third, while recognizing that acts of nurturing life are distinct from acts of generating life and that acts of nurturing are included within the meaning of parenthood, they also affirm that acts of generating life are parental in nature and carry with them responsibilities for nurturing the life generated.

In the following discussions of specific reproductive interventions, and in the analysis of the arguments employed, the presuppositions of the two groups will become more manifest and will be subjected to critical scrutiny.

Artificial Insemination

Since artificial insemination among humans, though known and performed in the nineteenth century, did not become common until the twentieth century, the ethical discussion of the procedure is heavily located in this period.

1. Artificial insemination by donor. In this section attention will center on the arguments offered by those who belong to the second group of authors previously mentioned. Their presuppositions will become evident in the exposition of their arguments.

Roman Catholic appraisals. Within the Catholic community, there never was and still is not much wavering on AID, although occasionally individual authors manifest doubts or even endorse it as ethically acceptable. It was and still generally is seen as morally wrong, and for several reasons, not all of equal weight. First, and above all, it violates the marriage covenant wherein exclusive, nontransferable, inalienable rights to each other's bodies and generative acts are exchanged by spouses. Even the more personalistic approaches to marriage subsequent to the Second Vatican Council have not substantially altered that appraisal. Second, as Pius XII worded it, "So it must be, out of consideration for the child. By virtue of this same bond, nature imposes on whoever gives life to a small creature the task of its preservation and education. Between the marriage partners, however, and child which is the fruit of the active element of a third person—even though the husband consents—there is no bond of origin, no moral or juridical bond of conjugal procreation."[11] Third, once conceded the right, even by their own husbands, to be inseminated artificially by the seed of another man, wives might too easily conclude that it would be preferable to receive the seed in the natural way (sexual intercourse). Thus adulteries would be multiplied to the detriment of marriage. Fourth, the human stud-farming mentality toward marriage would be fostered. (These last two considerations are but supportive teleological arguments—that is, arguments built on possible and probable consequences.)

One of Catholicism's leading theologians, Karl Rahner, has put the matter as follows:

> Now this personal love which is consummated sexually has within it an essential inner relation to the child, for the child is an embodiment of the abiding unity of the marriage partners which is expressed in marital union. Genetic manipulation [Rahner means AID here], however, does two things: It fundamentally separates the marital union from the procreation of a new person as this permanent embodiment of the unity of married love; and it transfers procreation, isolated and torn from its human matrix, to an area outside man's sphere of intimacy. It is this sphere of intimacy which is the proper context for sexual union, which itself implies the fundamental readiness of the marriage partners to let their unity take the form of a child.[12]

[11] Pope Pius XII, "To Catholic Doctors: An Address by His Holiness to the Fourth International Convention of Catholic Doctors, Castelgondolfo, Italy, September 29, 1949," *Catholic Mind*, 48 (1950), 252.

[12] Karl Rahner, "The Problem of Genetic Manipulation," *Theological Investigations, 9: Writings of 1965–67*, (1), trans. Graham Harrison (New York: Herder and Herder, 1972), 246.

Rahner adds other confirmatory arguments. For example, the donor remains anonymous, thus refusing his responsibility as father and infringing the rights of the child so conceived. Furthermore, AID commonly practiced would lead to two new races—the technologically bred supergroup and the ordinary, unselected group—and this at the very time we are attempting to dismantle all other forms of discrimination.

Jewish appraisals. Most rabbinic opinion sees AID as an abomination. With arguments very similar to those used in Catholic literature, Jakobovits summarizes the rabbinic attitudes: "By reducing human generation to stud-farming methods, AID severs the link between the procreation of children and marriage, indispensable to the maintenance of the family as the most basic and sacred unit of human society. It would enable women to satisfy their craving for children without the necessity to have homes and husbands."[13] Other reasons are also offered for regarding AID as prohibited: possibility of incest, lack of genealogy, problems of inheritance.

However, while that is the dominant rabbinic view, it is not universal. Dr. Soloman B. Freehof writes: "My own opinion would be that the possibility of the child marrying one of his own kin is farfetched, but that since according to Jewish law the wife has committed no sin and the child is 'kosher,' then the process of artificial insemination should be permitted."[14] Rabbinic opinion continues to be divided on whether AID should be regarded as adultery and the child illegitimate.

Protestant appraisals. The ethical analysis in the Protestant community reveals several diverging points of view. Joseph Fletcher argues that AID is not a violation of the marriage bond because (1) marriage is not a physical monopoly, and mutual consent by husband and wife protects AID against the accusation of broken faith, and (2) the donor's relationship to the wife is completely impersonal.[15]

13 Immanuel Jakobovits, *Jewish Medical Ethics: A Comparative and Historical Study of the Jewish Religious Attitude to Medicine and Its Practice* (New York: Philosophical Library, 1959), 248.
14 Cited in Benjamin Freedman, "Symposium on Artificial Insemination: The Religious Viewpoints: Jewish," *Syracuse Law Review*, 7 (1955), 104.
15 Joseph F. Fletcher, *Morals and Medicine: The Moral Problems of the*

Contrarily, Helmut Thielicke argues that the psychophysical totality of the marriage is threatened by the presence of the AID child, which is a factual incarnation of the division of the one-flesh unity of husband and wife. He states: "The problem is presented by the fact that here a third person enters into the exclusive psychophysical relationship of the marriage, even though it is only his sperm that 'represents' him."[16] Similarly, Paul Ramsey utterly rejects AID on the theological grounds that it separates what may not be separated: "To put radically asunder what God joined together in parenthood when He made love procreative, to procreate from beyond the sphere of love . . . or to posit acts of sexual love beyond the sphere of responsible procreation (by definition, marriage) means a refusal of the image of God's creation in our own."[17] Thus the spheres of responsible procreation and personal love must be held together if our conduct would reflect the creative love of God.

While accepting the substance of Ramsey's argument and giving a qualified "no" to AID, others add further practical objections. For example, in light of the demographic and ecological facts of our time, adoption serves the common good better than AID. Furthermore, when done for eugenic reasons, AID creates the enormous problem of deciding what qualities we should breed for and who decides this.[18] Still others note that both AID and adoption involve sacrifice and risks. However, adoption and AID enjoy a markedly different status and acceptance in the community. For adoption there is a "more complete supportive network helping the parents to adjust emotionally to their sterility and evaluate themselves as parents."[19] This, plus the radical asymmetry of the parents' relationship to the AID child and the psy-

---

Patient's Right to Know the Truth, Contraception, Artificial Insemination, Sterilization, Euthanasia (Princeton, N.J.: Princeton University Press, 1954), 139.

[16] Helmut Thielicke, The Ethics of Sex, trans. John W. Doberstein (New York: Harper & Row, 1964), 259.

[17] Paul Ramsey, Fabricated Man: The Ethics of Genetic Control (New Haven, Conn.: Yale University Press, 1970), 39.

[18] Harmon L. Smith, Ethics and the New Medicine (Nashville, Tenn.: Abingdon Press, 1970).

[19] Richard P. Richards, "Ethical and Theological Aspects," Soundings, 54 (1971), 323.

chological difficulties involved in that asymmetry, means AID is
the riskier of the two options and ought to be rejected as such.

2. Artificial insemination by husband. When AIH is under discussion, the matter is remarkably different.

Developments within Roman Catholicism. Within Catholicism
AIH was for years defended by some as at least probably permissible, if semen was obtained in a licit (nonmasturbatory) way.
The reasons adduced against AID were not there, and the method
seemed a defensible way of overcoming the sterility problems of
the couple. In 1949 Pius XII intervened and said AIH "must be
absolutely eliminated." In support of his rejection he noted:

> We must never forget this: It is only the procreation of
> a new life according to the will and plan of the Creator
> which brings with it—to an astonishing degree of perfec-
> tion—the realization of the desired ends. This is, at the
> same time, in harmony with the dignity of the marriage
> partners, with their bodily and spiritual nature, and with
> the normal and happy development of the child.[20]

In 1951 Pius XII returned to the subject in more detail. He
stated:

> To reduce the cohabitation of married persons and the
> conjugal act to a mere organic function for the trans-
> mission of the germ of life would be to convert the do-
> mestic hearth, sanctuary of the family, into nothing
> more than a biological laboratory. . . . The conjugal act
> in its natural structure is a personal action, a simulta-
> neous natural self-giving which, in the words of Holy
> Scripture, effects the union "in one flesh." This is more
> than the mere union of two germs, which can be
> brought about artificially—that is, without the natural
> action of the spouses. The conjugal act as it is planned
> and willed by nature, implies a personal cooperation, the
> right to which the parties have mutually conferred on
> each other in contracting marriage.[21]

20 Pope Pius XII, "To Catholic Doctors," 250–53.
21 Pope Pius XII, "Apostolate of the Midwife: An Address by His Holiness
to the Italian Catholic Union of Midwives, October 29, 1951," *Catholic Mind*,
50 (1952), 61.

The argument, then, of Pius XII, was that even AIH is immoral, because the child so born is not the fruit of an act *of itself* the expression of personal love. The hidden assumption in this argument would seem to be that the child must always be conceived of an act *of itself* a personal expression of love if marriage is not to be converted into a biological laboratory. That is the import of the phrase "willed by nature." Recently Catholic theologians have suggested that this is only generally true—that is, if procreation were commonly and routinely to occur via AIH, a long step would have been taken toward biologizing and mechanizing marriage, thus undermining it. However, if AIH is not a substitute for sexual intercourse, but in relatively rare cases its complement, the reasoning would not seem to support the absolute prohibition. This has led a number of theologians to maintain the probable moral licitness of AIH, at least in some instances of infertility—for example, Häring, Curran, Lobo, Rahner, Gründel, Mahoney, etc.

Protestant and Jewish approaches. A tolerant attitude is certainly dominant in the Protestant and Jewish communities. The very ethicists who most clearly and sometimes severely condemn AID—for example, Ramsey, Thielicke, Smith, and Jakobovits—have little problem with AIH as a morally legitimate intervention to overcome infertility. For at least many ethicists the self-stimulation that produces the semen is not seen as problematic, either because it is not an invariably necessary procedure or because it does not (as finally procreative in purpose) fall within the class of prohibited masturbatory acts. Furthermore, there is no foreign (donor) intrusion into the marital covenant or the psychophysical totality that is marriage.

Analysis of the arguments. It is clear, then, that the ethical aspects of artificial insemination have been approached from the dominant perspective of the meaning of marriage, parenthood, and the family. Furthermore, the majority opinion of ethicists has been that AID, by the introduction of donor semen, separates procreation from marriage, or the procreative sphere from the sphere of marital love, in a way that is either violative of the marriage covenant or likely to be destructive of it and the family.

Here it is opportune to examine in more detail the views of those writers, previously referred to, who operate with a different set of presuppositions. Obviously they would not agree with this approach to the question. Some argue that sexual intimacy and procreation are and should be distinct human acts each governed by "totally distinct ethics."[22] Still others would argue that "the demand of love in relation to parenthood is fulfilled in ensuring that all children born into this world, *by whatever means* [emphasis added], be reared in a family."[23] This position rests on the conviction that parenthood is, in its deepest sense, not principally a matter of biological begetting but a more broadly human function —a man and a wife accepting responsibility for caring for and rearing a child.

A possible counterstatement to that approach would be one that argues that in Christian conviction the same sexual love that generates ought to become *in principle* the parental love that nurtures.[24] Parents do not love their children simply because the children are there and need love. They ought to love them because they have loved each other and because the children are the visible fruits and extensions of that love—that is, it has been said (sometimes clumsily, to be sure) that conjugal love is by its very nature "ordained for the procreation and education of children, and finds in them its ultimate crown."[25] Just as education is, in a sense, a continuation of procreation, so there ought to be a basic identity and continuity in the love that procreates and the love that nurtures. Therefore to separate the acts that nurture from the acts that generate, and then to associate parental love only with the former, is to undermine the very foundation of the love that nurtures. To limit the notion and love of parenthood to "caring for and rearing a child" is therefore a radical attack on several basic humano-Christian values (the meaning of human sexuality, the meaning of marriage and parenthood).

This argument must be properly understood; otherwise it could

[22] Robert T. Francoeur, *Utopian Motherhood: New Trends in Human Reproduction* (Garden City, N.Y.: Doubleday & Company, 1970), 109.

[23] Michael Hamilton, "New Life for Old: Genetic Decisions," *Christian Century*, 86 (1969), 743.

[24] Richard A. McCormick, S.J., "Current Theology: Notes on Moral Theology: January–June 1969 (Genetic Engineering)," *Theological Studies*, 30 (1969), 680–92. See previous chapter.

[25] Vatican Council II, "Pastoral Constitution on the Church in the Modern World (*Gaudium et spes*)," in Walter M. Abbot (ed.), *The Documents of Vatican II* (New York: Herder and Herder/Association Press, 1966), 199–308, esp. Pt. 2, Chap. 1, Sec. 48, p. 250.

be used to show that adoption is an attack on some basic humano-Christian values. The argument is that we ought not to separate *in principle* the acts that generate from the acts that nurture, that the notion of parenthood ought *in principle* to include both. Obviously, conceptions occur *in fact* where marriage is impossible or inadvisable, and adoption offers the best resolution of the situation. Just as obviously, marriages *in fact* break up and remarriage occurs. In these situations it is clear that the child can be (and ought to be) loved, cared for, and protected within a family context wherever possible. The argument insists only that these are surrogate arrangements and that we ought to try to avoid them in principle insofar as possible.

The Hamilton approach holds that parenthood is not a biological but a human function. It identifies the human function with accepting responsibility for rearing a child. Summarily, caring for and rearing a child is human, procreating him is biological. But since parenthood and parental love are obviously human, procreation as such does not pertain to them.

Here, it might be argued, we are face to face once again with an all too familiar and destructive dualism, where persons love and care in many ways, but not in their sexual intercourse or procreation. Ultimately such an attitude is rooted in a principle that depreciates the body and disallows its participation in the specifically human. This is the area and these are the concepts and arguments that have by and large surrounded discussion of AID. It is important because it sets the stage for some of the ethical arguments that will be used in assessing *in vitro* fertilization and cloning.

There has been little discussion of AID where the husband is fertile but the wife sterile. That would involve an anonymous (preferably) ovum, and perhaps uterus, donor to provide the husband his self-fulfillment as a father. It is not properly AID as it has been discussed but represents a reproductive intervention that raises some of the problems associated with AID. Thus on the very principles espoused where artificial insemination is concerned, those against AID would be a fortiori opposed to such procedures, for they involve an even greater intrusion into or threat to the marital covenant and family. In this light sperm banks and ovum banks whose *sole purpose* is some form of AID

would share in the moral acceptance or rejection attributed to the
AID procedure itself. (It is possible, of course, that such storage
could serve other therapeutic purposes—for example, research on
infertility problems.)

Ultimate factors in decision-making. At this point it is important to make a methodological point about the arguments and
analyses used in the discussion of artificial insemination, because
such a methodological consideration will be operative in the
assessment of other reproductive interventions.

The point to be underlined is the relationship of an ultimate
moral judgment to the reasons used to express it. Some theologians involved in the discussion of reproductive interventions insist that there is a "moral instinct of faith" (Rahner). The "instinct" under discussion can be called by any number of names;
but the point is that there is a component to moral judgment that
cannot be adequately subject to analytic reflection. But it is this
component that is chiefly responsible for one's ultimate judgments in concrete moral questions. In that sense the ultimate
judgments are not simply the sum of the rational considerations
and analyses one is capable of objectifying. For that reason
Rahner states explicitly that "all the 'reasons' which are intended
to form the basis for rejecting genetic manipulation," such as
AID, "are to be understood, at the very outset, as only so many
references to the moral faith-instinct (and as so many appeals to
it, to have the courage to take a clear decision). For in my view
the moral faith-instinct is aware of its right and obligation to
reject genetic manipulation, even without going through (or being
able to go through) an adequate process or reflection."[26]

Something very similar to this is used by scientist Peter Medawar. What is the line between a humanizing use of technology
and a dehumanizing one? The answer we give in practice "is
founded not upon abstract moralizing but upon a certain natural
sense of the fitness of things, a feeling that is shared by most kind
and reasonable people even if we cannot define it in philosophically defensible or legally accountable terms."[27]

This nondiscursive element in ethical discourse is important.
One of the central assertions of those who regard AID (and, a for-

26 Rahner, "The Problem of Genetic Manipulation," 243.
27 Medawar, *The Hope of Progress*, 84.

tiori, more drastic reproductive interventions) as morally wrong is that procreation of a human being ought not occur outside the covenanted relationship of marriage. While various warrants (some biblical, some teleological) can be gathered to support that assertion, it remains true that it cannot be proved by rational arguments or analytic reasoning in a totally satisfactory way. This will be viewed as a fatal weakness only if one fails to realize that in all moral judgments concerned with basic human values there is a prethematic and instinctive component that cannot be totally recovered in analytic discourse; for our knowledge of those values or goods is not first of all discursive.

In that sense the arguments pro and con AID, *in vitro* fertilization, etc., important as they are, are always more or less imperfect, more or less incomplete, more or less persuasive. They only externalize, rationalize, and communicate a spontaneous sense of the rightness or wrongness of things. To think otherwise would almost invariably convert moral judgments in this area into technological judgments. It is in this sense that the "natural sense of the fitness of things" (Medawar) or "moral instinct of faith" (Rahner) underlies and animates the positions and arguments on reproductive interventions.

"In vitro" Fertilization

R. G. Edwards notes that there are three areas of medicine that could benefit greatly from the studies surrounding *in vitro* fertilization: (1) Some forms of infertility (blockage of the oviduct) could possibly be cured. (2) Knowledge useful for contraceptive technology could be gained. (3) Knowledge and methods could be obtained leading to the alleviation of genetic disorders and even other deformities.[28]

The simplest instance of *in vitro* fertilization is extraction of the wife's oocytes by laparoscopy, fertilization with husband's sperm followed by laboratory culture to the blastocyst stage, then embryo transfer (implantation) into the wife's uterus. The procedure would be aimed at overcoming sterility due to obstruction of

[28] R. G. Edwards, "Reproduction: Chance and Choice," in David Paterson (ed.), *Genetic Engineering* (London: British Broadcasting Corporation, 1969), 27.

the fallopian tubes. This is the "simplest" instance because it does not raise the further issues of donor sperm, host wombs, and totally artificial gestation.

The ethical issues involved in such a procedure are multiple, even if only this simplest form is in question. They involve considerations of justice, the beginning of human life, and the value of life, in addition to the questions of parenthood and sex. First, there is the question of embryo wastage. Only one or two of the eggs taken from the mother would be transferred back into her. The remaining embryos would be discarded although such discarding is not essential to the procedure. Those who are convinced that human personhood begins with fertilization would reject *in vitro* fertilization on that ground alone, for apparently it would involve the deliberate destruction of human life to achieve a pregnancy.

However, other ethicists argue that there is a genuine doubt about whether we are dealing with a human person at this stage of development. The existence of such a doubt leads to a variety of conclusions. Some say that the very probability of human personhood constitutes "an absolute veto against this kind of experimentation."[29] Others, while remaining basically negative, argue that given such a positive doubt, "the reasons in favor of experimenting might carry more weight, considered rationally, than the uncertain rights of a human being whose very existence is in doubt."[30] Finally, there are some who would undoubtedly agree with Joseph Fletcher that the product of *in vitro* fertilization is but human tissue, "fallopian and uterine material."[31]

Edwards' response to these serious ethical concerns seems unconvincing. He notes that in discarding embryos experimenters are doing nothing more than women who use intrauterine contraceptive devices. However, rather than an argument supporting embryo wastage, this could be viewed as an objection against intrauterine devices—to the extent that they achieve contraceptive effectiveness by expelling embryos. The same response could be made to his assertion that "in a society which sanctions the abortion of a fully formed fetus, the discarding of such a minute,

29 Häring, *Ethics of Manipulation*, 198.
30 Rahner, "The Problem of Genetic Manipulation," 236.
31 Joseph F. Fletcher, *The Ethics of Genetic Control: Ending Reproductive Roulette* (Garden City, N.Y.: Anchor Press/Doubleday & Company, 1974), 88.

undifferentiated embryo should be acceptable to most people."[32] Such an argument says nothing of the moral rightness or wrongness of abortion, but only of a particular society's toleration or sanctioning of it. As a form of ethical argument, it is equivalent to saying that a society that tolerates obliteration bombing of cities should not object to a little selective torture of enemy prisoners. While that may be true in terms of ethical consistency, it says nothing about the moral rightness or wrongness of either procedure.

The second serious ethical problem with *in vitro* fertilization is its experimental character. It has been argued that, given the unknown hazards associated with laboratory culture and embryonic transfer, and the inability to overcome such unknown hazards, *in vitro* fertilization with subsequent implantation constitute potentially hazardous experimentation with a human subject without his consent[33]—that is, risks are chosen for the future human being without his consent. More concisely, the experimental phase of this technology can be shown to be risk-free only by exposing a certain number of subjects to unethical experiments. Therefore we can never get to know how to perform such procedures in an ethical way. The argument does not rest on ascription of personal status to the embryo who is eventually discarded during development of the technology (though, as noted above, some ethicists would see a serious problem here too). Rather, it points to the possible harm to be inflicted on living children who come to be born after *in vitro* fertilization and laboratory culture. There is at present no way of finding out whether the viable progeny of these procedures will be deprived or retarded. Nor would a willingness to practice abortion on the deformed solve the problem, since many such deformities cannot and will not be identifiable by amniocentesis.

Others contend that this argument is not altogether persuasive, for procreation by natural processes produces a certain percentage

<hr>

[32] Edwards, "Reproduction: Chance and Choice," 28.
[33] See Paul Ramsey, "Shall We 'Reproduce'? I. The Medical Ethics of *in Vitro* Fertilization," *Journal of the American Medical Association*, 220 (1972), 1,346–50; Ramsey, "Shall We 'Reproduce'? II. Rejoinders and Future Forecast," *Journal of the American Medical Association*, 220 (1972), 1,480–85; and Leon Kass, "Babies by Means of *in Vitro* Fertilization: Unethical Experiments on the Unborn?" *New England Journal of Medicine*, 285 (1971), 1,174–79.

of deformed, crippled, or retarded children. Thus the natural process of sexual intercourse also imposes serious hazards on future children without their consent and is no less "experimental" in this sense than laboratory fertilization with embryo transfer. Thus the problem is to bring the dangers associated with *in vitro* fertilization procedures to an acceptable level. No one has insisted that "natural" procreation be completely safe for the fetus before it is undertaken. Even in the most severe cases (women with phenylketonuria, whose offspring are virtually certain of receiving damage during gestation), it is argued that we do not constrain such couples from procreating except by moral suasion. "If we accept the morality of couples making this childbearing decision, can we deny the needs of a couple childless because of the woman's blocked oviducts?"[34]

A possible double response could be made to this argument. First, we have no way of knowing the comparative risk ratios of the two methods of reproduction, since discovering the percentage of risk of *in vitro* procedures would expose a certain, perhaps very large, number of human subjects to serious risk without their consent. Second, when it is known that husband and wife are carriers of the same severe recessive, genetic disease, the course of moral responsibility demands that they not run the hazards of procreation. Therefore, when faced with the possible deformities from *in vitro* technology, the proper response is not to point to similar deformities in natural processes as justification for creating them by technology, but to use that technology to diminish them in the natural processes.

At some point, then, this discussion opens on the morality of risk-taking even within so-called natural procreative processes. What is the responsible course for couples who are carriers for the same deleterious recessive disease (for example, phenylketonuria) when there is a one-in-four chance that the child will be afflicted? Many, if not all, philosophers and theologians who have discussed the problem hold that running such a risk is morally irresponsible, and indeed that partners with such recessive defects ought not as a general rule to marry. As Medawar puts it: "If anyone thinks or has ever thought that religion, wealth, or color are matters that

[34] Marc Lappé, "Risk-taking for the Unborn," *Hastings Center Report*, 2 (Feb. 1972), 1–3.

may properly be taken into account when deciding whether or not a certain marriage is a suitable one, then let him not dare to suggest that the genetic welfare of human beings should not be given equal weight."[35] The problem remains, however, of where to draw the line where risk-taking is involved. Some would argue that a one-in-four chance of a seriously afflicted child is a tolerable risk. Others would disagree.

Here, however, several points must be made to structure the ethical discussion. First, even though abstention from childbearing may be the only responsible decision in these cases, it is another matter altogether whether this abstention should be compelled by law. Second, there is a line to be drawn where inherited defects are involved. Some diseases are relatively minor and manageable; others are enormously crippling and catastrophic for the child. Finally, in a highly technological and comfort-oriented society, the fear of having a defective child can easily become pathological. That is particularly possible in a society unwilling (unable?) to adjust itself to the needs of its most disadvantaged citizens.

The third set of arguments against *in vitro* fertilization concerns what it is likely to lead to, especially through the mentality it could easily foster. For instance, if *in vitro* fertilization is successfully (with safety and normality) introduced to treat sterility *within a marriage*, will there not be extensions beyond the marriage if either husband's sperm or wife's ovum is defective? And this raises all the ethical and theological problems associated with AID. Furthermore, the standard use of *in vitro* fertilization for infertility involves viewing infertility as a disease. But the accuracy of that description has been challenged not only because sterility is not a disease in the ordinary sense (since it is the incapacity or dysfunction of a couple, not of an individual), but above all because viewing it as a disease tends to undermine, in thought and practice, the bond between childbearing and the marriage covenant.[36] Those who have no problem with AID would see little force in this type of argument, or would see it overridden by the

[35] Medawar, *The Hope of Progress*, 93.
[36] Kass, "Making Babies—the New Biology and the 'Old' Morality," *The Public Interest*, 26 (1972), 18–56.

value of providing the couple with their own child. But that is
where the issue is.

If these arguments are overcome, there remain other issues of
ethical relevance. For instance, would children conceived by *in
vitro* fertilization suffer any identity or status problems? Would
they experience a possibly harmful pressure to research their mental, physical, and emotional development? If the technology were
widely used, would that distort the priorities of the health-care system in a way that would do harm by neglect in other, more urgent
areas?

In vitro fertilization can also be undertaken with donor sperm,
to be followed by embryonic transfer to the wife of the sterile husband, or to a host womb. Or it could occur with the sperm of the
husband and an egg of another woman to be implanted in the
wife (adopted embryo). Where donor sperm or ovum is used, not
only is there the issue of unknown hazards imposed without consent, but once again the relation of procreation to marriage becomes the focus of concern. The issue is intensified when a host or
surrogate womb (not the wife's) is used for the pregnancy, for not
only does one of the agents of fertilization come from outside the
marriage, but also the entire period of pregnancy and delivery is
outside the marriage.

Such a rather exotic arrangement raises further formidable problems. What if the surrogate "mother" were to become disen-
chanted with the pregnancy and desire an abortion? What if the
genetic parents desired such an abortion and tried to force the surrogate mother to undergo one? What if the genetic husband and
wife are determined to have a healthy child and refuse to accept
the deformed or retarded child that is born of the surrogate
mother? There are additional ethical problems with the social
identity of the child. Who is truly the child's mother? Who has
rights and responsibilities with regard to such a child? A society, it
can be argued, that already has enormous problems with marital
stability would be unwise in the extreme to add freely to those
problems.

My own view is that at the level of the individual couple's decision, there seems to be no argument that shows with clarity and
certainty that husband-wife *in vitro* procedures using their own
sperm and ovum are necessarily and inherently wrong, if abortion

of a possibly deformed child is excluded and the risks are acceptably low. This is not to say that *in vitro* procedures are without
problems and dangers. They are not. But such dangers issue only
in a prudential caution, not necessarily a moral judgment that
each instance is morally wrong. Let me take each of the major arguments once again in systematic form to make this clear.

1. *Technologizing marriage.* There are two forms this argument
takes. The first is associated with Pius XII and his statements on
artificial insemination by husband. The Pope excluded this, and
especially on the grounds that it separated the "biological activity
from the personal relation of the married couple." Rather, "in its
natural structure, the conjugal act is a personal act. . . ." In summary, Pius XII viewed the conjugal act as having a natural and
God-given design that joins the love-giving dimension with the
life-giving dimension. On this basis he excluded both contraception and artificial insemination—and a fortiori *in vitro* fertilization with embryo transfer. It is safe to say that this structured
the negative responses of some theologians and bishops when they
spoke of the "unnatural."

I believe that this is substantially the approach of Donald
McCarthy.[37] He refers to the "integrity of the procreative process" and argues that artificial fertilization is among those "actions
that violate human dignity or the dignity of human procreation."
Such actions are inhuman in themselves.

The second form of this argument is a softer form. It is a general concern that too much technology introduced into a highly
personal context (parenting, family) can mechanize and depersonalize the context. The argument issues in a prudential caution,
not necessarily a moral judgment that each instance is morally
wrong on this account alone—as noted earlier. This argument is
also justifiably concerned with objectifying the child into a consumer item ("what sex?" "what color eyes?" etc.).

What might be said of these arguments? I shall comment on
only the first, since the second is a dictate of common sense, and
leaves the question fairly well open. It is clear that at least very
many theologians have not been able to accept "the natural . . .
design of the conjugal act" as this was interpreted by Pius XII—

[37] Donald McCarthy, letter to the editor of *Hospital Progress,* 59 (Sept.
1978), 6.

that is, they have not viewed it as an inviolable value. Thus they can allow for contraception at times.

Similarly, and in some consistency,[38] they have not been able to see that artificial insemination by the husband is necessarily a violation of nature. Gründel states it well when he says that the child must be the expression and embodiment of love, but that sexual intercourse is not the only or necessary source for this expression and embodiment.[39] Many would respond in a similar fashion to Donald McCarthy's assertion that artificial fertilization always attacks the integrity of the procreative process. How can one establish that plausibly? We can intuit it, but intuitions notoriously differ. And in this case, such dehumanization has not been perceived by at least very many commentators (most recently Bernard Häring, George Lobo, Roger Troisfontaines, Karl Rahner *et al.*).

That is not to say that the separation of procreation from sexual love-making is a neutral thing. To say that would be to minimize the physical aspects of our being in a dualistic way. Rather the artificial route to pregnancy is a disvalue and one that needs justification. John R. Connery, S.J., has caught this well (though by saying this I do not imply that he should necessarily be associated with the analysis as one approving it).[40] Whether it can find such justification is the burden of some of the other arguments—especially that of the "slippery slope" involving possible undesirable future developments.

In summary, it seems very difficult to reject *in vitro* fertilization with embryo transfer on the sole ground of artificiality or the sepa-

---

[38] Note the following from the *National Catholic Register* (Aug. 13, 1978): "It comes as anything but a surprise that moral theologians who reject *Humanae vitae* have difficulty explaining why laboratory conception is morally wrong, or that they are not even sure it is wrong, or they may even think it justified. Father Richard McCormick admits to a certain uncertainty, says that since Pope Pius XII there has been 'a long second look, a rethinking that it can be justified,' and counsels caution. Fr. Bernard Häring observes that Pope Pius condemned test-tube fertilization 'a long way back,' but thinks the Church 'takes a long time to come to positions on these matters.'" The *Register* has it just right, but *praeteritio* is called for in the face of statements such as that those who condemn "laboratory concoction" of babies are "faithful Catholics."

[39] Johannes Gründel, "Zeugung in der Retorte—unsittlich?" *Stimmen der Zeit*, 103 (1978), 675–82.

[40] John R. Connery, S.J., in a letter to the editor of *America*, 139 (1978), 145.

ration of the unitive and the procreative in that sense—unless one accepts this physical inseparability as an inviolable value.

2. *Abortion and discarded zygotes.* It is admitted that at present in the process of *in vitro* fertilization with embryo transfer more than one ovum is fertilized.[41] Those not used will perish.[42] As I noted there are those who view zygotes as persons with rights and therefore condemn the procedure outright as abortion. Others see them as simply "human tissue" and find no problem in their creation and loss, the more so because so many fertilized ova are lost in *in vivo* attempts at pregnancy. Still a third group would assess the zygote as somewhere in between these alternatives—not yet a person, but a living human being deserving of respect and indeed protection. How much protection is the key question.

With no claim of saying the last word, I would suggest the following for consideration. First, the discussion ought not to center around the personhood of the fertilized ovum. It is difficult to establish this, and there are reputable theologians and philosophers in large numbers who deny such an evaluation at this stage. Moreover, it is unnecessary; for many of those who deny personhood insist that the zygote is not just a thing, but also deserves our respect and awe.

Second, it is one thing to fertilize *in vitro* in order to experiment and study the product of conception. It is quite another to do so in order to achieve a pregnancy. It seems to me that the respect due nascent life, even if not yet personal life, rubs out the first alternative at least as a general rule. Some research is necessary, of course, prior to implementation of transfer technology. I do not see this, given our strong doubts about zygote status, as incompatible with respect. This is, however, *the* gray and most difficult and controversial area. Kass has stated that the "presumption of ignorance ought to err in the direction of not underestimating the basis for respect."[43] That seems correct, and it is the

[41] It is not absolutely essential to the procedure as such. *In vitro* fertilization could be done either by freezing ova in advance or, during successive cycles, by doing (most unlikely) successive laparoscopies.

[42] Furthermore, it is generally accepted that the parties ought to be willing to abort during the pregnancy if something goes wrong. I put this in a footnote because it is not necessary to the procedure as such.

[43] Leon Kass, " 'Making Babies' Revisited," *The Public Interest*, 54 (Winter 1979), 32–59.

same as the traditional principle that states that in factual doubts life generally deserves the preference.

Third, the term "abortion" must be carefully used when there is question of discarded zygotes. We know that a very high percentage of naturally fertilized ova never implant, are lost. This means that there is a tacit acceptance on the part of the couple that their normal sexual relations will lead to this as the price of having a child.

The response often given to this explanation is that we may not reproduce by artifice everything that happens in nature. Thus, though people inevitably die, we do not kill them. Though there are life-taking earthquakes in nature, we ought not manufacture life-taking earthquakes. Perhaps a distinction is called for here between replicating nature's disasters and replicating nature's achievements. Is there anything particularly wrong about achieving artificially—*faute de mieux*—what occurs otherwise naturally? We are not exactly replicating disasters, but rather achievements even with unavoidable disvalues. If it is by no means clear that couples engaging in normal sexual relations are "causing abortions" because foreseeably many fertilized ova do not implant, it is not clear that the discards from artificial procedures must be called "abortions," especially if the ratio of occurrence is roughly similar.[44]

Put this in the language of rights to life on the supposition that the zygote is a person. It is not a violation of the right to life of the zygote if it is spontaneously lost in normal sexual relations. Why is it any more so when this loss occurs as the result of an attempt to achieve pregnancy artificially? The matter of discards is serious, indeed crucial for those of us who believe that human life must be protected and respected from its very beginning. These reflections are meant only as probes into a difficult area.

3. *Harm to the possible child.* The argument here is that the very procedure that gives life is inseparable from risks, physical and psychological. These may be small risks, but even so it is mor-

---

[44] It might be well to recall here that we do not object to tubal reconstructive surgery. Yet it is well known and foreseen that such surgery leads to a marked increase in ectopic pregnancies that will have to be reluctantly terminated—and at a later stage than the zygote stage.

ally wrong to induce for a nonconsenting child even a small risk of great harm. This seems to be Ramsey's key argument.

On the other hand, the counterstatement (by Kass and others) is that the risk of harm need not be positively excluded. It is sufficient if it is equivalent to or less than the risks to the child from normal procreation.

The response to this assertion, as I noted, is that we could never get to know *that* without exposing a certain number of children to unknown risk to get the statistic. This seems to some to be an insuperable argument for ever starting the *in vitro* procedures. However, once this statistic is had, is the objection any longer telling? In other words, even though Steptoe and Edwards may have acted wrongfully (in ignorance of the risks), after it is clear that the risks are equivalent to normal conception, are those who follow necessarily acting wrongfully?[45]

4. *The extension beyond marriage.* This reasoning takes two forms. First, once *in vitro* fertilization is used successfully in marriage, it will go beyond marriage to third-party donors (semen, ovum), host wombs, etc.[46] This extension is seen as a radical attack on marriage, the family, human sexuality, personal identity, and lineage of the child. The argument is one of inevitability, given the cultural acceptance by many of AID (donor insemination) already. As Kass says: "There will almost certainly be other uses involving third parties."[47] However, possible abuses need not morally indict legitimate uses. With discretion and judgment human beings are, I believe, capable of drawing lines. Abuses, therefore, are not inevitable, though it would be naïve to think that some will not occur.

The second form of the argument, an extension of the first, is

[45] In this respect it should be noted that some of the experts testifying before the Ethics Advisory Board thought factually that (1) not enough animal work had preceded and (2) the risks for humans have not been sufficiently assessed.

[46] That this is not an idle fear is clear from the testimony given before the Ethics Advisory Board by Drs. Randolph W. Seed and Richard G. Seed. They propose to inseminate a third party, then wash out the fertilized ovum to be reimplanted in the wife. Moreover, Dr. Landrum Shettles, waiting to testify in the Del Zio case, stated: "I have cloned three human eggs from testicular tissue. They lived for three or four days." See *Medical Moral Newsletter*, 15 (Sept. 1978), 28. In the words of Nobel Laureate James Watson, there is potential for "all sorts of unsettling scenarios" (*Reader's Digest*, 113 [Nov. 1978], 103).

[47] Kass, " 'Making Babies' Revisited," 32–59.

that the wedge argument is primarily a matter of the logic of justification—that is, the principles now used to justify husband-wife *in vitro* fertilization already justify in advance other procedures. The strict validity of this second argument, it seems to me, depends on the "principles now used to justify." If the principle is that an infertile couple, using their own gametes, may licitly use artificial means, that is one thing. If, on the other hand, it is less precise (for example, couples may licitly overcome their sterility with *in vitro* procedures), then all the problems involved in the second form of the argument strike home.

In summary, then, at the level of the individual couple's decision, there seems to be no argument that shows with clarity and certainty that *in vitro* procedures using their own sperm and ovum are necessarily and inherently wrong, if abortion of a possibly deformed child is excluded and the risks are acceptably low.[48] This is not to say that such procedures are without problems and dangers. They are not.

I would conclude, therefore, that *in vitro* fertilization with embryo transfer is ethically acceptable under a fourfold condition: (1) the gametes are those of husband and wife; (2) embryo wastage is not significantly higher in the artificial process than it is *in vivo*; (3) the likelihood of fetal abnormality is no greater than it is in normal procreation; (4) there is no intention to abort if abnormality does occur.

Another, and an extremely interesting, moral problem is the question of government funding of *in vitro* research. In my own—at this time very tentative—judgment, public policy should not support *in vitro* fertilization where research alone (not embryo transfer) is the purpose. Respect for germinating life calls for at least this. Granted, there is potentially a good deal to be learned from study of fertilized ova (genetic disease, contraception, fertility). But I do not see how this can be done without stripping nascent life of the minimal respect we owe it. Some research is necessary, of course, prior to implementation of transfer technology. I

---

[48] In saying this, I am in substantial agreement both in method and in content with the ethical committee of the Guild of Catholic Doctors (London). See "*In Vitro* Fertilization," *Catholic Medical Quarterly*, 24 (1972), 237–43. But note the words "seems" and "certainty."

do not see this, given our doubts about zygote status, as incompatible with respect.

As for *in vitro* fertilization with embryo transfer at the research stage (I mean clinical *trials*—for I think it quite clear that government should not support clinical *practice*), this should not be supported with government funds *in the present circumstances* (compare below) though it should not be prohibited by law or policy. Why "not be supported"? Because of the cumulative impact of many arguments: The dangers of going beyond marriage are almost certainly unavoidable in our present atmosphere; the distorted priorities of medicine this introduces (for example, prenatal care for children already *in utero* is unavailable to very many); the almost unavoidable dangers of proceeding to independent zygote research and the manipulation of the implanted fetus (compare our abortion culture) with the assault on nascent life that this involves; the readiness to abort that this procedure presently entails; the trauma this would visit on an already deeply divided nation (on abortion) by asking that tax money be used for purposes against the consciences of many and not necessary to the public good; the disproportion of benefits (to a relatively few) with costs; the growing neglect of more radically therapeutic (oviduct reconstruction) and preventive (of gonorrhea) interventions; government reinforcement of the dubious, perhaps noxious, notion that women's lives are unfulfilled if they cannot have their "own children."

It should be remembered that funding implies fostering. Whether it is appropriate to foster depends on what is being fostered. And that depends to some extent on the circumstances. Thus if we cannot fund *in vitro* fertilization between husband and wife without *in our circumstances* funding (and fostering) practices beyond that, we should not do so. I believe this to be the case. *In other circumstances* we could draw a different conclusion.

Cloning

The reproductive technology known as cloning represents the most intense intervention of all. At the present, cloning in the human species still pertains to the area of science fiction. Were it to occur at some future date it would involve removing insemination and fertilization from the marriage relationship, and it would also remove one of the partners from the entire process. Its purported advantages are eugenic in character (removal of deleterious genetic material from the gene pool, and programming the genotype in such a way as to maximize certain desirable traits—for example, intelligence, creativity, artistic ability).

There are those who judge such procedures as desirable and moral in terms of their consequences and advantages.[49] If such manipulative reproduction would heighten the intelligence (or artistic, or creativity) quotient of the race, or provide solutions to some particularly difficult and intractable human problems, it is good. To the objection or at least suspicion that there might be something inhuman in laboratory reproduction of human beings, it is asserted that "man is a maker and a selector and a designer, and the more rationally contrived and deliberate anything is, the more human it is."[50] On this basis it is concluded that "laboratory reproduction is radically human compared to conception by ordinary heterosexual intercourse. It is willed, chosen, purposed, and controlled, and surely these are among the traits that distinguish *Homo sapiens* from others in the animal genus."[51]

Whether such value judgments are the only ones capable of supporting the ethical character of cloning may be debatable. However, they do suggest that there comes a point in the moral discourse surrounding reproductive interventions when one must step aside from the casuistry of individual interventions and view the future possibilities and directions in aggregate and in the light of over-all convictions about what the "human" is. When that is done, some of the following questions arise. Will such reproductive interventions, even if they provide certain short-term remedies or advantages, actually improve the over-all quality of human life? If so, how is the improvement to be specified? What is the notion of the human that functions in the description of an "improvement"? And who decides this? If the development and application of such technology are likely to be humanly destructive, why will they be such? And if the more advanced forms of reproductive technology threaten some profoundly cherished human

[49] Fletcher, "Ethical Aspects of Genetic Controls," 776–83.
[50] Ibid., 779–81.
[51] Ibid., 781.

values and institutions (parenthood, marriage, the family), and are therefore something to be avoided, or at least stringently controlled, how are these values threatened, and where was the first wrong step or threatening one taken? Those are the questions that will be asked for decades as technology becomes increasingly sophisticated.

If the questions surrounding basic values are not asked, not asked seriously, not asked publicly, not asked continually, and in advance of the use of reproductive technologies, the danger is that we will identify the humanly and morally good with the technologically possible. That is why so much is at stake in reproductive interventions—not only in the conclusions that are drawn, but also in the criteria and form of moral reasoning involved.

SECTION VI

THE PRESERVATION OF LIFE

17. To Save or Let Die: The Dilemma of Modern Medicine

On February 24, 1974, the son of Mr. and Mrs. Robert H. T. Houle died following court-ordered emergency surgery at Maine Medical Center. The child was born February 9, horribly deformed. His entire left side was malformed; he had no left eye, was practically without a left ear, had a deformed left hand; some of his vertebrae were not fused. Furthermore, he was afflicted with a tracheal esophageal fistula and could not be fed by mouth. Air leaked into his stomach instead of going to the lungs, and fluid from the stomach pushed up into the lungs. As Dr. André Hellegers recently noted, "It takes little imagination to think there were further internal deformities."[1]

As the days passed, the condition of the child deteriorated. Pneumonia set in. His reflexes became impaired, and because of poor circulation, severe brain damage was suspected. The tracheal esophageal fistula, the immediate threat to his survival, can be corrected with relative ease by surgery. But in view of the associated complications and deformities, the parents refused their consent to surgery on "Baby Boy Houle." Several doctors in the Maine Medical Center felt differently and took the case to court. Maine Superior Court Judge David G. Roberts ordered the surgery to be performed. He ruled: "At the moment of live birth there does exist a human being entitled to the fullest protection of the law. The most basic right enjoyed by every human being is the right to life itself."

[1] André E. Hellegers, *Obstetrical and Gynecological News* (Apr. 1974).

"Meaningful Life"

Instances like this happen frequently. In a recent issue of the *New England Journal of Medicine,* Drs. Raymond S. Duff and A. G. M. Campbell[2] reported on 299 deaths in the special-care nursery of the Yale-New Haven Hospital between 1970 and 1972. Of these, 43 (14 per cent) were associated with discontinuance of treatment for children with multiple anomalies, trisomy, cardiopulmonary crippling, meningomyelocele, and other central nervous system defects. After careful consideration of each of these 43 infants, parents and physicians in a group decision concluded that the prognosis for "meaningful life" was extremely poor or hopeless, and therefore rejected further treatment. The abstract of the Duff-Campbell report states: "The awesome finality of these decisions, combined with a potential for error in prognosis, made the choice agonizing for families and health professionals. Nevertheless, the issue has to be faced, for not to decide is an arbitrary and potentially devastating decision of default."

In commenting on this study in the Washington *Post* (October 28, 1973), Dr. Lawrence K. Pickett, chief of staff at the Yale-New Haven Hospital, admitted that allowing hopelessly ill patients to die "is accepted medical practice." He continued: "This is nothing new. It's just being talked about now."

It has been talked about, it is safe to say, at least since the publicity associated with the famous "Johns Hopkins case"[3] some seven years ago. In this instance, an infant was born with Down's syndrome and duodenal atresia. The blockage is reparable by relatively easy surgery. However, after consultation with spiritual advisers, the parents refused permission for this corrective surgery, and the child died by starvation in the hospital after fifteen days, for to feed him by mouth in this condition would have killed him. Nearly every one who has commented on this case has disagreed with the decision.

[2] Raymond S. Duff and A. G. M. Campbell, "Moral and Ethical Dilemmas in the Special-care Nursery," *New England Journal of Medicine,* 289 (1973), 890–94.

[3] James J. Gustafson, "Mongolism, Parental Desires, and the Right to Life," *Perspectives in Biology and Medicine,* 16 (1973), 529–59.

It must be obvious that these instances—and they are frequent —raise the most agonizing and delicate moral problems. The problem is best seen in the ambiguity of the term "hopelessly ill." This used to and still may refer to lives that cannot be saved, that are irretrievably in the dying process. It may also refer to lives that can be saved and sustained, but in a wretched, painful, or deformed condition. With regard to infants, the problem is: Which infants, if any, should be allowed to die? On what grounds or according to what criteria, as determined by whom? Or again, is there a point at which a life that can be saved is not "meaningful life," as the medical community so often phrases the question? If our past experience is any hint to the future, it is safe to say that public discussion of such controversial issues will quickly collapse into slogans such as "There is no such thing as a life not worth saving" or "Who is the physician to play God?" We saw and continue to see this far too frequently in the abortion debate. We are experiencing it in the euthanasia discussion. For instance, "death with dignity" translates for many into a death that is fast, clean, and painless. The trouble with slogans is that they do not aid in the discovery of truth; they co-opt this discovery and promulgate it rhetorically, often only thinly disguising a good number of questionable value judgments in the process. Slogans are not tools for analysis and enlightenment; they are weapons for ideological battle.

Thus far, the ethical discussion of these truly terrifying decisions has been less than fully satisfactory. Perhaps this is to be expected, since the problems have only recently come to public attention. In a companion article to the Duff-Campbell report, Dr. Anthony Shaw[4] of the Pediatric Division of the Department of Surgery, University of Virginia Medical Center, Charlottesville, speaks of solutions "based on the circumstances of each case rather than by means of a dogmatic formula approach." Are these really the only options available to us? Shaw's statement makes it appear that the ethical alternatives are narrowed to dogmatism (which imposes a formula that prescinds from circumstances) and pure concretism (which denies the possibility or usefulness of any guidelines).

[4] Anthony Shaw, "Dilemmas of Informed Consent in Children," *New England Journal of Medicine*, 289 (1973), 885–90.

Are Guidelines Possible?

Such either-or extremism is understandable. It is easy for the medical profession, in its fully justified concern with the terrible concreteness of these problems and with the issue of who makes these decisions, to trend away from any substantive guidelines. As *Time* remarked in reporting these instances: "Few, if any, doctors are willing to establish guidelines for determining which babies should receive life-saving surgery or treatment and which should not."[5] On the other hand, moral theologians, in their fully justified concern to avoid total normlessness and arbitrariness wherein the right is "discovered," or really "created," only in and by brute decision, can easily be insensitive to the moral relevance of the raw experience, of the conflicting tensions and concerns provoked through direct cradleside contact with human events and persons.

But is there no middle course between sheer concretism and dogmatism? I believe there is. Dr. Franz J. Ingelfinger, editor of the *New England Journal of Medicine*, in an editorial on the Duff-Campbell-Shaw articles, concluded, even if somewhat reluctantly: "Society, ethics, institutional attitudes and committees can provide the broad guidelines, but the onus of decision-making ultimately falls on the doctor in whose care the child has been put."[6] Similarly, Frederick Carney of Southern Methodist University, Dallas, and the Kennedy Center for Bioethics stated of these cases: "What is obviously needed is the development of substantive standards to inform parents and physicians who must make such decisions."[7]

"Broad guidelines," "substantive standards"; there is the middle course, and it is the task of a community broader than the medical community. A guideline is not a slide rule that makes the decision. It is far less than that. But it is far more than the concrete decision of the parents and physician, however seriously and conscientiously this is made. It is more like a light in a room, a light

[5] *Time* (Mar. 25, 1974).
[6] Franz J. Ingelfinger, "Bedside Ethics for the Hopeless Case," *New England Journal of Medicine*, 289 (1973), 914.
[7] Washington *Post* (Mar. 20, 1974).

that allows the individual objects to be seen in the fullness of their context. Concretely, if there are certain infants whom we agree ought to be saved in spite of illness or deformity, and if there are certain infants whom we agree should be allowed to die, then there is a line to be drawn. And if there is a line to be drawn, there ought to be some criteria, even if very general, for doing this. Thus, if nearly every commentator has disagreed with the Johns Hopkins decision, should we not be able to distill from such consensus some general wisdom that will inform and guide future decisions? I think so.

This task is not easy. Indeed, it is so harrowing that the really tempting thing is to run from it. The most sensitive, balanced, and penetrating study of the Johns Hopkins case that I have seen is that of the University of Chicago's James Gustafson.[8] Gustafson disagreed with the decision of the Hopkins physicians to deny surgery to the mongoloid infant. In summarizing his dissent, he notes: "Why would I draw the line on a different side of mongolism than the physicians did? While reasons can be given, one must recognize that there are intuitive elements, grounded in beliefs and profound feelings, that enter into particular judgments of this sort." He goes on to criticize as too simplistic the assessment made of the child's intelligence, and he proposes a much broader perspective on the meaning of suffering than seemed to have operated in the Hopkins decision. I am in full agreement with Gustafson's reflections and conclusions. But ultimately, he does not tell us where he would draw the line or why, only where he would *not* and why.

This is very helpful already, and perhaps it is all that can be done. Dare we take the next step, the combination and analysis of such negative judgments to extract from them the positive criterion or criteria inescapably operative in them? Or more startlingly, dare we *not* if these decisions are already being made? Gustafson is certainly right in saying that we cannot always establish perfectly rational accounts and norms for our decisions. But I believe we must never cease trying—in fear and trembling, to be sure. Otherwise we have exempted these decisions in principle from the one critique and control that protects against abuse. Exemption of

---

[8] Gustafson, "Mongolism, Parental Desires, and the Right to Life," loc. cit.

this sort is the root of all exploitation, whether personal or political. Briefly, if we must face the frightening task of making quality-of-life judgments—and we must—then we must face the difficult task of building criteria for these judgments.

Facing Responsibility

What has brought us to this position of awesome responsibility? Very simply, the sophistication of modern medicine. Contemporary resuscitation and life-sustaining devices have brought a remarkable change in the state of the question. Our duties toward the care and preservation of life have been traditionally stated in terms of the use of ordinary and extraordinary means. For the moment and for purposes of brevity, we may say that, morally speaking, ordinary means are those whose use does not entail grave hardships to the patient. Those that would involve such hardship are extraordinary. Granted the relativity of these terms and the frequent difficulty of their application, still the distinction has had an honored place in medical ethics and medical practice. Indeed, the distinction was recently reiterated by the House of Delegates of the American Medical Association in a policy statement. After disowning intentional killing (mercy killing), the AMA statement continues: "The cessation of the employment of extraordinary means to prolong the life of the body when there is irrefutable evidence that biological death is imminent is the decision of the patient and/or his immediate family. The advice and judgment of the physician should be freely available to the patient and/or his immediate family."[9]

This distinction can take us just so far—and thus the change in the state of the question. The contemporary problem is precisely that the question no longer concerns only those for whom "biological death is imminent" in the sense of the AMA statement. Many infants who would have died a decade ago, whose "biological death was imminent," can be saved today. Yesterday's failures are today's successes. Contemporary medicine with its team approaches, staged surgical techniques, monitoring capabilities, ventilatory support systems, and other methods, can keep almost any-

[9] *Journal of the American Medical Association*, 227 (1974), 728.

one alive. This has tended gradually to shift the problem from the means to reverse the dying process to the quality of the life sustained and preserved. The questions, "Is this means too hazardous or difficult to use?" and "Does this measure only prolong the patient's dying?" while still useful and valid, now often become, "Granted that we can easily save the life, what kind of life are we saving?" This is a quality-of-life judgment. And we fear it. And certainly we should. But with increased power goes increased responsibility. Since we have the power, we must face the responsibility.

A Relative Good

In the past, the Judaeo-Christian tradition has attempted to walk a balanced middle path between medical vitalism (that preserves life at any cost) and medical pessimism (that kills when life seems frustrating, burdensome, "useless"). Both of these extremes root in an identical idolatry of life—an attitude that, at least by inference, views death as an unmitigated, absolute evil, and life as the absolute good. The middle course that has structured Judaeo-Christian attitudes is that life is indeed a basic and precious good, but a good to be preserved precisely as the condition of other values. It is these other values and possibilities that found the duty to preserve physical life and that also dictate the limits of this duty. In other words, life is a relative good, and the duty to preserve it is a limited one. These limits have always been stated in terms of the *means* required to sustain life. But if the implications of this middle position are unpacked a bit, they will allow us, perhaps, to adapt to the type of quality-of-life judgment we are now called on to make without tumbling into vitalism or a utilitarian pessimism.

A beginning can be made with a statement of Pope Pius XII in an allocution to physicians delivered on November 24, 1957. After noting that we are normally obliged to use only ordinary means to preserve life, the Pontiff stated: "A more strict obligation would be too burdensome for most men and would render the attainment of the higher, more important good too difficult. Life, death, all temporal activities are in fact subordinated to spiritual ends."[10] Here it would be helpful to ask two questions. First: What are these spiritual ends, this "higher, more important good"? Second: How is its attainment rendered too difficult by insisting on the use of extraordinary means to preserve life?

The first question must be answered in terms of love of God and of neighbor. This sums up briefly the meaning, substance, and consummation of life from a Judaeo-Christian perspective. What is or can easily be missed is that these two loves are not separable. St. John wrote: "If any man says I love God and hates his brother, he is a liar. For he who loves not his brother, whom he sees, how can he love God, whom he does not see?" (1 Jn. 4:20–21). This means that our love of neighbor is in some very real sense our love of God. The good our love wants to do Him and to which He enables us, can be done only for the neighbor, as Karl Rahner has so forcefully argued. It is in others that God demands to be recognized and loved. If this is true, it means that, in Judaeo-Christian perspective, the meaning, substance, and consummation of life are found in human *relationships*, and the qualities of justice, respect, concern, compassion, and support that surround them.

Second, how is the attainment of this "higher, more important (than life) good" rendered "too difficult" by life supports that are gravely burdensome? One who must support his life with disproportionate effort focuses the time, attention, energy, and resources of himself and others not precisely on relationships, but on maintaining the condition of relationships. Such concentration easily becomes overconcentration and distorts one's view of and weakens one's pursuit of the very relational goods that define our growth and flourishing. The importance of relationships gets lost in the struggle for survival. The very Judaeo-Christian meaning of life is seriously jeopardized when undue and unending effort must go into its maintenance.

I believe an analysis similar to this is implied in traditional treatises on preserving life. The illustrations of grave hardship (rendering the means to preserve life extraordinary and nonobligatory) are instructive, even if they are outdated in some of their particulars. Older moralists often referred to the hardship of moving to

---

[10] Pope Pius XII, *Acta Apostolicae Sedis*, 49 (1957), 1,031–32.

another climate or country. As the late Gerald Kelly, S.J., noted of this instance: "They (the classical moral theologians) spoke of other inconveniences, too: for example, of moving to another climate or another country to preserve one's life. For people whose lives were, so to speak, rooted in the land, and whose native town or village was as dear as life itself, and for whom, moreover, travel was always difficult and often dangerous—for such people, moving to another country or climate was a truly great hardship, and more than God would demand as a 'reasonable' means of preserving one's health and life."[11]

Similarly, if the financial cost of life-preserving care was crushing—that is, if it would create grave hardships for oneself or one's family—it was considered extraordinary and nonobligatory. Or again, the grave inconvenience of living with a badly mutilated body was viewed, along with other factors (such as pain in preanesthetic days, uncertainty of success), as constituting the means extraordinary. Even now, contemporary moralist M. Zalba, S.J.,[12] states that no one is obliged to preserve his life when the cost is "a most oppressive convalescence" (*molestissima convalescentia*).

The Quality of Life

In all of these instances—instances where the life could be saved—the discussion is couched in terms of the means necessary to preserve life. But often enough it is the kind of, the quality of the life thus saved (painful, poverty-stricken and deprived, away from home and friends, oppressive) that establishes the means as extraordinary. *That* type of life would be an excessive hardship for the individual. It would distort and jeopardize his grasp on the over-all meaning of life. Why? Because, it can be argued, human relationships—which are the very possibility of growth in love of God and neighbor—would be so threatened, strained, or submerged that they would no longer function as the heart and meaning of the individual's life as they should. Something other

[11] Gerald Kelly, *Medico-Moral Problems* (St. Louis: Catholic Hospital Association of the United States and Canada, 1957), 132.

[12] M. Zalba, *Theologiae Moralis Summa*, 3 (Madrid: La Editorial Catolica [1957]), II, 71.

than the "higher, more important good" would occupy first place. Life, the condition of other values and achievements, would usurp the place of these and become itself the ultimate value. When that happens, the value of human life has been distorted out of context.

In his *Morals in Medicine*, Thomas O'Donnell, S.J., hinted at an analysis similar to this.[13] Noting that life is a relative, not an absolute good, he asks: Relative to what? His answer moves in two steps. First, he argues that life is the fundamental natural good God has given to man, "the fundamental context in which all other goods which God has given man as means to the end proposed to him, must be exercised." Second, since this is so, the relativity of the good of life consists in the effort required to preserve this fundamental context and "the potentialities of the other goods that still remain to be worked out within that context."

Can these reflections be brought to bear on the grossly malformed infant? I believe so. Obviously there is a difference between having a terribly mutilated body as a result of surgery, and having a terribly mutilated body from birth. There is also a difference between a long, painful, oppressive convalescence resulting from surgery, and a life that is from birth one long, painful, oppressive convalescence. Similarly, there is a difference between being plunged into poverty by medical expenses and being poor without ever incurring such expenses. However, is there not also a similarity? Cannot these conditions, whether caused by medical intervention or not, equally absorb attention and energies to the point where the "higher, more important good" is simply too difficult to attain? It would appear so. Indeed, is this not precisely why abject poverty (and the systems that support it) is such an enormous moral challenge to us? It simply dehumanizes.

Life's potentiality for other values is dependent on two factors: those external to the individual, and the very condition of the individual. The former we can and must change to maximize individual potential. That is what social justice is all about. The latter we sometimes cannot alter. It is neither inhuman nor un-Christian to say that there comes a point where an individual's condi-

[13] Thomas J. O'Donnell, *Morals in Medicine* (Westminster, Md.: Newman Press, 1957), 66.

tion itself represents the negation of any truly human—that is, relational—potential. When that point is reached, is not the best treatment no treatment? I believe that the *implications* of the traditional distinction between ordinary and extraordinary means point in this direction.

In this tradition, life is not a value to be preserved in and for itself. To maintain that would commit us to a form of medical vitalism that makes no human or Judaeo-Christian sense. It is a value to be preserved precisely as a condition for other values, and therefore insofar as these other values remain attainable. Since these other values cluster around and are rooted in human relationships, it seems to follow that life is a value to be preserved only insofar as it contains some potentiality for human relationships. When in human judgment this potentiality is totally absent or would be, because of the condition of the individual, totally subordinated to the mere effort for survival, that life can be said to have achieved its potential.

Human Relationships

If these reflections are valid, they point in the direction of a guideline that may help in decisions about sustaining the lives of grossly deformed and deprived infants. That guideline is the potential for human relationships associated with the infant's condition. If that potential is simply nonexistent or would be utterly submerged and undeveloped in the mere struggle to survive, that life has achieved its potential. There are those who will want to continue to say that some terribly deformed infants may be allowed to die *because* no extraordinary means need be used. Fair enough. But they should realize that the term "extraordinary" has been so relativized to the condition of the patient that it is this condition that is decisive. The means is extraordinary because the infant's condition is extraordinary. And if that is so, we must face this fact head-on—and discover the substantive standard that allows us to say this of some infants, but not of others.

Here several caveats are in order. First, this guideline is not a detailed rule that pre-empts decisions; for relational capacity is not subject to mathematical analysis but to human judgment. However, it is the task of physicians to provide some more concrete categories or presumptive biological symptoms for this human judgment. For instance, nearly all would very likely agree that the anencephalic infant is without relational potential. On the other hand, the same cannot be said of the mongoloid infant. The task ahead is to attach relational potential to presumptive biological symptoms for the gray area between such extremes. In other words, individual decisions will remain the anguishing onuses of parents in consultation with physicians.

Second, because this guideline is precisely that, mistakes will be made. Some infants will be judged in all sincerity to be devoid of any meaningful relational potential when that is actually not quite the case. This risk of error should not lead to abandonment of decisions, for that is to walk away from the human scene. Risk of error means only that we must proceed with great humility, caution, and tentativeness. Concretely, it means that if err we must at times, it is better to err on the side of life—and therefore to tilt in that direction.

Third, it must be emphasized that allowing some infants to die does not imply that "some lives are valuable, others not" or that "there is such a thing as a life not worth living." Every human being, regardless of age or condition, is of incalculable worth. The point is not, therefore, whether this or that individual has value. Of course he has, or rather *is* a value. The only point is whether this undoubted value has any potential at all, in continuing physical survival, for attaining a share, even if reduced, in the "higher, more important good." This is not a question about the inherent value of the individual. It is a question about whether this worldly existence will offer such a valued individual any hope of sharing those values for which physical life is the fundamental condition. Is not the only alternative an attitude that supports mere physical life as long as possible with every means?

Fourth, this whole matter is further complicated by the fact that this decision is being made for someone else. Should not the decision on whether life is to be supported or not be left to the individual? Obviously, wherever possible. But there is nothing inherently objectionable in the fact that parents with physicians must make this decision at some point for infants. Parents must make many crucial decisions for children. The only concern is that the decision not be shaped out of the utilitarian perspectives so deeply sunk into the consciousness of the contemporary world. In a highly technological culture, an individual is always in danger of being valued for his function, what he can do, rather than for who he is.

It remains, then, only to emphasize that these decisions must be made in terms of the child's good, this alone. But that good, as fundamentally a relational good, has many dimensions. Pius XII, in speaking of the duty to preserve life, noted that this duty "derives from well-ordered charity, from submission to the Creator, from social justice, as well as from devotion toward his family."[14] All of these considerations pertain to that "higher, more important good." If that is the case with the duty to preserve life, then the decision not to preserve life must likewise take all of these into account in determining what is for the child's good.

Any discussion of this problem would be incomplete if it did not repeatedly stress that it is the pride of Judaeo-Christian tradition that the weak and defenseless, the powerless and unwanted, those whose grasp on the goods of life is most fragile—that is, those whose potential is real but reduced—are cherished and protected as our neighbor in greatest need. Any application of a general guideline that forgets this is but a racism of the adult world profoundly at odds with the gospel, and eventually corrosive of the humanity of those who ought to be caring and supporting as long as that care and support has human meaning. It has meaning as long as there is hope that the infant will, in relative comfort, be able to experience our caring and love, for when this happens, both we and the child are sharing in that "higher, more important good."

Were not those who disagreed with the Hopkins decision saying, in effect, that for the infant, involved human relationships were still within reach and would not be totally submerged by survival? If that is the case, it is potential for relationships that is at the heart of these agonizing decisions.

[14] Pope Pius XII, AAS, 1,031–32.

18. Saving Defective Infants: Options for Life or Death

Infant Doe, a Down's Syndrome baby with a tracheoesophageal fistula who was left unfed and untreated in a Bloomington, Ind., hospital for eight days until he expired of "natural causes," died on April 16, 1982. The first anniversary presents the occasion to reflect on the moral implications of that case. Two Monroe County Courts and the Indiana Supreme Court heard arguments on the issue and each determined not to intervene against the parents' determination to let the child die. Some called the parents' actions "infanticide"; others labeled it "an acceptable moral opinion."

The full facts in the case will never be known because the courts have sealed the records to protect the family. The press reports and comments from various involved parties are highly contradictory. Andrew Mallor, the family attorney, reported that "the parents were informed that there was evidence the baby had an enlarged heart and had an esophagus that wasn't attached to his stomach. They were told it would take more than one operation and would mean multiple traumas for the infant, and that his chance of survival was 50-50 at best." Mr. Mallor also claims that the parents were told the child would never have even a minimally acceptable quality of life if he survived. As he summarized the case, "This body was doomed by God before it was born."

Dr. James Laughlin, the consulting pediatrician who has treated a number of similar cases, insisted that other than the two major problems noted at birth, there were no clinically evident symptoms. He specifically ruled out evidence of congenital heart disease or other physical defects. Rather than the high risk of death quoted by the family attorney, Dr. Laughlin believed Infant Doe had a 90 percent chance of successful surgery. Further, he reminded us, it is impossible to predict the intelligence in a Down's case at that early state.

Whatever the facts, and they were twice debated by some six physicians before the lower courts, Chief Justice Richard Givan of the Indiana Supreme Court maintained the parents were loving, caring people who "wanted only what was best for the child." In his view, "The Down's Syndrome was 'a fact not a factor' in the death of the child." "It was the need for extensive surgery which was not thought to be productive that determined the case," he said. (The autopsy revealed only Down's Syndrome coupled with a malformed esophagus. No other medical problems were noted.)

The case of Infant Doe, as did the murder trial of Dr. Leonard Arthur for the nontreatment of a "normal Down child" in Leicester, England, just a year earlier, stirred a raging national debate over the policies of doctors and hospitals on the treatment of severely defective newborns. This debate revealed a wide diversity of views and expectations. Some saw the action as homicide, others as "letting nature take its course," still others as an occasion for permitting a "mercy killing."

The general response to the thought of allowing an infant with a correctable defect to starve to death because of retardation was outrage. The New York *Times* editoralized: "Because he had been inadvertently robbed of perfections, he was deliberately robbed of life." The Washington *Post*, reflecting on the classical distinction between ordinary and extraordinary care due a patient observed: "The Indiana baby died not because he couldn't sustain life without a million dollars worth of medical machinery, but because no one fed him." Columnist George Will, himself the father of a 10-year-old Down son, in a forceful and widely reproduced essay, charged: "The baby was killed because it was retarded."

The Reagan Administration responded to the public outcry with a memorandum sent at the President's direction by the Department of Health and Human Services to 6,800 hospitals warning that they could lose Federal funds if they "withhold from a handicapped infant nutritional sustenance or medical or surgical treatment required to correct a life-threatening condition" solely because of the handicap.

That memorandum, which caused widespread consternation and

fear of Government intrusion into medical practice, was but the
first in a series of responses to the Infant Doe case. For example,
Congressman John N. Erlenborn (R., Ill.) introduced a bill (H.R.
6492) that would allow an individual to bring suit in Federal
court against anyone who "deprives a handicapped infant of nutri-
tion which is necessary to sustain life, or . . . medical treatment
which is necessary to remedy or ameliorate a life-threatening medical condition."

These actions, however, pale in comparison to the politically
responsive prosecutorial threats that now surround nontreatment
decisions. In the same press release in which he announced the
warning to the institutions receiving Federal funds, then Health
and Human Services Secretary Richard Schweiker announced that
his department had sent an investigator to Crawford Memorial
Hospital in Robinson, Ill., to check a complaint by national and
local "right-to-life" groups that surgical treatment was being withheld from a baby born with spina bifida. And in June, Connecticut
State Senator Regina R. Smith, chairman of that state's Public
Health Committee, wrote a letter to the U.S. Attorney demanding
a criminal investigation of deliberate nontreatment or lethal over-
dosing of defective newborns at Yale-New Haven Hospital.

Commenting on such moves, John R. Robertson of the University of Wisconsin Law School observes: "Prosecutors may still be
reluctant to prosecute. . . . (But as) anti-abortion and right-to-life
groups . . . become interested in the issue and . . . generate support
for prosecution . . . prosecutors may lose more politically from
nonprosecution than they will from bringing charges." The reality
of that situation is strikingly evident in the observation made to a
large group of physicians and lawyers at a statewide conference on
"Ethical and Legal Aspects in the Treatment of Terminally and
Critically Ill Patients" held last fall in New York City. Robert L.
Adams, first assistant district attorney of New York's Rensselaer
County announced: "As things now stand, withdrawal of life support is homicide." The shock waves that reverberated through the
audience were intensified when Mr. Adams continued, "there are
D.A.'s in this state anxious to pursue such a charge. One told me
he would see how many are enrolled in the Right-to-Life Party in
his country. And he'd go from there."

We believe that such an approach to complex and trying issues of appropriate care of seriously impaired newborns is not the way to proceed. The delicate and multifaceted issues in such cases require tact, concern, openness and compassion. A politicized prosecutorial or legislative attack is not only overtly blunt; it reduces difficult and tragic moral choices to a crusade of slogans.

The highly charged atmosphere of criminal proceedings raises more emotional ire and physician angst than need occur. And as juries are notoriously unwilling to convict in "mercy killing" trials, such trials are highly unlikely to result in successful prosecution. Further, unlike civil proceedings or appellate reviews, criminal trials do not result in a reasoned opinion. "Guilty" or "not guilty" is the only verdict. As a result, a search-and-litigate approach is more likely to satisfy a cry for vengeance than it is to provide a balanced guide for future practice.

The issue is not quite so novel or unexamined as comments on Infant Doe would have us believe. A year earlier in Britain, Lord Justice Templeman of the Court of Appeal rendered judgment in a case similar to that of the Bloomington baby. A child was born suffering from Down's Syndrome and an intestinal blockage. Without the operation the child would die, with it she most likely would have a life expectancy of 20 to 30 years. Her parents, believing it would be kinder to allow her to die, refused to consent to the operation. The surgeon decided that the wishes of the parents should be respected and refused to operate. The local authorities sought a court order for the surgery which was denied. They appealed.

The case brings out one significant fact: The surgeon, who at first agreed to the relatively routine operation, changed his mind when he learned from the parents that the child was mongoloid. In his words: "I decided to respect the wishes of the parents and not to perform the operation, a decision which would, I believe (after about 20 years in the medical profession), be taken by the great majority of surgeons faced with a similar situation." Two other surgeons advised that the operation should be carried out.

Much like the parents' attorney in Bloomington, the family attorney here argued: "This is a case where nature had made its own arrangements to terminate a life which would not be fruitful."

He maintained: "In this kind of decision the views of responsible and caring parents . . . should be respected."

Lord Justice Templeman, while noting that great weight ought to be given to the views of the parents and doctors, observed: "They are not the views which necessarily must prevail." He put it baldly: "The choice before the court is this: whether to allow the operation to take place which may result in the child's living for 20 to 30 years as a mongoloid or (and I think this must be brutally the result) to terminate the life of a mongoloid child because she has an intestinal complaint." Faced with that choice —and not of a child so severely impaired that "the life of the child is so bound to be full of pain and suffering that the court might be driven to a different conclusion"—Lord Justice Templeman ruled: "I have no doubt it is the duty of this court to decide that the child must live." We agree.

These issues, as the High Court indicated, ought be framed not in terms of the emotional or financial burden on the family nor the philosophical predisposition of the physician, but in terms of the best interests of the child. That interest may or may not demand treatment. We do not share that technological view—one now becoming all too politicized—that if something can be done, it must be done. As we have written previously (see above, pp. 339-51), there are cases of dying patients or those so submerged in suffering and the struggle to survive that the best treatment may be no treatment.

We do not believe, as does Attorney Mallor, that these decisions are "private matters" to be left to the family and physician. Despite the obvious love and concern of the parents in all three of the cases noted here, loving parents can and do make mistakes. To think otherwise is to confuse the goodness of the decision-maker with the rightness of the decision. That we believe is to destroy both ethics in principle and sound public policy.

A further caution to be observed from these cases is the danger of leaving the formation of social policy exclusively in the hands of practitioners. The medical profession is little trained in and not particularly adept at setting social values. As evidence we need but review the surveys done of physician attitudes toward care of Down's Syndrome infants with an intestinal atresia. In a national study conducted by Anthony Shaw and his associates and published in *Pediatrics* in 1974, 76.8 percent of the pediatric surgeons polled reported that they, like the surgeon in England, would "acquiesce in parents' decisions" not to treat. When asked whether, if they were the parents of a Down infant with an intestinal obstruction, they would consent to intestinal surgery, 66.7 percent of the pediatric surgeons replied, "No." Interestingly, the percent of pediatricans answering "no" was significantly lower—37.4 percent. When factored for occupational and religious differences the disparity is even more pronounced: "Catholics in the (pediatrician group) are the most likely to say they would request operations on their own child (83 percent said 'yes'), while Jews in the (surgeon group) are least likely (7 percent)."

These data, which are similar to the findings in David Todres's study of attitudes of Massachusetts pediatricians, published in *Pediatrics* in 1977, are widely divergent from the outlook not only of such liberal sources as the editorial board of The New York *Times* and the Washington *Post*, but of the overwhelming majority of moral analyses and legal commentaries written on this subject.

Where, then does this leave us? The editors of *Lancet* correctly observe that the simplest, though not necessarily the right, course for doctors—and one with the greatest potential for pain and burden to patient and family—would be to do everything possible to save all lives. That, we believe, would be a tragic mistake, one which would violate good ethical practice and produce poor public policy.

In the preceding chapter, one of us proposed certain guidelines that might be helpful in determining which seriously impaired infants should live and which should be allowed to die. Here we would like to expand on that framework and explore a way of using those guidelines that would protect the interests of the infant and those of society without the need of costly, cumbersome and traumatic court interventions.

First, we would note that these are not private matters. What life-saving treatment is provided or not to the incompetent and handicapped is a matter of the gravest public concern. At stake, after all, is the life of a human being, and by consistent extension, the lives of many human beings. Second, some have argued that these decisions are medical decisions, that they are made according to "medical indications." That approach makes it appear as if these are exclusively scientific judgments. As the surveys of Anthony Shaw and David Todres show, they are no such thing. They are value judgments involving assumptions about the origin, destiny and meaning of life and death.

If the above approaches are inadequate, what are the proper positive criteria to be applied? In 1980 the Vatican issued its "Declaration on Euthanasia." When discussing the means to be used to preserve life, it stated: "It will be possible to make a correct judgment as to the means by studying the type of treatment to be used, its degree of complexity or risk, its cost and the possibility of using it and comparing these elements with the result that can be expected, taking into account the state of the sick person and his or her physical and moral resources."

Here the Vatican has identified the two elements that ought to anchor our judgments in life-sustaining decisions: burden and benefit. This means that life-sustaining interventions are not morally obligatory—for handicapped infants or anyone else for that matter—if they are either gravely burdensome or useless. These are, of course, value judgments, not mathematical judgments. The evaluation of burden and benefit is not always easy. Indeed, it can be borderline and controversial.

The earlier guideline we developed for dealing with handicapped newborns focused on the potential for human relationships associated with the infant's condition. If that potential was simply nonexistent or would be utterly submerged and undeveloped in the mere struggle to survive, that young life had achieved its potential and no longer made life-sustaining claims on our care.

That standard was admittedly general. It could clearly be misused and stretched beyond recognition. But we are convinced that it is fundamentally sound and that if further specified and concretized, can be helpful to families, physicians and society in making decisions in future situations. We suggest the capacity for human relationships—as a summary of the burden-benefit evaluation —can be further specified as follows:

1. Life-saving interventions ought not be omitted for institutional or managerial reasons. Included in this specification is the

ability of this particular family to cope with a badly disabled baby. This is likely to be a controversial guideline because there are many who believe that the child is the ultimate victim when parents unsuited to the challenge of a disadvantaged baby must undertake the task. Still, it remains an unacceptable erosion of our respect for life to make the gift of life once given depend on the personalities and emotional or financial capacities of the parents alone. No one ought to be allowed to die simply because these parents are not up to the task. At this point society has certain responsibilities. To face these agonizing situations by allowing the child to die will merely blunt society's sensitivities to its unfulfilled social responsibilities.

2. Life-sustaining interventions may not be omitted simply because the baby is retarded. There may be further complications associated with retardation that justify withholding life-sustaining treatment. But retardation alone, as both Chief Justice Givan of the Indiana Supreme Court and Lord Justice Templeman of the English Court of Appeals made clear, is not an indication for non-treatment. To claim otherwise is a slur on the condition of the retarded, one that would mandate fundamentally unequal treatment of equals.

3. Life-sustaining intervention may be omitted or withdrawn when there is excessive hardship on the patient, especially when this combines with poor prognosis (e.g., repeated cardiac surgery, low prognosis transplants, increasingly iatrogenic oxygenization for low birthweight babies).

4. Life-sustaining interventions may be omitted or withdrawn at a point when it becomes clear that expected life can be had only for a relatively brief time and only with the continued use of artificial feeding (e.g., some case of necrotizing enterocolitis).

These norms, we believe, provide some guidance for the types of cases under discussion. Here the term "some guidance" must be emphasized. Concrete rules such as these do not make decisions. They do not replace prudence and eliminate conflicts and doubts. They are simply attempts to provide outlines of the areas in which prudence should operate. They do not replace parental-physician responsibility, but attempt to enlighten it. If even good and loving parents can make mistakes—and they can and have—then there ought to be some criteria (even if general) by which we can

judge the decision to be right or wrong. For ethical persons ought
to be reason-giving persons.

But doubts and agonizing problems will remain. Hence a certain range of choices must be allowed to parents, a certain margin
of error, a certain space. Guidelines can be developed which aid us
to judge when parents have exceeded the limits of human discretion. They cannot cover every instance where human discretion
must intervene to decide. The margin of error tolerable should reflect not only the utter finality of the decision (which tends to
narrow it), but also the unavoidable uncertainty and doubt (which
tends to broaden it).

It is clear that the judgments of burden and benefit are value
judgments, moral choices. They are judgments in which, all things
considered, the continuance of life is either called for or not worthwhile to the patient. Such judgments are, as is clear from remarks
made above, the onerous prerogative of those primarily responsible
for the welfare of the family—the parents. When parents exercise
this prerogative in a way that is questionably no longer in the best
interests of the infant, especially by allowing the infant to remain
untreated, society has the duty to intervene. That intervention
can take many forms, like legislation, criminal prosecution or a
child-neglect hearing. The purpose of such proceedings is to guarantee that the primary decision-maker acts in a responsible way,
one that should be able to sustain public scrutiny. We believe that
public accountability and review, a review that guarantees that the
values of the society are respected and adhered to, can be invoked
short of judicial intervention.

One approach to achieving that goal is found in the "Decisions
to Forgo Life-sustaining Treatment" Report of the President's
Commission for the Study of Ethical Problems in Medicine
(March 21, 1983). The Commission argues that the judicial responsibility to protect incompetent patients is not necessarily best
fulfilled by judges taking upon themselves the role of principal
decision maker. Remoteness from the clinical situation and inability to keep pace with the on-going fluctuations in the patient's
condition, particularly in a neonatal intensive-care setting, are
strong arguments in support of that thesis. The report favors having the parents' decision in difficult cases reviewed by an inplace,
broadly based, multidisciplinary hospital ethics committee that

would be familiar both with the medical setting and with community standards. That consultative body, which would have an ongoing charge of establishing standards of treatment and issuing guidelines for the institution, would provide a framework for impartial but sensitive review of hard choices. It would guarantee that the interests of the patient were being considered without the formality and intensely adversarial character of a court proceeding.

If after all this, irreconcilable disagreement still persists, the report recommends referral to the court for the appointment of a legal guardian who would be empowered to evaluate the options and make a decision "in the best interest of the infant." The decision, of course, would be subject as a last resort to judicial scrutiny.

We agree that this approach, one that guarantees a discussion of the issues with a concerned and distinterested "representative of the public" while at the same time insulating the agonizing and tragic decision from the glare of publicity and the distortions of political posturing, is a sensible and desirable way to proceed. It is also a way of insuring that as a society we distinguish between acceptable medical options and infanticide.

19. The Moral Right to Privacy

In attempting to relate law and morality when dilemmas of life and death are involved, one could consider many aspects—for example, living wills, organ donation, definition of death, and euthanasia, to mention but a few. I wish to address myself to several of the moral implications of the Quinlan case, especially as that case was decided on March 31, 1976, by the Supreme Court of New Jersey. I do so in an effort to get at a key issue in that decision—the right to privacy. The essentials of that decision were as follows:

1. The right to privacy is "broad enough to encompass a patient's decision to decline medical treatment under certain circumstances."

2. "Certain circumstances" refer to situations wherein "bodily invasion increases and prognosis dims." In other words, the state's interest *contra* weakens and the individual's right to privacy grows in these circumstances. (This implies that the right to privacy asserted is not absolute and unrestricted.)

3. Karen Quinlan should not be deprived of this right simply because she is incompetent. Thus Karen's guardian and family should be permitted to render their best judgment as to whether Karen would exercise her right.

4. If they decide that she would so exercise her right, their decision should be accepted "by a society the overwhelming majority of whose members would . . . exercise such a choice in the same way for themselves or for those closest to them." Why? Because there is no real possibility that Karen would return from a "comatose condition to a cognitive, sapient state."

5. The use of an "ethics committee or some like body" should be made to support the physicians' judgment that there is "no reasonable possibility of Karen's emerging from this state."

6. Such withdrawal of treatment is not to be considered legal

homicide. There is a real difference between "self-infliction of deadly harm and a self-determination against artificial life support or radical surgery. . . ."

7. This ruling should not be understood as implying that comparable decisions must be brought to court for their determination.

The reaction to this decision is important because it expresses the public attitudes and degree of sophistication with which the decision will be read and implemented in other cases. Mildred Jefferson, M.D., chairperson of the National Right to Life Committee, attacked the decision as extending to parents and a team of doctors the "private right to kill." She continued: "I don't believe that anyone has the right to end the life of anyone who is still functioning."[1] The use of the terms "kill" and "end the life" unfortunately identify noninstigation or withdrawal of life supports with killing.

There were also misgivings expressed about the decision's use of "cognitive" and "sapient." As one critic put it: "This sounds as if decisions are to be based on the patient's 'capacity for meaningful life' and this is a dangerous . . . principle."[2] I grant that "meaningful life" is a dangerous term; but that does not mean we can avoid the substance of the notion in our decision-making. It means only that we must proceed with great caution. In a letter written in the name of Pope Paul VI to the National Federation of Catholic Doctors on October 3, 1970, Cardinal Villot used a very similar phrase. He wrote: "The duty of a doctor consists principally in applying the means at his disposal to lessen the suffering of a sick person instead of concentrating on prolonging for the longest time possible—using any methods and under any circumstances—*a life which is no longer fully human* (emphasis added) and which is drawing naturally to its end."[3]

The major focus of criticism of the New Jersey decision centered around the "right to privacy." Columnist Joseph Breig asserted that "the so-called right to privacy has absolutely nothing to do with the Karen Quinlan case." He considers privacy a "silly

[1] National Catholic News Service.
[2] Ibid.
[3] Cardinal Villot, *Tablet*, 230 (1976), 385–87.

notion" and believes instead that the case involves "the right to die when God calls."[4]

This finesses the real problem of when God should be said to be calling. The first time a surgeon took scalpel in hand, he took a long step in making it difficult for us to know who is doing the calling—God or man—and how we know the difference. The very fact that we can do so many things to preserve life means that the "call of God" increasingly comes to us through human voices and human hands. For instance, is God calling all patients who cannot live without hemodialysis, without a respirator? Or is he calling only those who *choose* not to use such supports? Is he calling Karen Ann even though she can be kept alive for many more months? Serious decisional problems are rarely illumined by invoking circular catechetical simplicities.

Monsignor James T. McHugh stated that the decision contains some dangerous principles, one of which is the right to privacy, "a penumbral right that is still very ambiguous."[5]

The Miami archdiocesan newspaper *The Voice* rejected the use of privacy in this decision. It stated: "The New Jersey Supreme Court is saying that Karen's body can die because of the right to privacy. This is at best an ivory-tower legalism and does not base the ruling squarely on the ultimate issues of life and death."[6] The editorial continued: "The court only added weight to the already overloaded catch-all of the right to 'privacy' which is becoming an excuse for too many other practices which may occur privately but whose effects on society do not necessarily remain private." The editorial lamented that "the most fundamental thing of all—life—has been thrown into that constitutional limbo called 'privacy.'" It concluded: "We believe in the ordinary principle of privacy in everyday living, but not as the basis for deciding the future of all terminally ill patients."

The Catholic Standard and Times, Philadelphia, had problems with the appeal to privacy. It stated: "It seems to us that there can be a danger of exaggeration of the right to privacy. . . . In fact, we believe that the United States Supreme Court has already erroneously asserted the right to privacy as superior to the right to

---

[4] *Catholic Chronicle* (Apr. 30, 1976).
[5] National Catholic News Service.
[6] *The Voice* (Apr. 9, 1976).

life in declaring unconstitutional most laws which restrict abortion. We wonder how long it will take for some to assert the right to privacy in cases of suicide or the direct taking of the lives of the old, the deformed, the retarded, and the sick. Thus the right to privacy can have an innocent sound but a dangerous message."[7]

Law professor Surgio Cotta, University of Rome, sees the ruling as moving toward proclaiming the right to suicide. He stated: "The reasons given by the court seem to me to be an exaggeration of the tendency in American courts to affirm the right to privacy as the right to be able to make any decision whatsoever."[8]

Thomas A. Shannon, writing in *Commonweal*, complained about the broad use of the right to privacy to cover both Karen Ann Quinlan's predicament and a woman's decision to terminate her pregnancy. Shannon considers this broad application unfortunate: "The court has opened itself unnecessarily to the possibility of a strong attack by extreme right-to-life groups who argue a moral domino theory with respect to the practice of abortion and euthanasia." The court, he says, has not only waffled on euthanasia but also "has done so by using the same reasons which justify abortion."[9]

The Idaho *Register*, in an article by news editor Frederic M. Lilly, faulted the use of the so-called right to privacy. It stated: "This 'right to privacy,' carried just a little further by another court decision or legislative action, could open the door for euthanasia."[10]

Eugene J. Schulte, director of government and legal services of the Catholic Hospital Association, made a similar complaint. The verdict is faulty, he argued, because of its use of the right to privacy, "the same right used to support the abortion decisions. We have now extended the right of privacy into the area of death." According to Schulte, "this leaves the door open to conclude that there is a right to suicide and a right to euthanasia."[11]

America magazine editorialized against the notion of privacy.

---

[7] *Catholic Standard and Times* (Apr. 8, 1976).
[8] National Catholic News Service.
[9] Thomas A. Shannon, "The Court's Verdict," *Commonweal*, 103 (1976), 293–94.
[10] National Catholic News Service.
[11] Ibid.

"In recent years," the editors said, "courts have shown a disturbing tendency to confuse 'privacy' with 'self-determination.'" What is objectionable about this? *America* says: "By categorizing as 'private' certain acts of self-determination, the courts obscure the balancing of personal and public interests that their judicial function imposes on them."[12]

In summary, then, many reactions have criticized the right-to-privacy reasoning of the court and on several grounds: (1) It is vague and ambiguous. (2) It was in the *Wade* and *Bolton* abortion decisions. (3) Therefore it too easily leads to euthanasia and suicide.

Since the court was speaking of a constitutional right (a right in law), the criticisms of the New Jersey Supreme Court must be seen as criticisms of the basis of a *legal* right. The constitutional basis for the so-called right to privacy is, according to constitutional experts, vague and dissatisfying. This vagueness appeared clearly in *Griswold* v. *Connecticut* and was possibly the basis for the misuse of privacy in the *Wade* and *Bolton* abortion decisions. However, ultimately I agree with the statements of well-known moral theologian Fr. John R. Connery, who has said that "the decision of the court in no sense opens the door to euthanasia" and that "while one may have legitimate misgivings about the application of the right of privacy to abortion by the U. S. Supreme Court, there can hardly be objection to the reasoning of the New Jersey Supreme Court in this case."[13] In other words, Connery is saying that the abuse of the right to privacy by making it so unlimited that it takes precedence over human life is no reason to attack the right to privacy as such. It is reason for properly limiting it. In still other words, it seems to me that most of the criticisms leveled against the Quinlan decision's reasoning are not valid against the right to privacy as such, but against the contemporary atmosphere in which that right is interpreted.

My thesis is that, the New Jersey Supreme Court's decision being the right decision for the right reason, our best and most constructive response to it is *not* to attack it on the admittedly vague and even possibly erroneous constitutional grounds, but to bring forth more clearly the underlying *moral* tradition upon

12 "Karen Quinlan and the Right to Die," *America*, 134 (1976), 327.
13 National Catholic News Service.

which it rests. By doing this I believe we will be able to clarify a key point that forms the basis for the constitutional criticism— namely, that use of privacy as the basis for the decision will lead to legal acceptance of suicide and euthanasia just as it has led to legal acceptance of abortion. In the realm of constitutional law, that may be correct, given both the vague and penumbral character of the constitutional right to privacy and the abuse to which it has been put in *Wade* and *Bolton*. In the realm of moral reasoning, it certainly is not correct, as I hope to show.

Since good law and good morality are all but identical in areas concerned with justice considerations surrounding a basic human good like life, our most creative and constructive response to constitutional vagueness and abusive interpretation is not simply to note it and criticize it, but to recover and reassert the underlying moral tradition. In doing so we provide the moral antidotes to vagueness and abusive interpretation, and, in my judgment, show why the New Jersey Supreme Court was right both in its conclusion and in its reasoning. We show why that decision was not an example of the vagueness and abusive interpretation we criticize elsewhere.

In summary, then, it may be of help to examine the right to privacy as a *moral* right. If such an analysis will clearly reveal the foundation of this right as well as the basis for limitations on it, then it will suggest the outline of such limitations in the *legal* sphere, and aid us in removing the notion of privacy from the "penumbra of ambiguity" that, in the opinion of many, surrounds it.

As I understand Catholic moral tradition, the so-called right to privacy or self-determination (I realize that there is a difference in these concepts, but for the purpose of stating a general moral tradition, I shall use them as if they were synonymous) in health care and the preservation of life originates through the following steps.

1. Human life, as a gift of God and the condition of all other achievements, is a basic good. Our flourishing both as individuals and as a society depends on the adequacy of our attitudes and actions with regard to this basic good. Any number of more specific modes of obligation spell out the meaning of "adequacy of our at-

titudes and actions." Certainly one mode of obligation is that we ought to preserve life.

2. An individual has the primary obligation to preserve this basic good in himself or herself, to preserve his or her own life. The first and most obvious reason for this is that it is his or her good at stake. The individual is a free and responsible agent. If this obligation did not fall primarily on the individual, how could we ascribe any other obligation to him? Furthermore, the individual himself is the only one who can most of the time take the steps to preserve life and avoid those things that threaten life. Thus it is the individual who is primarily charged with feeding himself properly, clothing himself, avoiding unjustifiable dangers, recognizing threatening disease processes, and seeking remedies. If this duty were not the individual's primarily, who else would do it? (I say "primary" obligation because it is clear that as social and dependent beings, we do depend on others in securing our own well-being.)

3. This obligation to preserve one's life and care for one's health is a *limited* one in Christian perspective. For instance, Christian convictions have never allowed one to do something immoral to preserve one's life. There are also limitations where there is no question of sin. Not all means must be used, otherwise we would convert life from a basic value to an absolute and unconditioned one, and in the process subvert some profound Christian convictions about the meaning of life. No one has stated this more clearly than Pius XII.

4. The limits on one's duty to preserve life are very relative to time, locale, personal biography, personal position, personal perspectives, outlooks, achievements, and recovery prospects.

5. The person himself or those closest to him or her have the best knowledge or understanding of these personal considerations. The individual has the best knowledge of what may be called a "reasonable benefit" to the patient, or of what may be too much of a burden to him, all things considered.

6. Therefore, one has the *right* to those means that make personal execution of this duty possible, and to those means that best provide for the practical admission of limits on this duty.

7. But self-determination with regard to the means of preserving life is a necessary means.

In summary, as I read Catholic moral tradition on this matter, there is first a *duty* to preserve one's life, and following on that a right not to be interfered with in making moral decisions with regard to this duty. The right of privacy or self-determination is a necessary means because, given the personal or individual character of the considerations that limit this duty and given the personal character of the situations that activate this duty, it is the person himself or herself who is best situated to implement decisions. Or again, the underlying supposition for self-determination in the acceptance or refusal of treatment is that the *over-all good of the patient will best be served* if treatment is controlled in this way.

Perhaps we could summarize further as follows. A moral right is always with regard to a good. The good in question is self-determination in the acceptance or rejection of medical treatment. This self-determination (or privacy) is a conditional or instrumental good—that is, it is a good precisely insofar as it is the instrument whereby the best interests of the patient are served by it. If, for example, the best over-all good of patients would be better achieved without self-determination, it would be senseless to speak of self-determination as a right.

By putting the matter in this way—namely, by seeing the good underlying the right of privacy as *the over-all good of the patient* —we see two immediate limitations on this right. First, when the exercise of this right is *de facto* and in the circumstances no longer to the over-all good of the person involved, then the very reason for self-determination or privacy has disappeared. For example, if the person is going to exercise self-determination in a way commonly regarded as destructive to self, then the underlying good that founds the right no longer supports it. Concretely, if the exercise of privacy is going to be—in common opinion— suicidal, then one can argue that the right has met its limits. Or at least, at this point self-determination ceases to be an instrumental good. (The "over-all good of the patient" is a notion that is complicated at times by religious beliefs—for example, Jehovah's Witnesses and blood transfusion.)

Second, self-determination as a means to the over-all good of the person or patient says nothing about the exercise of this right to the detriment of others. That is another judgment altogether—

that is, how the over-all good of the patient is related to and perhaps limited by the good of other patients is simply not to be
derived from the notion of privacy or self-determination itself.
The U. S. Supreme Court, of course, said that such derivation is
possible. But in order to make that as a *moral* judgment, one
would have to assume that the fetus is not a patient (person) or
at least not one to be evaluated as such. Absent that assumption,
and the *prima facie* implication is that the fetus also has a
right of privacy or self-determination, to be exercised, of course, by
proxy in the fetus' best interest.

From the moral point of view these two conclusions point to
the traditional understanding of the limitation of rights. Rights
are limited in two ways. First, there is the limitation *on the right
itself.* And such limitations are rooted in the nature of the good at
stake. For instance, our right to private property is limited by the
extreme need of others, for the primary destination of material
goods is the need and good of all persons. Private property is but
the best way of realizing this primary destination. Where, in rare
circumstances, it hinders rather than realizes this purpose, the
right to private property meets its limits. Thus if I take food from
another because I am in a state of extreme need (my life is at
stake), this is not to be viewed morally as theft.

Second, there can be limitations *on the exercise of rights.* Such
limits are rooted in the social nature of man and concretely in the
rights of others. Thus no one has the right to use his own right
such that it would injure the right of another. For example, it
would be unjust to play with my gun if another person would be
thereby endangered. Or more to our point, granted that we have a
right to privacy (or self-determination) where health care is concerned, we may not use such a right in a way that violates the
rights of others (for example, the fetus).

This is, I believe, the moral tradition on the right to self-determination. It is an instrumental right in service of and subordinate
to a good—the *best interests of the person.* By saying that, we say
also thereby that such a right (1) does not extend, as instrumental
to a good, to actions not comprehended in that good, not in the
best interests of the patient (and here moral tradition would include suicide and euthanasia), and (2) asserts or implies nothing
about the exercise of his right in a way detrimental to others, for
the right is rooted in the best interests of the person in question.

If these best interests conflict at times with the best interests of others, then we must appeal to principles other than the right to privacy to resolve such conflicts.

In the language of medical ethics, this moral right gives birth to the professional requirement of informed consent. The decision of Judge Robert Muir that treatment in the Quinlan case is a "medical decision, not a judicial one" and that "it may be concurred in by the parents but not governed by them" was seen by the vast majority of commentators as a basic assault on the venerable doctrine of informed consent, and thereby on its moral rootage, the right to privacy or self-determination. As Norman L. Cantor, professor of law at Rutgers University School of Law, stated of Muir's wording: "This blueprint for decision-making completely reverses normal procedures."[14] Robert Veatch of the Kennedy Institute referred to Muir's decision as a "fundamental analytical mistake."[15]

The New Jersey Supreme Court reversed this and put the decision for treatment where it belongs—with the patient, or if the patient is incompetent, with those who presumably have the patient's best interest at heart, the parents or nearest of kin. It was, I am convinced, essential that this reversal take place. The court used the right of privacy to argue and convey this reversal. If there are constitutional problems to appeal to such a right, there are, I believe, no moral problems. And it is in reasserting the moral tradition, not only in complaining about constitutional vagueness and past interpretive abuse, that we will best clarify this vagueness and correct these abuses. That is how I see law and morality relating in this particular dilemma of life and death. That is why I think the critics of the New Jersey Supreme Court decision were both right and wrong. They were right that the vehicle, the right to privacy, in its present constitutional status and in the present destructive atmosphere, is a wobbly vehicle. They were wrong in failing to show how and why that need not be the case. In other words, they were wrong because they only criticized a constitutional vehicle when they could also have corrected it. And that correction is, I am convinced, to be found in the *moral* tradition.

[14] Norman L. Cantor, "Quinlan Case: An Analysis," New York *Law Journal* (Dec. 22, 1975).
[15] Robert Veatch, "The Quinlan Case: A Tragedy of Faulty Analysis," *Bioethics Northwest*, 1 (1976), 2.

20. The Case of Joseph Saikewicz

Joseph Saikewicz, aged sixty-seven in 1976, was profoundly mentally retarded. He had an IQ of 10 and a mental age of approximately two years, eight months. He could communicate only by gestures and grunts, and was deeply disoriented when out of his familiar environment. Mr. Saikewicz had lived in state institutions since 1923, and in Belchertown State School since 1928.

On April 19, 1976, Saikewicz was diagnosed as suffering from acute myeloblastic monocytic leukemia. This blood disease results from the body's production of excessive white blood cells, and is associated with enlargement of organs (spleen, lymph glands, bone marrow), internal bleeding, and, in acute stages, with severe anemia and vulnerability to infection. The disease is unavoidably and invariably fatal.

Chemotherapy can produce remission of the disease (temporary return to normal) in around 30 to 50 per cent of cases, but this remission lasts typically between two and thirteen months. With patients over sixty the prognosis is somewhat poorer. If left untreated, Saikewicz would die within a matter of several weeks or months. Should he receive the chemotherapy? The authorities at Belchertown thought so and, on April 26, 1976, petitioned the Probate Court of Hampshire County, Massachusetts, for the appointment of a guardian *ad litem* with authority to make medical decisions. The guardian *ad litem* was appointed on May 5. The very next day the guardian filed a report that "not treating Mr. Saikewicz would be in his best interests." At the hearing on May 13, 1976, the probate court agreed in essence with that recommendation. Chemotherapy was not administered. On September 4, 1976, Joseph Saikewicz died at the Belchertown State School hospital from bronchial pneumonia, a complication of leukemia.

The "no chemotherapy" decision of the probate judge was referred to the Massachusetts Supreme Court. Two questions were put for appellate review: (1) Does the probate court have the authority to order in certain circumstances the withholding of treatment, when withholding may lead to a shortening of life? (2) Was its judgment correct in the Saikewicz case? On July 9, 1976, the Supreme Court of Massachusetts answered both questions in the affirmative and said that its opinion would follow. That opinion was issued on November 28, 1977.

We think the decision of the Massachusetts Supreme Court to be of enormous importance to all of us. Therefore, we propose to review the reasoning of the decision, its implications, and our objections to that decision.

The court first admits that human dignity requires that individuals have a general right to self-determination where medical decisions are involved. We say "general right" because there are certain state interests that can take precedence over this right. The court mentions four state interests that may override the right: (1) the preservation of life; (2) the protection of the interests of innocent third parties (for example, where children would suffer "abandonment" by the death of the parent if the parent refused treatment, as in the case of a Jehovah's Witness); (3) the prevention of suicide; and (4) the maintenance of the integrity of the medical profession. When one of these interests competes with the individual's right of self-determination, the court must engage in a balancing process to determine which is more important. The most important of these interests (and the one on which all others depend) is the preservation of life. Here the court is sensitive and balanced. It states: "Recognition of such an interest, however, does not necessarily resolve the problem where the affliction of disease clearly indicates that life will soon, and inevitably, be extinguished. The interest of the State in prolonging a life must be reconciled with the interest of the individual to reject the traumatic cost of the prolongation."[1]

Applying these consideratios to Saikewicz, the court concluded that two state interests (prevention of suicide, protection of innocent third parties) had no relevance. The other two did not override the right to decline treatment because Saikewicz was a dying

[1] *Superintendent of Belchertown State School* v. *Saikewicz*, 370 N. E. Rep., 2d Ser., 417–35 (Mass. 1977).

patient whose life could be only "briefly extended" (hence the *preservation* of life is not precisely the issue) and because it is fully within accepted medical standards to withhold treatment when the expected outcome is merely prolongation of dying.

The Massachusetts Supreme Court developed its analysis in terms of the rights of the competent patient. But since Saikewicz was incompetent, it turned next to this factor. Does a choice to refuse treatment exist even if the person is incompetent, or must the court always order life-prolonging treatment? If a choice exists, what considerations enter the decision-making process? The court agreed that a choice does exist, because the best interests of incompetents are not always served by imposing on them what competent persons may rightfully choose to omit. "To presume that the incompetent person must always be subjected to what rational and intelligent persons may decline is to downgrade the status of the incompetent person by placing a lower value on his intrinsic worth and vitality." Rather, incompetent persons have the same rights here as competent persons—that is, they may at times refuse treatment.

But how are incompetents to exercise this right? Here the court explicitly accepts the doctrine of substituted judgment. In short, with an eye to the patient's best interests and preferences, "the decisions in cases such as this should be those which would be made by the incompetent person if that person were competent. . . ."

What, then, would Saikewicz himself choose? Weighing the factors both for and against chemotherapy, the Massachusetts Supreme Court concluded that Saikewicz would reject chemotherapy, for such a decision best serves "his actual interests and preferences."

Thus far, we agree with this conclusion and analysis. Saikewicz was a dying patient in the court's opinion—though it is not always that easy to determine who should be said to be dying and who should not. He had a terminal disease; an optimistic prognosis would extend his life from two to thirteen months at most. Furthermore, any extension of life he gained would be associated with continuing painful and distressing side effects and disorientations due to chemotherapy. Therefore, we believe with the court that his over-all best interests would not be served by this treatment, and hence that he would not choose to undergo it.

In arriving at this same judgment, the court was careful to distinguish a factor adduced by the lower court: "the quality of life available to him even if the treatment does bring about remission." If this phrase ("quality of life") is taken to refer to Saikewicz's retardation, the court stated that "we firmly reject it." If, however, it refers to the continuing state of pain and disorientation associated with chemotherapy, the court accepts it. We agree and strongly underline this distinction. Substituted judgments about acceptance or rejection of treatment should not be made merely on the basis of the retarded condition. This is not to say, however, that quality-of-life considerations have no place in such judgments.

But here our agreement with the court ends and profound misgivings arise, for the court then turned to the procedures appropriate for decision-making in cases of using or withholding life-prolonging treatment for a "person allegedly incompetent." In the Karen Ann Quinlan case, the New Jersey Supreme Court entrusted the decision whether to continue artificial life support to the patient's guardian (her father, Joseph Quinlan), in consultation with physicians and a badly named "Ethics Committee" (as its functions were described by the court, it was really a prognosis committee). The Massachusetts court rejected "the approach adopted by the New Jersey Supreme Court in the *Quinlan* case." Rather, the questions of life and death require a "detached but passionate investigation and decision that form the ideal on which the judicial branch of government was created." Achievement of this ideal is the responsibility of the courts and "is not to be entrusted to any other group." Briefly, the proper and only tribunals for determining the best interests of all incompetent persons are the courts.

The implications of this are enormous, and, we think, highly questionable. What are the immediate implications? As Richard A. Knox wrote in the Washington *Post:* "The new Massachusetts ruling essentially holds that issues of both withholding and terminating critical care—for the elderly stroke victims or cancer patients, as well as for severely ill newborns—are matters for the probate courts to decide, not for the families, doctors, nurses, social workers, priests, committees, or anyone else."[2]

Why are these the implications of the decision? For two reasons: First, the term "incompetent" includes the mentally retarded, insane, comatose, unconscious, infants, etc. Second, the court made it clear that it regarded Saikewicz as a *dying* incompetent patient. Therefore, its ruling extends in principle to all dying incompetents. This is of crucial importance. Thus the court distinguished preserving life from prolonging life. It stated: "There is a substantial distinction in the State's insistence that human life be saved when the affliction is curable, as opposed to the State interest where, *as here* [emphasis ours], the issue is not whether, but when, for how long and at what cost to the individual that life may be briefly extended." Furthermore, the court referred to the Saikewicz case with the following phrases: "a brief and uncertain delay in the natural process of death"; "life-saving treatment is available—a situation unfortunately not presented by this case"; "treatment which . . . may increase suffering in exchange for a possible yet brief prolongation of life." And finally: "Nor was this a case in which life-saving, as distinguished from life-prolonging, procedures were available."

In this connection, it should be noted that Paul Ramsey's discussion of the Saikewicz case in his recent book, *Ethics at the Edge of Life*, was composed before the court's November 28 analysis.[3] Therefore, it remains incomplete and even flawed. Professor Ramsey did not view Saikewicz as a *dying* patient, at least not in the same way the court did, although at one point he describes him as "dying, without treatment." Thus Professor Ramsey is fearful throughout his treatment that the court's decision may have been based on Saikewicz's retardation. The fear is legitimate, but unjustified.

In support of the court's decision, George Annas, assistant professor of law and medicine at the Boston University School of Medicine, has argued in the *Hastings Report* that a correct resolution of the case of the incompetent "is more likely to come from a judicial decision after an adversary proceeding in which all inter-

2 Washington *Post* (Feb. 18, 1978).
3 Paul Ramsey, *Ethics at the Edges of Life* (New Haven, Conn.: Yale University Press, 1978).

ested parties have fully participated . . . than from the individual decisions of the patient's family, the attending physician, an ethics committee or all of these combined."[4]

We disagree. Indeed, we find this intolerable. It is one thing to recognize that the cases of certain incompetent persons are doubtful, agonizingly ambiguous, extremely difficult, and vulnerable to abusive decision. These cases in dispute might appropriately call for judicial overview. But it is something else to say that all cases of life-prolonging treatment or withholding of treatment from the incompetent must be routinely decided in probate court.

Our disagreement with Professor Annas and the Massachusetts Supreme Court is rooted in several considerations. First, we disagree with the contention that it is "only by using the admittedly difficult machinery of a legal proceeding" that the best interests of the incompetent can be promoted. This contention assumes that the ordinary consultative process involving family, physicians, nurses, and so-called ethics committees is insufficient or is likely to be widely abused. We know of no such evidence to justify Professor Annas' implied assertion. Furthermore, a careful and conscientious consultation by the concerned parties will contain the very virtues and cautions he attributes to an adversary procedure. We have seen this happen repeatedly. To say that a more correct decision is likely to come from a judicial proceeding (after all the interested parties have been consulted) denies to concerned people the very discernment, wisdom, and prudence attributed to the probate judge. This is contrary to our experience. For example, we agree with the decision of the probate judge and the Massachusetts Supreme Court in the Saikewicz case; but we think that conclusion was not terribly difficult to arrive at in the light of the pros and cons that went into its making.

At some point, then, there is an unintentional but undesirable arrogance in the court's assumption that a probate judge can determine, better than anyone else, the best interests of desperately ill patients. We do not deny the wisdom of appeal to the courts when concerned parties are in dispute about these interests. But when such appeal becomes a mandatory routinized procedure, it makes a new priesthood of the judiciary. Treatment and manage-

[4] George Annas, "The Incompetent's Right to Die: The Case of Joseph Saikewicz," *Hastings Center Report*, 8 (Feb. 1978), 21–23.

ment decisions are not mere medical decisions; nor are they mere legal decisions. They are above all human decisions. To shift them routinely to the courts tends to undermine this fact. What evidence is there to support the idea that probate judges are the only persons who can safely make such decisions? Indeed, the assumption that the courts do a better job is challenged by some recent history. In the Quinlan case, for example, Judge Muir and the New Jersey Supreme Court came to diametrically opposite conclusions on the same facts. We agree with the court that these questions of life and death demand a "detached but passionate investigation," but we believe that families, physicians, nurses, and moral advisers consulting together should not be presumed incapable of such investigation and decision.

Second, the ruling and its language mean that everybody must be resuscitated, and that all incompetents must be kept on respirators until the probate judge decides otherwise, for the court's language ("Life may be briefly extended . . . a brief and uncertain delay in the natural process of dying . . . a possible yet brief prolongation of life") encompasses these cases. What we have in mind is that the physician is now forced to start the treatment in order to find out from the probate court whether he should have started it. Therefore, the procedural requirements of the court force the initiation of therapies that the court itself might deem unnecessary and would indeed countermand.

This is highly problematic. For instance, what is to happen to the incompetent patient (baby, elderly, retarded, etc.) while this "admittedly difficult machinery of a legal proceeding" is grinding into action? Do we simply continue life supports in the interim, a perhaps long, drawn-out interim? Or do we withhold them pending judicial intervention? Much that is at best inappropriate, at worst abusive, could happen to a patient as the adversary procedure unfolds. The result is that patients are now to be made to suffer, often needlessly, for the purposes of the court's procedures.

Moreover, in the sometimes long process of dying, conditions and prognoses change. The intent of the court could only be met if physicians and family returned to the probate court on several occasions. The Massachusetts Supreme Court seems to be ignorant of the fact that therapies are often started on a trial basis, only to be discontinued if a desired effect is not obtained or adverse results are obtained. The idea is intolerable and absurd that, as prognoses change, all should have to return to the probate court. This is to set up the court as cophysician. We do not see the physician as the master of the patient, but neither do we see judges as masters of physicians who can decide which therapies should be tried and which not, which stopped and which not.

The immediate impact of this ruling, then, will inevitably be a renewed vitalism, a never-say-die policy. This is threatening in itself, because it is at odds with the cherished convictions of many people about the meaning of life and death. But it is also subtly threatening in its implications, for the prospect of such end-stage treatment will all but force us to support legislation that recognizes living wills. We have already stated our serious misgivings about such legislation.[5] One of the major objections is that legislated living wills are a reinforcement of the idea that physicians (or the medical system) are masters of the patient, who must then extract himself by making such a will. Embedded in this notion is a subtle shift from the medicomoral axiom *primum non nocere* (first do not harm) to *primum non nocere societati* (first do no harm to society).

The practical consequence of all this may well be a policy that leads to what we call the "undertreatment-overtreatment syndrome"—a kind of safe policy; that is, foreseeing the demand of a legal procedure, some hospitals will prevent the cumbersome problem from arising by failing to resuscitate where perhaps the patient is resuscitable. Other hospitals, from fear of malpractice suits or criminal liability, will keep incompetents on life-prolonging equipment when such treatment is not indicated.

Third and finally, the Massachusetts Supreme Court seems to have no idea about the number of cases of incompetence that occur each day. These cases (involving what the court called "a brief and uncertain delay in the natural process of dying") are not simply occasional. They occur by the hundreds on a daily basis. The courts simply will be incapable of dealing with the problem. Hospital personnel, aware of this sheer impracticality, will quietly ignore the ruling—a practice that not only undermines

[5] Richard A. McCormick, S.J., and André E. Hellegers, "Legislation and the Living Will," *America*, 136 (1977), 210–13. See the final chapter of this book.

the integrity of the legal system, but also intensifies the liability and malpractice atmosphere that already plagues American hospitals. Or, if they do not ignore it, they will keep every incompetent person alive, regardless of the condition, prospects, and circumstances of that individual.

There is a long and honored moral and legal tradition that medical-treatment decisions are the prerogatives of the patient (which the court admits when the patient is competent) or of those who presumably have the best interests of the patient at heart (for example, the family) when the patient is incompetent. This is as it should be, always saving right of appeal where abuses are judged to be present or very likely. We could accept the court's solution for wards of the state or patients restricted to institutions even before their dying had begun (for example, prisoners, the mentally retarded in state institutions). In brief, if the court had restricted its decision to the abandoned, where it could not be assumed that anyone had their interest at heart, we could have thought of the decision as a prudential one, designed for the protection of a small segment of the population. But to apply it to all incompetents is to fail to understand the process of dying in an age of high technology and to misconceive the court's role as *parens patriae.*

Treatment decisions are utterly personal. They must be made in terms of the individual's history, aspirations, achievements, age, family, beliefs, etc. They are a glove fitting an individual hand. For this reason they have been appropriately made within the patient-family-physician context of health care. When these decisions are routinely (*all* incompetents) removed from this matrix, they are handed over to two impersonal forces: technology and the law. Individual and personal decisions begin to be made by impersonal forces. That is a threat to our well-being. If technology and the law were largely to usurp the patient-family-physician prerogatives in management decisions, we would all be worse off. Impersonal considerations would too easily replace personal ones and preprogram our treatment. That is always the root of oppression and depersonalization, in medicine as well as in other areas. That is why the case of Joseph Saikewicz remains not simply an individual case, but also a threatening specter.

21. The Preservation of Life and Self-determination

On October 2, 1979, Brother Joseph Charles Fox, an eighty-three-year-old member of the Society of Mary (Chaminade High School, Mineola, N.Y.), underwent hernia surgery. During the surgery he suffered severe cardiorespiratory arrest, which resulted in diffuse cerebral and brain-stem anoxia. Brother Fox lost spontaneous respiration and had to be maintained on a respirator. His physicians concluded that he was in a "permanent vegetative state."

Rev. Philip K. Eichner, president and religious superior at Chaminade High School, after consulting the only surviving relatives (ten nieces and nephews), requested removal of the respirator. Nassau Hospital refused and Eichner sought judicial relief. Three *amici curiae* briefs (New York State Right to Life Committee, Human Life Amendment Group, the diocesan Catholic Lawyers' Guild) supported Eichner and Brother Fox's relatives. The Nassau County district attorney opposed any such relief.

On December 6, New York Supreme Court Judge Robert Meade rendered his decision. In brief, the relief was granted—as in our opinion it should have been. Indeed, we are convinced that the appropriate decision is so clear that it need not have gone to court, and ought not to do so in similar cases.

However, it is not the decision itself that is our concern; it is rather its reasoning. In his petition for termination of "extraordinary life-support systems," Eichner argued that "to maintain the life-support system of an unwilling patient is an invasion of his constitutionally guaranteed right of privacy." In urging the right of privacy, the petitioner was relying on two highly publicized precedents, *In re Quinlan* and *Superintendent of Belchertown State School v. Saikewicz*. In the well-known Karen Ann Quinlan case, the New Jersey Supreme Court recognized the constitutional right of privacy and stated that it is "broad enough to encompass a patient's decision to decline medical treatment under certain circumstances." The Massachusetts Supreme Court argued very similarly in the Saikewicz case,[1] referring to "the unwritten constitutional right of privacy found in the penumbra of specific guarantees of the Bill of Rights."

Judge Robert Meade refused to pass on the applicability of the right of privacy to the Fox case. He had misgivings about it. For instance, since the right of privacy is protected by the Fourteenth Amendment's concept of personal liberty and restrictions upon state actions, "is it not necessary to the establishment of a violation of that right that 'State action' be involved?"[2] Furthermore, Meade felt that the right of privacy is so insufficiently defined but so attractively worded that it invites "unrestrained applications."

Rather than basing relief on the right to privacy, Judge Meade turned to the common-law notion of the right of self-determination. After examining preceding decisions,[3] Meade concluded that there is a common-law right to bodily self-determination "which includes the right of a competent adult to refuse life-sustaining medical treatment." Even though there are limits to this right, Meade concluded that these limits (countervailing state interests) were not germane in Brother Fox's case. For instance, the state interest in the preservation of life is not at stake because Fox's condition is "hopeless" and further treatment "serves only more or less briefly to extend the process of dying."

Now clearly, since Brother Fox could not exercise such a right for himself, Eichner was seeking to do so for him, relying once again on the Quinlan and Saikewicz cases. In both cases a substituted judgment was allowed—that is, a judgment made for one person by another. The substance of such a judgment, of course, must be the best interests of the incompetent, what the incompetent would do were he or she able to choose for himself or herself. Judge Meade rejects this approach: "Respectfully this court is

1 Confer chapter 19.
2 Citations here and hereafter from Meade's decision are taken from the manuscript (No. 21,242-I/79) kindly provided by Rev. Philip K. Eichner, S.M.
3 For instance, *Union Pacific Railway Co.* v. *Botsford* (1891), *Erikson* v. *Dilgard* (1962), *Palm Springs General Hospital, Inc.* v. *Martinez* (1971), *In re Long Island Jewish-Hillside Medical Center* (1973).

unable to accept the analyses adopted in those [*Quinlan, Saike-wicz*] decisions." Meade argued that *by its very nature* the right to decline life-saving treatment can be exercised by the individual alone, for it is "a right of the individual to make up his or her own mind." Karen Quinlan could not do this, and even less so could Joseph Saikewicz, who had never been competent.

Even though he rejected the analyses of *Quinlan* and *Saikewicz* as involving a fiction (the use of a substituted or proxy judgment as if it were the concerned individual's), Judge Meade did not reject the relief requested. Why? He first noted that Brother Fox had clearly indicated that, under the circumstances and conditions that then surrounded him, he would not consent to continuation of the life-supporting respirator. Then comes his crucial reason: "If Father Eichner, his committee, were to request the termination of the respirator, then that request would be the decision of Brother Fox which Father Eichner would merely pass on as a conduit. Unlike *Quinlan* and *Saikewicz*, no fiction is created nor is the judgment of Father Eichner substituted for that of Brother Fox."

In other words, Judge Meade feels authorized to grant relief *only because* the decision is that of Brother Fox. It is the decision of Brother Fox *only because* he had seriously discussed the *Quinlan* case and made his views clear before his predicament. Any other analysis Judge Meade sees as substituted judgments, which must be disallowed because the right in question is that of *self*-determination.

We believe this analysis has great importance with regard to the moral duty of preserving life. We will first suggest its implications and possible consequences, then the broader issues it suggests.

The very first implication of this reasoning is that the vast majority of dying incompetent patients will be unable to have respirator (etc.) support discontinued where in balanced human and Christian judgment this is the thing to do. Why? Because most people will not have made their minds and preferences known through prior discussion, or if they have, witnesses of the fact may be lacking. For instance, how many people have discussed the *Quinlan* case in such a way that their clear preferences would be known and certifiable in their own incompetent, dying hour? If they have not, then there are no grounds for removing them from the respirator. We find reasoning that leads to such a conclusion self-defeating and ultimately very vulnerable.

Second, if Judge Meade disallows substituted judgments in cases of perpetual incompetency such as *Saikewicz* (he refers to any attempt to discern the actual interests and preferences of *Saikewicz* as "a ritualistic exercise, necessarily doomed to failure"), it is clear a fortiori that he would have to do the same for infants. That would imply that no dying infant could ever be withdrawn from life-sustaining equipment if such equipment could continue to keep that life going—regardless of condition or prognosis. This seems to us at odds with humane medical practice and good morality.

Third, Judge Meade's reasoning clearly is based on the notion of individual self-determination understood, as he says, as "the right . . . to do whatever its possessor desires irrespective of the views of the majority." "Whatever its possessor desires" is not necessarily coincident with the best interests of the possessor. Thus in deciding what is responsible medical treatment of the dying incompetent, Judge Meade has driven a wedge between true best interests and personal desires, favored the latter as the basis of treatment, and left certification of these desires in the hands of the nearest of kin. Does this not offer greater possibility for abuse than an analysis that attempts to link more closely personal desires with actual best interests, and allows public opinion ("the overwhelming majority," as *Quinlan* words it) some role in determining, at least broadly, the meaning of best interests?

Finally, if these indeed are the implications of Judge Meade's reasoning, they constitute a nearly unavoidable stimulus toward legislation of living wills. Judge Meade adverted to this when he noted that "some form of such legislation may perhaps be required if the cessation of artificial life-support systems is to be possible under other circumstances." Contrarily, we believe that most current laws legislating living wills may be unnecessary and even dangerous.[4] Furthermore, we believe that if any such legislation is called for, the most acceptable and least dangerous form is that whereby a person, in good health, deputes a proxy who will have

---

[4] Cf. André E. Hellegers and Richard A. McCormick, S.J., "Legislation and the Living Will," *America*, 136 (1977), 210–13.

decisive say in stating his best interests during incompetency. But this is precisely what Judge Meade denies can be done if the right in question is individual self-determination.

And that brings us to the substantive issue raised by his decision: the meaning of self-determination in this context and its relationship to guardianship.

We believe that the principle of individual self-determination is, at best, a limited, partial basis for an understanding of the appropriate resolution of conflict over decisions about the withdrawal of treatment from seriously or terminally ill persons. It perhaps provides an adequate basis for a policy of nonintervention on the part of the state, the medical community, and the family. Any adequate understanding of the moral basis for decisions in cases like that of Brother Fox, however, must move beyond the principle of individual self-determination. It is a sufficient but not necessary condition for decisions about the incompetent.

First, although the competent patient in a liberal society may have the legal right and even the ethical right of self-determination, this principle does not provide any moral basis for that individual to reach his or her own moral decision about whether it is appropriate to refuse or accept medical treatment; for that, some fuller moral basis for decision must be provided. Traditionally many moral frameworks have acknowledged two justifiable grounds for treatment refusal: the burdensomeness of treatment or the uselessness of treatment. Some such positive moral guidance beyond the principle of individual self-determination will be required for an individual to determine whether medical treatment is morally to be refused or accepted.

But for the incompetent patient there must also be some moral foundation beyond that of individual self-determination. Judge Meade is correct in his recognition that incompetent patients cannot at the time of incompetency exercise self-determination. We think he is also correct in recognizing that the clearly expressed and demonstrated views of formerly competent patients such as Brother Fox provide an acceptable basis for making decisions for such patients provided there is no evidence that the patient has rejected those views. Occasionally such cases may have to be adjudicated when there is doubt about the expressed wishes of the formerly competent patient or disagreement about whether those wishes remained in effect at the time of the patient's lapse into incompetency. In such cases the next of kin, other family members, or family surrogates such as Father Eichner are important and legitimate sources in reconstructing the formerly competent patient's actual wishes at the time of his lapse into incompetency.

Many patients, however, have never been competent or, if competent, have not formulated and expressed a consistent position about their treatment if seriously or terminally ill. Here individual *self*-determination is out of the question, but a fuller understanding of the principles of autonomy and benefit to the patient may still provide a basis for making responsible decisions about the care of such patients. In fact, we maintain that some decision simply must be made for such patients. To fail to make a decision seems impossible or at least morally irresponsible.

We suggest two principles that can replace the principle of individual self-determination as bases for forming social policy regarding the care of patients like Joseph Saikewicz, Karen Quinlan, and others who have either never been competent or who have not expressed themselves adequately while competent. The first principle is the principle of patient benefit. Incompetent patients and formerly competent patients who have not expressed themselves adequately while competent must be accorded full dignity as human beings. We must affirm the moral obligations placed upon others that this implies. Someone must have the responsibility of determining what is in such a patient's best interest. By confining withdrawal or withholding medical treatment within actual individual self-determination, Judge Meade makes it impossible (unless he says more) to get incompetents who have not expressed themselves or those who have always been incompetent off useless or gravely burdensome life-extending machinery. In other words, he makes it impossible for the best interests of many patients to be served by disallowing the only judgment (substituted, guardian) that could possibly serve such interests. In this we disagree. If some medical interventions are not in the best interests of the patient, it would be irresponsible to permit those medical interventions to continue. The patient-benefit principle, thus, leads to the conclusion that someone ought to have the responsibility for deciding both to provide and to withhold medical intervention.

We are left with the question of who this "someone" might be. There are two reasons why family members or family surrogates are in a good position to make the initial determination. First, the family is normally in the best position to judge the real interests of the incompetent patient. They know his or her life-style, preferences, and values. The family knows those treatments that might be particularly disturbing and those that the patient may have accepted without distress in the past.

Second, however—and we think this is the more important reason—our society places great value on the family. The family is a basic moral community affirmed to have not only rights, but also responsibilities in determining how best to serve the interests of its incompetent members. In fact, the principle of self-determination can best be understood to extend beyond the individual to encompass the notion of familial self-determination. This familial autonomy or self-determination is a value highly treasured. While it perhaps should not take precedence over individual autonomy or self-determination in cases where patients are or were competent, it certainly justifies a prominent role for family members in helping to assess what is in the best interests of the incompetent one. Family members are given enormous responsibility for moral nurture, theological and secular education, and decisions about the best interests of their incompetent members throughout the lifetime of the family unit. It should be no different in the case when the incompetent family member is seriously or terminally ill. Occasionally this may lead a family to decide that the incompetent one's interests can best be served by declining a medical intervention.

Even though the courts will approach the matter in a more secular way, there are sound theological warrants supporting the principle of familial self-determination. In Christian tradition the family is seen as a tightly bound unit with a sacramental ministry to the world. It is to mirror forth, by its own cohesiveness and solidarity, the love of Christ for his people. It is the school of love and caring, of nourishing and growth. It shares and deepens its values and spiritual life together as a unit. It determines what is to be its Christian life-style. It is the Church in miniature, and therefore like the Church has its own inner dynamics, priorities, and ideals. Since it lives and grows as a unit, its decisions in many important matters are, or ought to be, corporate decisions, directions taken as a result of its own familial self-determination.

Of course, the principle of familial self-determination cannot ride unchecked. Society's responsibility to assure that the interests of its incompetent members are served will place some limits on familial autonomy. In cases, however, where a family is willing to make such decisions, and they act to fulfill their responsibility in this regard, the state should intervene only when the familial judgment so exceeds the limits of reason that the compromise with what is objectively in the incompetent one's best interests cannot be tolerated.

When there is no family member or family surrogate willing to be appointed guardian for an incompetent one, then the principle of familial autonomy no longer has any significance for the specific case. The principle of patient benefit remains and becomes the exclusive principle for determining the case. Even then, however, when the only principle is that of choosing the course that will best serve the patient's best interests, someone will have to make that determination. In these most tragic cases often a public official such as a judge may have to be called upon. By this method due process will be provided to protect the interests of a most vulnerable group in our society. In some cases the choice of the single course that is most objectively in the patient's interests may be so obvious to all concerned that official judicial involvement may not be necessary. There will be a real risk in permitting such decisions to be made outside of public scrutiny for such patients, but our faith in the wisdom and objectivity of those providing care may justify such a risk.

In any case for such patients standing outside the arms of a loving and caring family structure, the goal must be to choose the single most objectively determined beneficial course.

A decision must be made in these cases. Apparently Meade's rejection of *Quinlan* and *Saikewicz* has led him to reject all substituted and guardian judgments. We disagree. There must be a principle for determining the best interests of the incompetent. The principle cannot be that of individual self-determination. When family members are available to lead in the decision, the principle of familial self-determination should grant them some discretion. They must determine what they consider to be in the best interests of their incompetent member based on their own system of familial beliefs and values. As long as those judgments do not deviate too far from what is most reasonably in the patient's best interests, the family's wishes should be controlling. If they do deviate so far that the principle of patient benefit is unacceptably compromised, then others involved—medical professionals, friends of the patient, or any others significantly associated with the patient—must seek review to determine the limits of familial autonomy.

SECTION VII

THE QUALITY OF LIFE

22. The Qualty of Life, the Sanctity of Life

The tragic case of Karen Ann Quinlan sent moral theologians and ethicists back to their traditions to re-evaluate the formulations that attempted to spell out and mediate traditional value judgments in an increasingly complex world. Conceptualization has always been very important to moral theology. Because times, circumstances, and perspectives change, sometimes dramatically, the viability of some of our most treasured value judgments depends on the accuracy of their formulation in our time.

The adequacy of our formulations is being challenged in the area of life preservation. The availability of powerful new technologies that can sustain life almost indefinitely has forced us to ask: What are we doing when we intervene to stave off death? What values are we seeking to serve? How should we formulate these values in our time if we are to maintain (individually and collectively) our grasp on the basic values that define our well-being? Ought we sustain life when the individual stands to gain nothing from such sustenance? And what does "stands to gain nothing" mean?

More concretely, did "right reason" (as informed by the perspectives of Christian faith) demand that we keep a person like Karen Quinlan on a respirator, or (once she was removed) on artificial feeding, or antibiotics? She was described by attending physicians as in a "persistent vegetative state" with no hope of return to a "cognitive and sapient state." If sound morality did not demand such efforts, why was this so? That is, how should we analyze or conceptualize our response? Should we say that the means are "extraordinary" or "heroic"? Or should we say that the life itself had achieved its human potential?

Cases like this are particularly difficult and decisions are especially awesome in neonatal intensive-care units. Here we are dealing with tiny patients who have no history, have had no chance at life, and have no say in the momentous decision about their treatment. Some are born with anomalies or birth accidents so utterly devastating (especially extensive brain damage) that they will never rise much above the "persistent vegetative state" used to describe Karen Quinlan—though accurate prognosis is often difficult and uncertain in the early weeks of infancy, the very times when a decision about life-sustaining intervention is necessary.

Our duties of life-preservation and care have for years been formulated in terms of the use of what has been called "ordinary" and "extraordinary" means. If the means could be characterized as "extraordinary," there was no obligation per se for the patient to use them, or for those with proxy rights (such as parents) to decide to use them for incompetents. If, all things considered, they were to be characterized as "ordinary," they were seen as obligatory. These phrases were always extremely flexible and had to be made concrete by reference to any number of variants. As Pius XII worded it: "But normally, one is held to use only ordinary means—according to circumstances of persons, places, times, and culture—that is to say, means that do not involve any grave burden for oneself or another. A more strict obligation would be too burdensome for most men and would render the attainment of the higher, more important good too difficult. Life, death, all temporal activities are in fact subordinate to spiritual ends."[1]

In 1973 this language (ordinary/extraordinary) officially moved into the secular realm when it was adopted by the House of Delegates of the American Medical Association. After rejecting "mercy killing," the statement continued: "The cessation of the employment of extraordinary means to prolong the life of the body when there is irrefutable evidence that death is imminent is the decision of the patient and/or his immediate family."[2]

The Ethical and Religious Directives for Catholic Health Care Facilities (United States Catholic Conference)[3] use this same lan-

[1] Pope Pius XII, *Acta Apostolicae Sedis*, 49 (1957), 1,031–32.
[2] *Proceedings, AMA House of Delegates* (Dec. 1973). Cited in James Rachels, "Active and Passive Euthanasia," *New England Journal of Medicine*, 292 (1975), 78–80.
[3] United States Catholic Conference, 1971.

guage. Bishop Lawrence Casey (Paterson, N.J.) repeated it on November 1, 1975, when he supported the Quinlan family's decision to remove Karen from the respirator. "Karen Ann Quinlan," he stated, "has no reasonable hope of recovery from her comatose state by the use of any available medical procedures. The continuance of mechanical (cardiorespiratory) supportive measures to sustain continuation of her body functions and her life constitute extraordinary means of treatment."[4] Bishop Casey's statement strongly implies that cardiorespiratory measures are extraordinary *because*, while sustaining life, they continue only a "comatose state." This relativity was explicitly noted by the New Jersey Supreme Court, which stated that the "record is somewhat hazy in distinguishing between 'ordinary' and 'extraordinary' measures."[5] The court went on to say that one or the other term is used depending on whether the patient is "possibly curable" or not.

Increasingly, then, decisions about life support are more narrowly focusing on a single element: the *kind of life* the patient experiences as a result of the employment of new life-support technologies. Moral theologian Margaret Farley of Yale University put it this way: If we are beginning to consider means more or less extraordinary in "relation to the capacities for fullness of life in an individual infant, then it is the case that we are basing decisions for treatment or nontreatment on 'quality of life' considerations."[6] Thus Bishop Lawrence Casey refers to death "beyond any hope other than that of preserving *biological life in a merely vegetative state*" (emphasis added).[7]

This trend sparked an interesting debate on how we ought to formulate the basic principles and criteria of life preservation in our time, especially (but not exclusively) where incompetents are concerned. After I present the ideas of several participants in this discussion, I will offer some personal reflections.

[4] *In the Matter of Karen Quinlan, an Alleged Incompetent*, A-116 (Mar. 31, 1976), 24.

[5] Ibid., 48.

[6] Margaret Farley, "A Response to Dr. Duff," *Reflection*, 72 (1975), 11–12.

[7] *In the Matter of Karen Quinlan*, 25.

Various Approaches

Paul Ramsey. In his most recent writing on this subject, the Princeton theologian refers to the terms "ordinary" and "extraordinary" as "incurably circular until filled with concrete or descriptive meaning."[8] Our task, he says, is to identify the morally relevant features of an action that leads us to put it under one of those terms. Ramsey identifies two such features to which the older language can be reduced "almost without remainder," and then urges that "the older language be abandoned."

The first feature is a comparison of treatments that are medically "indicated" and expected to be helpful. Where the dying are involved, that means that further *curative* treatment is not indicated. The second feature is the patient's right to refuse treatment. Once these elements have been identified as central to life-preservation decisions, we no longer need the language of ordinary/extraordinary.

But Ramsey hesitates. Thus he says that the meaning of ordinary/extraordinary can be reduced "almost without remainder" to these two components. Why this hesitation? Because Ramsey fears that abandonment of ordinary/extraordinary terminology means abandonment of *objective* considerations based on the patient's medical condition or human circumstances, and makes the decision too subjective—so that a decision is right solely *because* the patient makes it.

Thus, in Ramsey's judgment, the key substantive criterion and the language to formulate it is: treatment medically indicated, or curative treatment not indicated (for the dying). Behind this distinction would seem to stand the distinction between those who are dying and those who are not—the implication being that those who are not ought to be treated ("medically indicated").

The difficulty with Ramsey's terminology is that for terminology he calls "cumbersome, opaque, and unilluminating," it substitutes terminology that is hardly less cumbersome, opaque, and unilluminating! The difficulty is twofold. First, the terminology in no way indicates those objective features in light of

---

[8] Paul Ramsey, "Euthanasia and Dying Well Enough," *Linacre Quarterly*, 44 (1977), 43.

which the treatment is medically indicated. For instance, was continued use of the respirator "medically indicated" in Karen Quinlan's case? If not (as Ramsey believes), *why* not?

Second, Ramsey would answer that question by saying that "treatments that were potentially life-saving (or reasonably believed to be so) when first begun have now become means for aimlessly prolonging Karen's dying."[9] But that answer assumes clarity with regard to treatments that are "curative" and those that are not. It further assumes a definition of "dying." Both present problems. For instance, the notion of "curative" has any number of levels, one of which is simply staving off death. I know physicians who feel that they must continue life supports even when only *that* level of "cure" is possible. In other words, some treatments are indeed life-saving but at a level Ramsey would reject (for example, the case of Karen Quinlan). He makes the problem a bit too easy by referring to this as "aimlessly prolonging Karen's dying." Somewhat similarly, when should a person be said to be "dying," so that continuance of a respirator is said to be "aimlessly prolonging dying"? Increasingly, the notion of "dying" is dependent on the technology available. Some years ago a child born with certain anomalies was dying; but not now, because the condition can be corrected. Similarly, is a patient on dialysis dying or not?

The point about "cure" and its meaning comes out clearly in a pastoral by the bishops of the Federal Republic of Germany.[10] At one point the bishops pose the question about the moral duty to use indefinitely artificial supports such as the respirator. Their answer:

> As long as there is any possibility of the sick man recovering in this way, we will have to use all such means. Also, it is the duty of the state to ensure that even costly apparatus and expensive medicine are available for those who need them. It is quite another matter when all hope of recovery is excluded and the use of particular medical

[9] Paul Ramsey, "Prolonged Dying: Not Medically Indicated," *Hastings Center Report*, 6 (Feb. 1976), 16.
[10] "Das Lebensrecht des Menschen und die Euthanasie," *Herder Korrespondenz*, 29 (1975), 335–37.

techniques would only lengthen artificially a perhaps painful death. If the patient, relatives, and doctors decide after considering all the circumstances not to have recourse to exceptional measures and means, they cannot be accused of usurping illicitly the right to dispose of human life. The doctor must, of course, obtain first the consent of the patient or, if this is no longer possible, of his relatives.[11]

What is interesting here is the term "recovery." The probability of recovery determines, in the bishops' statement, whether certain life supports and interventions need be used or not. If recovery is possible, they should be used. However, it must be noted that the notion of "recovery" is not without problems. "Recovery" can mean at least three things: (1) return to the state of health enjoyed prior to illness, a full state of health; (2) return to a lesser state, perhaps one characterized by severe physical or mental disturbance (how severe?); (3) return to spontaneous vital functions without consciousness. All these represent forms of recovery in the sense that death has been stayed. It seems clear that if the bishops would not deem obligatory (for the patient) the medical interventions that produce the latter two categories—a point they explicitly make—then they would not include them under the term "recovery." This suggests that "recovery" implies a certain level of recovery or quality of life; for if the means need not be used by the patient and the reason is that they do not produce "recovery," then the term clearly means not just staving off death, but also preserving a certain quality of life. What the term "recovery" really means, then, in the pastoral is "*sufficient* recovery," and that is subject to quality-of-life assessment.

Ramsey is right, I believe, in rejecting the ultimate usefulness of the ordinary/extraordinary language. But while his suggested substitute ("medically indicated/not medically indicated") may verbally underline the objective conditions and circumstances of the patient, it does not in any way specify these objective conditions. Ramsey is reluctant to come to terms with—indeed, resolutely rejects—"quality of life" judgments. Can he avoid them for long if

11 Ibid., 336.

he is to improve on the "incurable circularity" of past terminology? I think not; for among the objective conditions of the patient to be considered, one of the most crucial is the *kind of life* that will be preserved as a result of our interventions, at least if the medical community is to have any voice in determining what is "medically indicated."

Robert Veatch. In his discussion, Robert Veatch of the Kennedy Institute of Ethics notes that the terms "ordinary" and "extraordinary" are "extremely vague and used inconsistently in the literature."[12] Beneath this confusion he finds three overlapping but fundamentally different uses of the terms: usual v. unusual, useful v. useless, imperative v. elective. All these elements function in determining what is the morally proper course of action, but no one description exhausts the notion. For instance, consider usualness. It does not seem reasonable to require a treatment just because it is usually provided. Similarly, adequate primary care is not expendable because it is unusual (for example, not present in urban ghettos).

The same type of objection, he argues, can be made against reducing the term "ordinary" to "useful." Some treatments that are useful are nonobligatory (because disproportionately expensive or otherwise burdensome). Contrarily, some that are useless for saving or prolonging life could be imperative for a patient's comfort.

In the end, then, Veatch states that the ordinary/extraordinary distinction "should be banned from further use. It is clearer simply to speak of morally imperative and elective means. . . ."[13]

What are the elements that go into distinguishing what is morally imperative from what is merely elective? At this point Veatch makes two moves. He argues first that we ought to adopt the patient's perspective. Second, we ought to adopt the language of reasonableness. On this basis, we ought to ask: What treatments is it reasonable to refuse?

Veatch's answer to that question distinguishes two situations: the competent patient and the incompetent patient. As for the first, he writes: "From the patient-centered perspective it should be sufficient for competent patients to refuse treatments for them-

[12] Robert Veatch, *Death, Dying, and the Biological Revolution* (New Haven, Conn.: Yale University Press, 1976).
[13] Ibid., 110.

selves wherever they can offer reasons valid to themselves—that is, out of concern about physical or mental burdens or other objections. . . ."[14]

As for the incompetent such as the child, the senile, the comatose, obviously "reasons valid to themselves" no longer apply as the criteria of reasonableness. Someone else must make the judgment. Veatch finds refusal of treatment morally acceptable if it would seem "within the realm of reason to reasonable people." But what would reasonable people find to be a reasonable or an unreasonable refusal? Veatch answers:

> A reasonable person would find a refusal unreasonable (and thus treatment morally required) if the treatment is useful in treating a patient's condition (though not necessarily life-saving) and at the same time does not give rise to any significant patient-centered objections based on physical or mental burden; familial, social or economic concern; or religious belief.[15]

Veatch's treatment is subtle and disciplined, and I find the notion of "reasonable means" a useful one, and the reasonable person a useful referrent. However, his study does raise two key questions. The first concerns his idea of patient-centered objections to treatment. He admits that concern for the welfare of others could be among a patient's concerns and be a basis for refusal of treatment. But he limits this to the *competent* patient. "Do we really want to say that the physician or the agent for an incompetent patient can judge a treatment unreasonable because it is a burden on persons other than the patient?"

Veatch's concern here is fully justified and highly sensitive. Yet it raises the following question: If the welfare of others is a legitimate concern of the *competent* patient justifying (making reasonable) refusal of treatment, why cannot a similar judgment be made at times of the incompetent patient? In other words, if the patient's own good is at some point inseparably related to the welfare of others where competent patients are concerned, why is this any less true—at least theoretically—where noncompetent patients

14 Ibid.
15 Ibid., 112.

are concerned? I raise this as a theoretical question only because I am in deep sympathy with the direction of Veatch's thought here —if for no other reason than that the danger of abuse is heightened where the patient is incapable of sharing in the determination of what is reasonable.

The second problem is Veatch's phrase "treatment . . . useful in treating a patient's condition" as a criterion of reasonableness. Is a treatment "useful" if it maintains biological life but in a noncognitive, nonsapient state? It may be useful to others (in providing the assuagement of guilt feelings, in expanding the availability of experimental subjects or organ donors). But is it "useful *in treating the patient's condition*"? This is, of course, the basic problem, especially where treatment of the newborn is involved. The patient may be kept alive in a noncognitive, nonsapient state, or with virtually no potential for anything more. I myself do not believe that that is "useful in treating a patient's condition" in any *human* sense, a perspective adopted by Bishop Casey. But in order to say that, one must be more specific about what is to count as "useful." In other words, one must at some point come to grips with the levels of human existence or quality-of-life assessments if the term "useful" is to be at all helpful where the problems are most severe.

Bernard Häring. Häring has faced this problem in several of his writings.[16] A single concern or criterion—freedom—constantly returns in his analysis. He cites with approval R. Kautzky: "Since human life is the condition for the realization of human freedom, it should be prolonged with all appropriate and reasonable means insofar as prolongation according to a competent estimate can serve this goal."[17] Häring uses phrases such as "*reasonable* use of his own freedom," "realization of *significant* liberty," "*reasonably* happy and significant existence," "truly a prolongation of *human* life" (emphasis added in each case). These quotes indicate that freedom as a criterion is subject to gradations. But Häring makes it clear that a fairly low level of freedom is *significant*, constitutes *human* life, and so on, for he rightly insists on protecting and supporting "bodily and mentally disabled children" and the like.

[16] Bernard Häring, *Medical Ethics* (Notre Dame, Ind.: Fides, 1973); *Manipulation* (Slough: St. Paul Publications, 1975).
[17] Häring, *Medical Ethics,* 142.

Having stated the criterion, Häring makes two key statements. First, he distinguishes prolonging a life artificially when "there is no hope whatever that health can be regained" (prolonging dying) and "when there is a *real* chance of serving human life." The two situations are distinguished precisely by the absence or presence of human freedom. Second, it is in the second instance only that the distinction between ordinary and extraordinary means enunciated by Pius XII maintains its validity and use-fulness—that is, even though there is a "real chance of serving human life," it might be too burdensome for the patient to do so.

It seems to me that implicit—and almost explicit—in Häring's treatment is a quality-of-life criterion where the perservation of the life of incompetents is concerned. For he (1) distinguishes (with Helmut Thielicke) between mere *biological* life and *human* life; (2) says the difference between the two is a "reasonable use of freedom"; (3) agrees that freedom "can be defeated by total lack of consciousness, grave defects and suffering of all kinds."[18] The only question remaining is: What is a *reasonable* degree of freedom (or *significant* liberty) and how do we determine it? By using the term *"reasonable* use of his own freedom," there is some indication that Häring would be content with the assessment of the reasonable person—a criterion that would put him very close to Veatch.

Albert R. Jonsen and Michael J. Garland. These authors, to-gether with their colleagues, face the problem of conceptualiza-tion concerning treatment of newborns.[19] They do not appeal to the language of ordinary and extraordinary means. Rather, the heart of their proposed moral policy reads as follows:

> The responsibility of the parents, the duty of the physi-cian, and the interests of the State are conditioned by the medicomoral principle, "do no harm, without ex-pecting compensating benefit for the patient." Life-preserving intervention should be understood as doing

18 Ibid.
19 A. R. Jonsen et al., "Critical Issues in Newborn Intensive Care: A Con-ference Report and Policy Proposal," *Pediatrics,* 55 (1975), 756–68. See also their *Ethics of Newborn Intensive Care* (Berkeley, Calif.: Institute of Govern-mental Studies, 1976).

harm to an infant who cannot survive infancy, or will live in intractable pain, or cannot participate even minimally in human experience.

If the court is called upon to resolve disagreement between parents and physicians about medical care, prognosis about quality of life for the infant should weigh heavily in the decision as to whether or not to order life-saving intervention.[20]

Thus the authors appeal explicitly to quality-of-life criteria and specify these criteria in a general way. They admit that their third condition (capacity to "participate even minimally in human experience") is likely to be the "most controversial." By this condition they understand "*some* inherent capability to respond affectively and cognitively to human attention and to develop toward initiation of communication with others" (emphasis added). They do not desire to quantify this but do give examples. "A baby with Down's syndrome would fulfill the criteria, whereas one with trisomy 18 will not."

Leonard Weber. Theologian Leonard Weber has devoted an entire book to the ethical aspects of treatment of the newborn.[21] He reviews the studies of several writers (Joseph Fletcher, David Smith, Richard McCormick, Warren Reich) and ultimately rejects the quality-of-life formulation. He feels that what he calls "the extraordinary-means approach" better provides "for some protection against an arbitrary decision being made on the basis of a judgment about the worth of a particular type of life."[22] To decide on the basis of quality is "to risk the danger of saying that one person is more valuable than another because of his condition." On the other hand, the extraordinary-means approach "puts the whole question in the context of the goodness of life and of our obligation to respect that goodness." Thus he contrasts a "sanctity-of-life ethic" with a "quality-of-life ethic."

Several things are interesting in Weber's sensitive study. First, he admits that our decisions are often factually based on quality-

[20] Jonsen et al., "Critical Issues in Newborn Intensive Care," 760–61.
[21] Leonard J. Weber, *Who Shall Live?* (New York: Paulist Press, 1976).
[22] Ibid., 85.

of-life assessments, but he is very reluctant to "move toward a quality-of-life language." This language, he believes, gives support to
the very values we ought to oppose.

Second, when he applies the ordinary/extraordinary distinction
to infants, he speaks in terms of two elements: reasonable hope of
success (the child can be kept alive for "more than just a few days
or weeks") and excessive burden. Under this latter category,
Weber includes, among others, treatments that demand a long
series of critical operations, or those that leave the child seriously
handicapped (for example, brain-damaged). He then writes very
interestingly:

> One can even talk about treatment imposing an exces-
> sive burden when it is the timing of the treatment that
> results in a burdensome life. If, for example, the oxygen
> supply to the brain has been stopped and the opportu-
> nity to resuscitate such a person only comes when it is
> probable that extensive damage has already been done to
> the brain, it should be considered an extraordinary
> means to attempt to restore normal blood circulation, no
> matter how common the procedure. By saving the life of
> the patient *at this time*, an excessive burden would be
> imposed. McCormick and others would probably say
> that the decision not to treat in such a case is based on
> concern for the quality of the life of the child. And, of
> course, they are largely correct.[23]

But Weber still wants to speak of the "treatment imposing a burden"—because the child "would not have this burden if it were
not for this treatment now."

To that it must be said, I believe, that the burden is precisely
the damaged condition. It is *that* which is the basis for the decision. And if that is so, we are—regardless of the language we use—
actually making quality-of-life judgments. Weber's application of
the ordinary/extraordinary conceptualization is, I believe, quite
strained. And such artificiality underlines the limited usefulness of
that terminology.

[23] Ibid., 93.

So much for some of the recent literature. Two quite distinct positions emerge: those who wish to abandon the terminology of ordinary/extraordinary (Ramsey, Veatch, Häring [by implication], Jonsen, and Garland), and others (notably Weber) who want to retain it.

Personal Reflections

Before spelling out the direction I believe this discussion ought to be taking in the future, let me note several introductory points that cling to it.

Life as a condition for other values and achievements. It is clear that before any human experiences, responses, or achievements are possible, there must be life. In this sense, life is a condition for all other values and experiences. Some theologians have stated therefore that life is a value to be preserved precisely because it makes other achievements possible. When, because of the condition of the patient, no experience or interrelation is possible, then (so the formulation goes) that life has achieved its potential. As Kautzky words it: "Since human life is the condition for the realization of human freedom, it should be prolonged with all appropriate and reasonable means insofar as prolongation according to a competent estimate can serve this goal."[24]

William May has leveled the following objection against this reasoning: "In other words . . . life itself, in the sense of physical or biological life, is what an older terminology would have called a *bonum utile*, not a *bonum honestum*."[25]

Two possible responses can be made. First, one could insist that to say life is a good to be preserved insofar as it contains some potentiality for human experience is not to make life a *bonum utile*, or merely a useful good, and therefore a kind of negotiable thing. Rather it is to talk about our duties—and especially the why of those duties—toward the preservation of a *bonum honestum*—that is, a good in itself, the dying human person, and to admit that these duties may differ depending on the conditions of that *bonum honestum*.

[24] R. Kautzky, "Der Arzt," *Arzt und Christ*, 15 (1969), 138.
[25] William May, "Ethics and Human Identity: The Challenge of the New Biology," *Horizons*, 3 (1976), 35.

Second, and perhaps even more to the point, it could be counterstated that the usage of "useful good" and "good in itself" plays upon the ambiguity of the term "life." "Life" can mean two general things: (1) a state of human functioning (or capacity thereof), of well-being; or (2) the existence of vital and metabolic processes with no human functioning or capacity. We do not, in Christian perspectives, preserve these functions *for their own sake*; we are not vitalists. In this second sense of "life," then, one could argue that it is indeed a useful good only, though it is not clear to me how such terminology illumines the matter. Where one draws the line between the two senses of "life" is crucial, of course. But once it is drawn, I have no problem with referring to life beyond that line as a useful good, though I see no gain in doing so.

Very close to this is the insistence of some discussants (such as Weber) that use of quality-of-life criteria means that "life is not good or worthwhile or meaningful anymore."[26] Similarly, this move is seen as implying that "life is not good in itself."[27] Or again, it is argued that for the infant "just to be alive may be a great success." Such statements are subject to the distinction made above. Concretely, if "life" means *only* metabolism and vital processes, then what is meant by saying that this is a "good in itself"? If that means a good to be preserved independently of any capacity for conscious experience, I believe it is a straightforward form of vitalism—an approach that preserves life (mere vital processes) no matter what the condition of the patient. One can and, I believe, should say that the *person* is always an incalculable value, but that at some point continuance in physical life offers the person no benefit. Indeed, to keep "life" going can easily be an assault on the person and his or her dignity. Therefore, phrases such as "the good of life in itself" are misleading in these discussions.

Sanctity of life v. quality of life. Some who compare "sanctity of life" and "quality of life" approaches see the former as the more satisfactory.[28] It focuses our attention on our obligations to preserve life and avoids degrees of discrimination in quality-of-life

[26] Weber, *Who Shall Live?*, 83.

[27] Ibid., 81.

[28] Leonard J. Weber (see below), and Eugene F. Diamond, " 'Quality' vs. 'Sanctity' of Life in the Nursery," *America*, 135 (1976), 396–98.

criteria. Actually, the two approaches ought not to be set against each other in this way. Quality-of-life assessments ought to be made within an over-all reverence for life, as an extension of one's respect for the sanctity of life. However, there are times when preserving the life of one with no capacity for those aspects of life that we regard as *human* is a violation of the sanctity of life itself. Thus to separate the two approaches and call one *sanctity* of life, the other *quality* of life, is a false conceptual split that very easily suggests that the term "sanctity of life" is being used in an exhortatory way.

Quality-of-life criteria and equality of value. It is argued that quality-of-life language implies "that not all lives are equally good or equally deserving of protection."[29] Thus it is essentially discriminatory. As Weber puts it: "Can one really use a condition-of-life criterion and still insist that every life is of equal value regardless of condition?"[30]

While speaking in terms of "every life" being of "equal value" reveals a legitimate concern (that medical treatment not be denied or withheld in a way violative of the rights of individuals), that is not the issue. Every *person* is of "equal value." But not every *life* (once again, the distinction noted above) is of equal value if we are careful to unpack the terms "life," "equal," and "value." If "life" means the continuation of vital processes but in a persistent vegetative state; if "value" means "a good to the individual concerned"; if "equal" means "identical" or "the same," especially of treatment, then I believe it is simply false to say that "every life is of equal value."

What the "equal value" language is attempting to say is legitimate: We must avoid *unjust* discrimination in the provision of health care and life supports. But not all discrimination (inequality of treatment) is unjust. *Unjust* discrimination is avoided if decision-making centers on the benefit to the patient, even if that benefit is described largely in terms of quality-of-life criteria.

The means approach and sanctity of life. It is occasionally argued that emphasis on means better protects the equal value of all lives because it stresses "*objective* indications" and "puts the

29 Weber, *Who Shall Live?*, 78.
30 Ibid., 82.

whole question in the context of the goodness of life."[31] Thus Weber states: "Focus on means is a constant reminder that we should not decide who should live or die on the basis of the worth of someone's life."[32]

Here it must be pointed out that the terms "ordinary" and "extraordinary" are so relative that they are equally capable of abuse as quality-of-life language. The famous Johns Hopkins case (in which a baby with Down's syndrome, needing minor surgery, was allowed to die on the grounds that the surgery would be extraordinary) is a well-known instance. What is important in these matters is that the line be drawn in the proper place. Language itself does not draw such lines. Both the "means approach" and "quality-of-life approach" can be abused. But they need not be. Indeed, if treatment decisions are often quality-of-life decisions, as Weber admits, then the greater danger may be to disguise this fact with the language of ordinary/extraordinary, for it means that we are not attending to the line-drawing process and its criteria. And not attending to it could easily lead to allowing that line to slip around in a way that is ultimately unfair to the incompetent patient. In sum, then, I would seriously question whether "means language" better protects human life.

This discussion is far from ended. Indeed, in a sense it is just beginning; for one thing is increasingly clear: Technological and medical advances bring, for some individuals, mixed blessings at best. In the contemporary literature one sees a move away from the language of ordinary/extraordinary means as being increasingly confusing, ambiguous, and circular. I myself, with Veatch, favor the terms "reasonable/unreasonable treatment." These terms are themselves of course empty, but they do achieve two things. First, and negatively, they move us away from a terminology (ordinary/extraordinary) that suggests too easily and to too many that "usualness" is the key and crucial factor in these decisions, whereas that notion very often disguises the real character of the decision.

Second, and more positively, the terms "reasonable/unreasonable" point in the direction of what will be in the future the crucial referrent in these decisions—the judgment of the reason-

[31] Ibid., 84.
[32] Ibid., 85.

able person. In the Quinlan case, the New Jersey Supreme Court argued: (1) that Karen Quinlan had a right to self-determination (the court said "privacy") where treatment is concerned; (2) that she is in a noncompetent and vegetative state, leaving her incapable of exercising her right to withdraw treatment; (3) that it may be exercised on her behalf by her family and guardian. Then most interestingly it stated: "If their [family] conclusion is in the affirmative their decision should be accepted by a society *the overwhelming majority of whose members would, we think, in similar circumstances, exercise such a choice in the same way for themselves or for those closest to them*" (emphasis added).[33] This is an appeal to what most of us, in similar circumstances, would do—as reasonable people with healthy outlooks on the meaning of life and death.

That is a formal criterion, of course, and in itself leaves untouched the criteria that reasonable people would use in making decisions. The judgment of reasonable people is not *constitutive* of the rightness of the decision. It is merely *confirmatory* that the criterion is close to the mark. In deciding what those criteria are, we must distinguish carefully with Veatch between competent and noncompetant patients. For competent patients, refusal of treatment may be considered reasonable "whenever they can offer reasons valid to themselves—that is, out of concern about physical or mental burdens or other objectives. . . ."[34] In other words, the appropriate mix of values during dying, how one shall live while dying, belongs to the patient. And here patients may and do differ within the range of morally acceptable options.

Of the three key values copresent (preservation of life, human freedom, lack of pain), some will choose to maximize freedom, others to minimize pain even with the diminution of freedom.[35] Still others will manage their dying with a controlling view of the financial and/or psychological condition of their dear ones. That is the meaning of "reasons valid to themselves." These cannot and need not be specified further. Treatment that conforms to such wishes and perspectives may be considered reasonable (morally

[33] *In the Matter of Karen Quinlan*, 24.
[34] Veatch, *Death, Dying, and the Biological Revolution*, 110.
[35] See the helpful article of Albert Ziegler, "Sterbehilfe—Grundfragen und 'Thesen,'" *Orientierung*, 39 (1975), 39–41, 55–58.

appropriate), always allowing for legal appeal by physician or hospital if a patient is judged to be frivolously jeopardizing life.

For the incompetent patient, obviously this decision must be made by proxy (family or guardian). When the incompetent (unconscious) person is an adult, there may exist warrants in past statements and clearly known perspectives that aid the proxies in determining what is reasonable treatment. When these are not present, I believe that the judgment of reasonable people may be used as an aid to a morally acceptable decision—that is, if the situation is such that most or very many of us would not want life-preserving treatment *in that condition*, it would be morally prudent (reasonable) to conclude that life-preserving treatment is not morally required for this particular patient. But once again, it is not the consensus that *constitutes* the reasonableness. Rather, reasonable people can be presumed to be drawing the line on the kind of life being preserved at the right place—in the best over-all interests of the patient.

The matter becomes even more difficult when the patient is an infant, for the simple reason that it is all but impossible for *healthy adults* to extrapolate backward on what kind of life will be acceptable to the infant. Yet, if we are to avoid vitalism in practice, these judgments must sometimes be made. I agree with Judson G. Randolph (surgeon in chief, Children's Hospital National Medical Center, Washington, D.C.) when he states: "I think it is well within the guidelines of right and wrong to make certain qualitative judgments about human life. . . ."[36] Randolph continues: "If a severely handicapped child were suddenly given one moment of omniscience and total awareness of his or her outlook for the future, would that child necessarily opt for life? No one has yet been able to demonstrate that the answer would always be 'yes.' " In my judgment, the perspectives of the Christian tradition on life and its meaning would suggest that in some instances the answer would be "no." In some cases the reason would be the continuing burden to the patient of treatment. But in others, the reason is that in this tradition mere life (vital processes, metabolism) has not been viewed as a value *in itself*.

[36] As cited by J. G. Randolph in "Ethical Considerations in Surgery of the Newborn," *Contemporary Surgery*, 7 (1975), 17–19.

This is the implication in the analyses of Häring, Veatch, Jonsen-Garland, and even Weber (though he resists the language).

I believe this is correct. Our main task is to discover as a community of reasonable persons where the line is drawn and why. When we do so, we will have discovered the differences between reasonable and unreasonable treatment, especially for those who cannot make the decision themselves but depend for their well-being on us. In other words, we will have made a quality-of-life judgment in a way that both expresses and reinforces our concern for the sanctity of life.

23. Legislation and the Living Will

Recently, Governor Edmund G. Brown, Jr., of California signed A.B. 3060, known as the Natural Death Act, a bill that had been introduced by State Assemblyman Barry Keene.[1] This historic act provides for the possibility of a written directive by an adult patient authorizing the "withholding or withdrawal of extraordinary life-sustaining procedures" in the situation of "terminal illness." The California Legislature explicitly stated the reasoning behind the motivation of the bill. It emphasized the right of adult patients to control decisions relating to their own medical care; the advance in powerful, modern life-sustaining devices; the hardships associated with some prolongation of life (loss of patient dignity, unnecessary suffering, unreasonable emotional and financial hardship on the patient's family); and, above all, the existing uncertainty in the medical and legal professions about the legality of terminating the use of life-sustaining procedures "where the patient has voluntarily and in sound mind evidenced a desire that such procedures be withheld or withdrawn." There can be little doubt that New Jersey's Karen Ann Quinlan case intensified this latter concern.

The effect of the bill is to relieve physicians, paramedical personnel, and health facilities from civil liability or criminal prosecution when they act according to the provisions of the bill. Furthermore, A.B. 3060 provides that action according to such provisions will not constitute a suicide.

In this Natural Death Act, we have the first legal recognition of the so-called living will. The California Conference of Catholic Health Facilities originally opposed the legislation. It argued, first, that the legislation was unnecessary, because patients, family, and

[1] California Health and Safety Code, Secs. 7,185–95. Approved by the governor on September 30, 1976.

physicians are presently free to exercise their respective preroga- tives and responsibilities without legislation, and the specter of legal action in these cases is more imagined than real. Further- more, legislation cannot resolve the conflicts arising from ques- tions regarding medical competence or the accuracy of prognosis, any more than it can guarantee that a patient's wishes will be ac- curately interpreted.

Second, the conference argued that the legislation was undesira- ble in several ways. For instance, the doctor-patient relationship is threatened by making the physician a servant of the statute, thereby losing his ability to be an advocate for his patient. Simi- larly, and very importantly, the conference feared the implications of the absence of a living will. Patients' rights could be threatened if physicians, seeking the security of the statute, refused to with- hold or withdraw artificial life sustainers from dying patients. Moreover, how can an individual make intelligent, informed deci- sions regarding specific and appropriate response to unknown events and detailed circumstances? And, if that is the case, is it desirable that public policy compel adherence to directives origi- nating in uninformed consent? Finally, the conference wondered how any statute could fully capture the specific meaning of termi- nology that relates more to the human dimensions of decision- making than to the practice of medicine. These and other serious fears led the conference to its original attitude of opposition to- ward A.B. 3060, even though it eventually adopted a position of neutrality toward the bill, since Assemblyman Keene was sensitive to, and highly responsible about, the criticisms and suggestions of the conference.

The Natural Death Act has been imitated in many other states. The main features of all such bills are: (1) the execution of a written document directing the withholding or withdrawal of ex- traordinary life sustainers when the individual is in a terminal con- dition; (2) definition of "terminal illness" as that which will end in natural death whether life sustainers are used or not; (3) the verification of the prognosis by one or more physicians; (4) provi- sions protecting the compliance of the physician and health facil- ity against liability.

All this seems to make good sense. But does it? Anticipating a vote on Maryland's Senate Bill No. 60, the Maryland Catholic

Conference, composed of William Cardinal Baum, Archbishop William D. Borders, and Bishop Thomas J. Mardaga, has stated in a recent pastoral that they are "strongly" opposed to Senate Bill No. 60 on "theoretical and practical grounds."[2] Much as had the California Catholic Conference, the Maryland Catholic Conference admits that the intention of the bill—to protect patients' rights—is good. But they also argue that "the basic reason advanced for passage of this law—protection—is ultimately the basic reason we offer for its rejection." The statement adduces two reasons for this rejection. First, the bill is unnecessary. Without the complication of law, the patient already has the right to refuse, either personally or through family or legal guardian, the use of extraordinary life-sustaining devices. Second, the bill is unduly restrictive. For "the immediate conclusion that can and will be drawn from this law is that the living will is the only way in which a person's God-given right may be exercised." This suggests that, in the absence of such a document, the patient risks being badly overtreated.

The Baum-Borders-Mardaga statement further notes: "In its [living will] absence, will the physician feel obliged to use extraordinary means? Will the family or legal guardian feel pressured into using extraordinary means at all costs? The rigidities and restrictions of human laws should not enter a field concerned with the delicate relationships of a dying person and his physician and family." Thus the Maryland conference concludes that such legislation is neither "necessary, effective, or desirable" in protecting the right of the person to refuse treatment.

We believe that the original misgivings and objections of the California Catholic Conference and those of the excellent Baum-Borders-Mardaga pastoral are well founded. They provide us with the occasion to state some of our own reactions to living-will legislation, reactions in some respects very similar to those of the documents mentioned. We concentrate on three considerations: the presuppositions of such legislation, the possible consequences, and an alternative solution.

The medical profession is the servant of patients, not their master. In one sense, the living-will legislation seeks to maintain

---

[2] I take these and the following citations from various news releases issued at the time (Jan. 1977) of the official statement.

this self-determination of the patient. But in another, it dangerously abdicates this patient control. The need to write a living will to prevent the use of so-called extraordinary means implies that in some way physicians are masters of their patients, unless patients take legal action in advance. Thus it raises the entire question of the locus of power in those cases where no living will has been written, either because the potential patient was too young to write a will (the child) or because the potential patient was not aware of the implications of writing, or not writing, such a will.

Our opposition, then, to living-will legislation does not stem from what such legislation seeks to achieve, namely the self-determination of the patient over his or her own fate in the face of a potentially abusive use of technology. Rather, we question whether such legislation may not result in precisely the opposite effect. We have no objection to the living will as a signal sent in advance by knowledgeable persons to their potential physicians. Indeed, such informal documents can be immensely helpful and reassuring. Our profound misgivings stem from the notion of living wills as law. The very fact that a law is deemed necessary to assure patients' rights implies, and therefore tends to reinforce, an erroneous presupposition about the locus of decision-making in the physician-patient relationship.

The Karen Ann Quinlan case is a dramatic example. In that case, the Quinlan family sought to subtract their daughter from the jurisdiction of her physicians. We believe the Quinlan parents were justified in asking that the use of the respirator be stopped. Dr. Jack E. Zimmerman, director of the intensive-care unit at Washington, D.C.'s George Washington University Medical Center, reflected what is widely regarded as the attitude of most physicians. If Joseph Quinlan had asked physicians at the intensive-care unit to turn off his daughter's respirator, Mr. Quinlan's request "would have been met." Contrarily, if her actual physicians believed the request of the Quinlan family to be frivolous, we believe the moral onus was upon those physicians to have resort to the courts to subtract Karen Ann from the guardianship of her parents. The way events developed in that case, the presumptions were that physicians have a right to treat a patient unasked—indeed, opposed. We reject that premise. We believe that, both philosophically and practically, proposed laws on death with dignity or living wills tend to enshrine the notion that physicians are masters of their patients and not their servants.

What is objectionable about such enshrinement? We believe it is both wrong in itself and threatening in its implications. It is wrong in itself because the individual, having the prime obligation for his own health care, has also thereby the right to the necessary means for such basic health care—specifically, the right of self-determination in the acceptance or rejection of treatment. When an individual puts himself into a doctor's hands, he engages the doctor's services; he does not abdicate his right to decide his own fate. Patients retain the right to refuse a physician's advice, however ill advised they might be in doing so.

No one has made that point more clearly than Pius XII. In an address to the International Congress of Anesthesiologists on November 24, 1957, the Holy Father stated: "The rights and duties of the doctor are correlative to those of the patient. The doctor, in fact, has no separate or independent right where the patient is concerned. In general, he can take action only if the patient explicitly or implicitly, directly or indirectly, gives him permission."[3] Furthermore, Pius XII stated that when the patient, of age and *sui juris*, is unconscious, it is the right and duty of the family to make decisions based on the presumed will of the unconscious patient. Thus he explicitly concluded that when attempts at resuscitation become too onerous, "they [the family] can lawfully insist that the doctor should discontinue these attempts, and the doctor can lawfully comply." This very same primacy of patient and proxy rights has been beautifully and forcefully restated by the Board of Trustees of the Catholic Hospital Association.[4] Any legislation that tends to make it necessary to write a living will in order to avoid unreasonable treatment during the dying process is a move toward undercutting patient rights.

Furthermore, such a subtle shift in the doctor-patient relationship is threatening in its value implications, for in lessening the patients' rights, it will tend to blunt those perspectives that are intended to inform the exercise of those rights. In the Catholic tradition and even more broadly in the Judaeo-Christian tradi-

---

[3] Pope Pius XII, *Acta Apostolicae Sedis*, 49 (1957), 1,031–32.
[4] "The Dying Patient," *Hospital Progress*, 58 (Jan. 1977).

tion, all life tends toward death. But just as values can be pursued in living, so also they can be pursued in dying. This tradition maintains that there are values more important than life in the living of life. So, it also holds that there are values more important than life in the dying. For this reason, the accumulation of minutes of life is not the moral guideline by which dying must be done. For instance, the justification for administering pain-killing drugs, even if they should shorten life, recognizes that there is a value in being pain free, which permits the pursuit of other values, such as prayer.

An individual makes his decision about how he will live while dying in terms of his basic perspectives on the meaning of life and death. For the Christian, especially the Catholic, those perspectives are rooted in a tradition that sees no difference in the purpose of living and in the purpose of dying. Both are well expressed in the answer to the age-old catechism question: "Why was I born?" The answer is: "To know, love, and serve God in this world and to be reunited with Him in the next." It was precisely these perspectives on the meaning and importance of life and death that led to the use of the moral terms "ordinary" and "extraordinary" means for preserving life. The former (defined by Pius XII in the allocution cited above as "means that do not involve any grave burden for oneself or another") must be used; the latter need not be. What is important is Pius's reason for this conclusion. Not only would a more strict duty be too burdensome, but also it would "render the attainment of the higher, more important good too difficult. Life, health, all temporal activities are in fact subordinate to spiritual ends."

What treatment renders "the attainment of the higher, more important good too difficult," what treatment distorts and destroys the subordination of life and health to spiritual ends, must, of course, be individualized according to the biography and condition of each patient. That is why the terms "ordinary" and "extraordinary" in their full moral sense remain so utterly personal. (That is also why, incidentally, we believe decisions about the means and treatment of dying patients are above all quality-of-life judgments—judgments about how a patient will live while dying, with what mix and balance of values.) But what is crucial is that in this view there is a subordination of life and health to spiritual ends, there is a higher good within which such an individualization may occur. We fear that legislation that implies and therefore reinforces the notion of physician mastery over patients will at the same time undermine those altogether balanced perspectives within which patient choice ought to occur, for the very notion that a dying patient has a moral choice as to how he will live while dying is an outgrowth of these basic perspectives. A policy that undermines the choice attacks, however subtly, the perspectives that generated it.

The intestate. The first consequence of the proposed legislation is the abandonment to codification of a right that human beings inherently have—that is, to refuse to be treated by any or all physicians. The very proposal to write such legislation easily suggests the practical conclusion that that right must be acquired. That immediately raises this issue: What does the law do to or for those who have written no will, as both the California and Maryland Catholic Conferences asked? Until now, no legislature has proposed the introduction of laws whereby potential patients can demand extraordinary therapy treatment, as most often legally depicted, that maintains circulation and respiration without being able to cure the disease. Must or may the physician assume, with or without a will, that his patient wants extraordinary means used, since the patient had an opportunity to write a will? At stake, then, is whether the onus is on the individual to write a will if he wishes to avoid excessive resuscitation.

Since the intestate—and they are likely to be the vast majority—are left unprotected in a medicomoral limbo, we fear the growth of the popular misconception that living-will legislation confers rights rather than recognizes them. This is particularly dangerous in our time because once the right to refuse treatment is construed as conferral, the traditional distinction between omission and commission (officially adopted by the American Medical Association in 1973)[5] is threatened. In other words, if the right is not viewed as basically a natural right—with inherent moral limitations—but a conferred right, then on such a view the law could also confer the right to be killed. It is a well-known fact that advo-

---

[5] *Journal of the American Medical Association*, 227 (1974), 728.

cates of mercy killing strongly support so-called death-with-dignity bills.

Family. The second effect of living wills is that they tend to exclude the family from any responsibility. Advocates of living wills see this as a desirable aim, for they argue that families tend to insist on excessive treatment. On the other hand, families are theoretically more likely to know the wishes of their relatives than physicians who may never have met them in health. Moreover, many physicians hold that it is very important for a family to participate in decision-making. They are, in a sense, both copatient and cophysician—copatient because they are afraid, cophysician because they would be the physician if they could. The living will essentially excludes the family from any decision-making for those people who have written one. As yet undetermined, even undiscussed, is the role of the family in the case of the intestate patient. If absence of a will is taken to be an indicator of the patient's desire for extraordinary means (or else he would have written a will), the family is again excluded.

Penalties and practice. In most living-will legislation, there is no penalty attached for violation. In this case, it is not clear why the legislation is written in the first place, for a medal, an armband, or even a written document without legal force would suffice to inform a physician of the patient's general philosophy of living or dying.

In some proposals, however, violation of the declarant's wishes is a misdemeanor. The effects of this on practice are rarely discussed. To underresuscitate a patient with a living will may lead to his death, but is unlikely to lead to a penalty, since it is against overtreatment that the will is directed. Conversely, to overresuscitate a patient with a will and to leave him in a state repugnant to him may save his life, but makes the physician liable for the penalty. In sum, then, where penalties are attached to the law, it is not inconceivable that those with wills will be needlessly underresuscitated and those without wills overresuscitated. Paradoxically, since it is likely that large numbers, through neglect or ignorance, will never write a will, it is not unlikely that the legislation will lead to an increase in excessive treatment rather than a decrease.

Emergencies. There is likely to be a practical problem in emergencies. It is a fact that fewer and fewer patients today have private physicians—about 25 per cent, by most estimates. Moreover, family physicians, with close ties to their patients, are not likely to be the ones at whom the legislation is aimed. Excessive treatment is a problem of patients outside primary care, in impersonal hospitals with modern technologies. Emergency rooms in hospitals are unlikely places in which to search for wills, while having to decide, almost instantaneously, whether to resuscitate or not. It is highly unlikely that a law on living wills can work in such an emergency setting in the way it is intended, unless physicians refrain from resuscitating to be on the safe side of being penalized.

Conscience clauses. In some states, it is proposed to add a "conscience clause" to death-with-dignity bills so that the physician need not comply. He then must transfer the patient to another doctor willing to comply. Paradoxically, unwise as we think living-will legislation is, the effect of conscience clauses only accentuates our first misgivings about such legislation. The conscience clause gives to a physician precisely those rights of possession of patients that we deny in the first place, yet that this legislation seems tacitly to assume. Physicians have always had the right to withdraw from a case if they are asked to perform acts that are incompatible with their conscience as physicians or as individuals. To codify this freedom changes by implication the onus and assumes that, without taking a legal provision, the physician has lost an inherent right. So the proposed legislation assumes, philosophically, that the traditional rights of physicians to withdraw from their patients, or vice versa, do not exist and must be asserted.

There are two main reasons why living-will legislation might, in theory, be written: (1) because without it, patients cannot subtract themselves from physicians who will overtreat them; (2) because without it, doctors are not free to render such treatment as they wish to give and patients desire to receive. We believe that legislation is not designed above all to protect patients against the excessive zeal of physicians, but to protect physicians against existing laws that hamper their freedom to omit extraordinary means of treatment when patients and their families do not wish to undergo such treatment. In a recent poll conducted by the American

Medical Association[6] 94.5 per cent of the physicians polled stated that they normally try to adhere to a terminally ill patient's expressed wishes about the nature and extent of care to be provided as death approaches. More concretely, most surveyed stated that when a patient had made a no-intervention decision, a doctor should respect it. The same poll indicated that legal constraints are most often mentioned by 67.5 per cent of doctors when they are asked what factors might keep them from acceding to a patient's wishes. Thus fear may exist among physicians that to omit or to cease a therapy could be construed under existing laws to constitute malpractice or even homicide.

If this be the case, we suggest that it is, both in discussion and in legislation, better to face directly the issue of physician protection from existing laws rather than to imply that the problem is one of protecting patients from excessive zeal in physicians. We suggest that such legislation can be written without the creation of the philosophical and practical problems alluded to above.

Without going into detail, we suggest that legislation could be written that simply states that, when a patient suffers from a fatal disease, a physician can register that fact with an appropriate hospital body that would have the right, but not the duty, to verify the fact. A mentally competent patient could then request in writing that no extraordinary treatment be applied to him. Where a patient was incompetent to act, by age or condition, the family could make a similar written request. Once the written request had been made, the legislation could stipulate that the treating physician was not subject to civil or criminal prosecution for omitting or ceasing treatment.

In those cases where it was the opinion of the physician that the patients, or their families, were needlessly or frivolously jeopardizing the patients' lives, the physician could notify the same committee, which could then have recourse to the courts to place the patient under guardianship. It should be noted that our proposal diametrically opposes the procedures followed in the Karen Ann Quinlan case, where the moral onus fell upon the parents to subtract their daughter from the jurisdiction of her physicians.

If the key problem is one of malpractice and homicide law, we

[6] *American Medical Association News* (Jan. 24, 1977).

suggest it be addressed directly. But we deplore the trend to do so by writing laws that too easily suggest that there is an inherent right of physicians over patients, unless those patients can assert their independence from unasked-for and uncalled-for ministrations by physicians through the mechanisms of writing a will in advance. Will not the freedom of physicians and patients be threatened by such an approach? We fear so.

24. Living-Will Legislation, Reconsidered

Technological advances have greatly increased modern medicine's ability to preserve and to save lives. Procedures which a decade ago were only dreams have now become a reality. However, like all human artifacts, sophisticated technology can be turned into an abuse; the very means used to preserve life may transform it into a hellish nightmare by reducing it to a sub-lethal extension of monitoring machines and sustaining apparatus.

That possibility has long been recognized by the church in its value judgments. Thus it is a centuries-old teaching that individuals need not undergo or be subjected to "extraordinary" means of preserving life. The teaching was reiterated in the Vatican's 1980 Declaration on Euthanasia, which notes the importance of protecting the dignity of the dying patient from a technological attitude that threatens to become an abuse. Today that potential, even at the hands of the well-intentioned physician, is becoming an ever more distinct possibility. The competent patient may avoid such difficulty by declining unwanted therapies. The more pressing issues involves the incompetent patient, who, unable to express his or her desires, may be subjected to treatments that at great expense and personal suffering serve only to prolong his or her dying.

Traditionally, it has been understood that these individuals retain their right to decline treatment and that the proxy exercise of the right belongs to the family or guardian. That understanding has led each of us to oppose "Living Will" legislation as unnecessary and a potential threat to the fundamental moral rights of those who have not executed a living will.[1] We continue to believe that individuals may express their desires on treatment regimes to their

---

[1] See above, pp. 412–22, and John J. Paris, "Brother Fox, the Courts and Death with Dignity." *America*, 143 (1980), 282–285.

physicians without specific enabling legislation, but several recent
state supreme court opinions have forced us to reconsider our
opposition to the legislation.

In the most recent of these cases, Eichner v. Dillon, the New
York Court of Appeals, the state's highest court, ruled that life-
sustaining treatment may be withheld from an incompetent dying
patient only if: 1) there is no hope of recovery and 2) there is "clear
and convincing" evidence that the patient when competent had
stated that in such circumstances he or she would not want treatment.

The Eichner ruling specifically excluded the possibility of proxy
consent on either a "reasonable basis" standard as in Quinlan or
in a Saikewicz style "substituted judgment." Further, it insisted
that the standard "forbids relief whenever the evidence is loose,
equivocal or contradictory" or if it emanates from "casual remarks
made at some social gathering" or made by one "too young to
realize or feel the consequences of his statements." What the court
insisted on was the kind of "solemn pronouncement" provided by
Brother Fox, the subject of the Eichner case, when in the context
of formal community discussions on Karen Ann Quinlan, he had
repeatedly stated he did not want "any of the extraordinary business."

How, one might ask, does the ordinary person provide such
evidence? The best and most reliable method, as the Eichner trial
court indicated, is a written statement given to the physician and
family spelling out the individual's values and desires. That such
a statement is not incompatible with basic Catholic values is evidenced by the testimony on living wills given to the Joint Committee on the Judiciary of the Massachusetts Legislature by Bishop
Timothy J. Harrington in March 1979 and repeated by Bishop
Thomas V. Daily on March 16, 1981: "The patient has the responsibility to inform his or her physician of the desire to be treated
in a way consistent with human dignity and the right to self-
determination. . . . In fact, every individual should be encouraged
to do so." The bishops, in a position consistent with our own
published views, then argued that there is no need for legislation
in this area.

Our experience of recent rulings by the Florida (Satz v. Perlmutter), Delaware (Severns v. Wilmington Medical Center), and New York (Eichner v. Dillon) supreme courts on the need for legislative direction on these questions, and the fact that an overwhelming number of physicians, attorneys and legislators continue to believe an individual's statement has no legitimacy without a statutory enactment, force us to revise our previous opposition to this legislation.

The major objections which we had to such legislation were: There is no need for it; the potential for misunderstanding about the proper locus of decision making in the patient-physician relationship; the danger that those without a living will are presumed to want all possible treatments; the exclusion of the family from participation in decision-making; and the possibility that the state, construing the right to refuse treatment as a conferral rather than a natural right—one with inherent moral limitations—could also confer the right to be killed. We believe these objections remain valid. However, they are overwhelmed by the recent involvement of the courts in these decisions, and the attitudes they engender.

Court rulings and the widespread perception that a law is necessary to provide adequate protection for the will of an incompetent, terminally ill patient have led many legislatures to consider living will proposals. Since the original California Natural Death Act in 1976, some 10 states have enacted statutes on this subject. Proposals in many other states, including Ohio, Virginia, Massachusetts and Connecticut, have been repeatedly defeated in great part because of the opposition from the Catholic Conference and various right-to-life groups.

Individual sponsors of legislation, anxious to overcome the repeated objections from the Catholic community, have structured their proposals to meet the criticisms expressed by the different Catholic Conferences. The 1981 bill of State Senator William Rogers of Connecticut is a good example of that concern. The preface of his text, drafted in part from the Vatican's Declaration on Euthanasia, expresses the legislature's recognition of "the fundamental right of adults" to determine the extent of their own medical care, a right founded in the "autonomy and sanctity of the person." It also recognizes the fact that artificial or extraordinary procedures of prolonging life "for persons where incurable death is imminent may cause loss of patient-dignity, and secure only a precarious and burdensome existence."

To meet the other major objections, Senator Rogers adopted at our suggestion the following provisions from the 1979 Kansas statute: "Nothing in this act shall be construed to condone, authorize or approve mercy killing or permit any affirmative or deliberate act or omission to end life other than to permit the natural process of dying as provided in this act.

"This act shall create no presumption concerning the intention of an individual who has not executed a declaration to consent to the use or withholding of life-sustaining procedures in the event of a terminal condition."

With the legislative recognition of the dignity and natural moral rights of the person and the carefully drawn provisions to protect those without living wills and to prohibit any form of active euthanasia, we find no substantial reason for continued opposition to living will legislation. Indeed, we believe that the probability of continued court involvement in this area makes it prudent to support well-delineated legislation rather than to leave the determination of patients' rights to the vagaries of conflicting court rulings.

A yet additional reason for a change in our position is the growing awareness that some of the opposition to the legislation by the more radical right-to-life advocates threatens the traditional Catholic position on the sanctity of life and the rights of the individual, in the Vatican's phrasing, "to refuse forms of treatment that would only secure a precarious and burdensome prolongation of life." Such a stance was evident in the Nassau County District Attorney's insistence on the continued respiratory treatment of the chronic vegetative 83-year-old Brother Fox; in the actions of the Bronx Municipal Hospital physicians who this April refused a family's request to remove the respirator from a 3-year-old meningitis victim whose neurological signs were all negative, but who continued to show residual E.E.G. activity; and in the recurring position of the physicians at New York's Nassau Hospital, the site of Brother Fox's hospitalization, who again refused a request of a family and the Rev. Philip Eichner (the principal of Chaminade High School and guardian for Brother Fox) for the removal of the respirator from a patient beyond all medical help.

This second Nassau Hospital case in which Father Eichner was involved concerned a 17-year-old Chaminade student who collapsed at school last May from a massive aneurysm in the brain. A CAT scan which revealed a huge herniated mass established that there was no possibility of recovery. E.E.G.'s which are confirmatory of clinical diagnosis showed some slight residual electrical activity, activity that the physicians informed the family would never be absent because of the electronic equipment surrounding the patient. Yet on that finding, the physicians refused to remove the respirator. Two days later the boy, whose family had desired to donate his kidneys in the hope of saving some other life, succumbed to uremic poisoning.

A final example of the life-at-any-cost mind-set involves a 23-year old Connecticut woman, Melanie Bacchiochi, who suffered cardio-respiratory arrest while having her wisdom teeth extracted. Resuscitated and rushed to the local hospital, she was placed on a respirator, and after several days of testing she was declared brain dead. Her physician then announced that he would never remove the machine without a court order. Some 43 days later, in response to the trial judge's admonition that the doctor should proceed on the basis of the appropriate medical response to the patient's physical condition, the physician removed the respirator. At that time a militant right-to-life spokesman commented: "Well, we lost that one, but we won't lose on the living will." (In fact, shortly thereafter Senator Rogers' bill, which had passed the Senate 27-9, was defeated by a close vote in the House after what the Hartford *Courant* described as "the offensive scare tactics and irresponsible distortions used by the Connecticut Right-to-Life Corporation.")

These examples and the recent statement of the wife of a Catholic New York City police officer, who was brain dead from a bullet wound to the head (I will "never, never remove the respirator. It is against my religion") convince us that there is a renewed need for the local churches to speak with clarity on the complex and sometimes overwhelming issue of the appropriate care of the dying.

It might be argued that the decisions of a few courts like those of New York, Florida and Delaware do not set national precedents. After all, it is often stated, physicians are making life and death decisions every day without the benefit of legislation. This overlooks two points. First, even though no physician has ever been prosecuted for removing a respirator from one whose death was imminent and unavoidable, still there exists a pervasive fear of liability in the medical world. This fear spawns a reluctance to discontinue treatment even when the patient can derive no possible benefit from it. Thus, commenting on the Bacchiochi case, Dr. Allen Douma, assistant director of health education for the American Medical Association, stated that because there is no law establishing a definition of death in Connecticut, doctors who would disconnect Miss Bacchiochi "would be open for a suit." Robert A. Burt, professor of medical law at Yale University, correctly labeled this "hysertia in the medical profession." Hysteria it may be, but it is there. Its probable sources are the repeated interpretations of what removal of life-sustainers would mean legally. For instance, Carol A. Smith, Assistant Attorney General of the State of Washington, gave this opinion (1977) regarding the law with respect to withdrawing or withholding life support from a dying patient: "Under the present law, an attempt to bring about death by the removal of a life sustaining mechanism would constitute homicide, first degree." As long as such statements from authoritative sources continue to be made, we are in trouble.

Second, we are concerned less with court decisions themselves than we are with the all too widespread vitalist attitudes symbolized and reinforced by these decisions. For instance, a directive in the policy statement of Worcester Hahnemann Hospital states: "No one, patient, family or physician, may consent to, direct or initiate the removal or withdrawal of care or treatment which may be considered in any way to be life sustaining to any patient, except as provided below." The "provision below" was that the patient be dead according to the so-called Harvard Criteria of Death and be declared so by the attending physician. In other words, no withdrawal of any life-sustaining technology unless the patient is dead!

Similarly, a memo from superintendent William E. Jones (Belchertown State School, Mass.) to all physicians and nursing personnel of the hospitals receiving Belchertown patients, reads: "Since it is our moral, legal and ethical duty to provide the highest quality of medical care to our clients, you are reminded that the Administration of this facility holds the preservation of life to be ultimate and expects that all known techniques to prolong the life of the client be utilized unless countermanded by Court decree." We see this as a threat to the best interests and rights of the incompetent and incompatible with what might be called a healthy and balanced Christian perspective toward life and death.

That such vitalist attitudes are broadly shared throughout the ranks of medical personnel is clear from some of the statements made to the President's Commission for the Study of Ethical Problems in Medicine and Biomedical and Behavioral Research (April 9, 1981). For instance, Dr. Marshall Brummer, a pulmonary specialist, at one point was asked: "Is it the duty of the physician to do everything for that patient until that patient is called to his or her reward?" The answer: "Yes." Furthermore, Dr. Brummer stated that he would not regard the permanent maintenance of a person on a respirator as "heroic." We find such attitudes, deplorable as they are, disturbingly widespread. Thus the need for local churches to speak clearly in what is increasingly a medical-legal fog.

A sensitive and balanced example of that form of teaching was the pamphlet on "Death and Dying" issued in 1976 by the Catholic Bishops of Connecticut. Such a convenient and well designed text, updated to cover the Vatican's 1980 Declaration on the sanctity of life and the care to be used in its preservation, and including a sample living will, if widely distributed in the parishes, would do much to dispel mistaken notions on the church's teaching and to protect the rights and values of human life.

There are many versions of living wills. Most that have been recognized in state legislation are quite narrow. They address only situations of imminent death whether or not life-sustaining procedures are used. We believe that in the present atmosphere such legislation should no longer be opposed.

In saying this, we believe two points should be underlined. First, since these "legislated living wills" are drafted to apply only to a very narrow set of circumstances, they can leave the impression that these are the only circumstances in which it is morally appropriate to forego life-sustaining measures. That is not the case, as the Vatican's Declaration on Euthanasia makes very clear. Therefore, in indicating directions to a physician for one's own treatment, a broader set of guidelines would be helpful.

Second, in order to safeguard one's right to refuse treatment, it can be very useful explicitly to authorize an acquaintance or friend to plan, accept or refuse treatment on one's own behalf.

Both of these concerns are provided for in the sample will drawn up by ethician Sissela Bok in *The New England Journal of Medicine* (August 12, 1976). We find this both helpful and fully Christian. It reads as follows:

Directions for My Care

I wish to live a full and long life, but not at all costs. If my death is near and cannot be avoided, and if I have lost the ability to interact with others and have no reasonable chance of regaining this ability, or if my suffering is intense and irreversible, I do not want to have my life prolonged. I would then ask not to be subjected to surgery or resuscitation. Nor would I then wish to have life support from mechanical ventilators, intensive care services, or other life prolonging procedures, including the administration of antibiotics and blood products. I would wish, rather, to have care which gives comfort and support, which facilitates my interaction with others to the extent that this is possible, and which brings peace.

In order to carry out these instructions and to interpret them, I authorize _____ to accept, plan and refuse treatment on my behalf in cooperation with attending physicians and health personnel. This person knows how I value the experience of living, and how I would weigh incompetence, suffering, and dying. Should it be impossible to reach this person, I authorize _____ to make such choices for me. I have discussed my desires concerning terminal care with them, and I trust their judgment on my behalf.

In addition, I have discussed with them the following specific instructions regarding my care:

(Please continue on back)

Date _____ Signed _____

Witnessed by _____ and by _____

Appendix

The Principle of the Double Effect

The "principle of the double effect" is a kind of code name to summarize the distinction between what is said to be directly willed and what is said to be indirectly willed in certain key areas of human life. This distinction has been used to face many practical conflict situations where an evil can be avoided or a more or less necessary good achieved only when another evil is reluctantly caused. In such situations the evil caused as one goes about doing good has been viewed as justified or tolerable under a fourfold condition: (1) The action from which evil results is good or indifferent in itself; it is not morally evil. (2) The intention of the agent is upright—that is, the evil effect is sincerely not intended. (3) The evil effect must be equally immediate causally with the good effect, for otherwise it would be a means to the good effect and would be intended. (4) There must be a proportionately grave reason for allowing the evil to occur. These conditions have been variously stated and qualified over the years,[1] but when all is said and done, if they (or their qualified versions) were fulfilled, the resultant evil was referred to as an "unintended by-product" of the action, only indirectly voluntary, and justified by the presence of a proportionately grave reason.

A classic example is the situation of a woman with a nonviable pregnancy who is diagnosed as having cancer of the uterus. If nothing is done, the cancer will (at least in many cases and in the case here envisaged) spread and bring death to both mother and child. If, however, the cancerous uterus is removed, the woman would be saved but the fetus would obviously perish. Uterine excision was judged permissible under the conditions detailed above.

[1] See, for example, A. Vermeersch, S.J., *Theologiae Moralis, Principia-Responsa-Consilia* (Rome: Gregorian University Press, 1947), I, 105 ff, for some qualifications.

Specifically, the action was seen as good or indifferent (removal of
the uterus); the intention is upright (removing the uterus to save
the mother's life); the good effect is equally immediate causally
with the evil effect (thus, for example, the uterus would be removed whether it were pregnant or not, an indication that the
death of the fetus is not exactly a means in the strict sense to the
attainment of the good); there is a proportionate reason.

This distinction has been used by theologians over the years, especially in three areas of concern: actions involving the sin of another (scandal), actions involving killing, and actions involving
the use of the sexual faculties. Because of the importance of these
areas and the almost limitless variety of human situations in
which they can occur, a huge casuistry concerning the double
effect built up over the centuries.

Furthermore, the so-called double-effect principle has been
taken over and used extensively in official documents of the magisterium, especially in recent decades. For example, in discussing
abortion, Pius XI asked: "What could ever be a sufficient reason
for excusing in any way the direct murder of the innocent (*direc-
tam innocentis necem*)?"[2] Pius XII repeatedly condemned the
"deliberate and *direct* disposing of an innocent human life"[3] and
argued that "neither the life of the mother nor that of the child
can be subjected to an act of *direct* suppression."[4] He also applied
the direct-indirect distinction to sterilizing drugs.[5] The most recent and authoritative use of this distinction is found in *Humanae
vitae*. Paul VI stated: "We must once again declare that the *direct* interruption of the generative process already begun, and
above all, *directly* willed and procured abortion, even if for therapeutic reasons, are to be absolutely excluded as licit means of
regulating birth." He immediately added: "Equally to be excluded, as the teaching authority of the Church has frequently declared, is *direct* sterilization, whether perpetual or temporary,
whether of the man or of the woman."[6]

The use of this distinction has had two general effects. First, it

[2] *Acta Apostolicae Sedis*, 22 (1930), 563. Hereinafter cited as AAS.
[3] AAS, 43 (1951), 838–39.
[4] AAS, 43 (1951), 857.
[5] AAS, 50 (1958), 735–36.
[6] AAS, 60 (1969), 481–518.

has reduced the intolerable consequences of adhering to a simple rule against taking any human life (or, respectively, the fertility of the sexual act). An unqualified rule against taking any human life offers little difficulty most of the time. But unrestricted adherence to it means that we are, for example, helpless in the face of aggressors who do not respect it. Thus over the centuries Catholic tradition restricted the rule to apply to *innocent* life. However, there are still other instances (especially obstetrical) where adherence even to the modified rule would cause greater loss of life. So another refinement was called for. That refinement is the distinction between direct and indirect killing. Thus in certain life-threatening situations it is possible to save the mother even though the fetus is "indirectly killed." The second result of this distinction is that by such a process of restrictive interpretation of the rule against killing, it has been possible not only to save life in some conflict situations, but also to preserve a strong deontologically interpreted rule against killing. The upshot, then, of such restrictive interpretation of the rule against killing has been the combination of a common-sense need to save life when possible, with a strongly felt need to maintain a strict rule against killing. In summary, as Schüller has shown,[7] the present "hard" (deontologically understood) rule against killing ("no *direct* killing of an *innocent* human being") is just as plausible as it has been teleologically modifiable to its present wording.

Historically the terms "direct" and "indirect" referred to the relationship of the will to the evil inextricably associated with the agent's action. Thus certain evil effects were said to be "indirectly *voluntary*" or "directly *voluntary*." As time passed, the terms became attached to certain physical actions that were regarded as necessarily entailing such voluntariety. Thus certain procedures were said to be "direct killings" or "direct sterilizations." In other words, the visible procedure began to define the intentionality, rather than the over-all intentionality defining the procedure. At any rate, once an action was said to be "*direct* scandal," "*direct* killing," "*direct* sterilization," it was regarded as morally wrong. The directness and the indirectness of the evil produced were decisive.

[7] Bruno Schüller, S.J., "Direkte Tötung-indirekte Tötung," *Theologie und Philosophie*, 47 (1972), 341–57.

It is interesting that this distinction, very crucial for so many centuries in Catholic tradition, is so generally unrecognized or ignored outside of this tradition. There are a few prominent moral theologians and philosophers who make use of it (for example, Paul Ramsey, Philippa Foot to a degree, and a few others) but by and large it does not function in most Protestant moral analysis. Any number of reasons are possibly responsible for this. For instance, the common-sense modifications of unqualified rules achieved through use of the double effect was achieved in other ways in non-Catholic traditions. Or again, it could be argued that non-Catholic ethical traditions often concerned themselves less with behavioral norms than with the broad biblical perspectives of the moral life. Whatever the reason, the fact remains that the use of double effect has not been and is not widely used outside the Catholic tradition.

What is the actual moral relevance of the double effect? In the past decade a lively literature has begun to explore this matter.[8] The discussion is still ongoing, and to that extent the question must be said to be unresolved. But a brief report of some of the literature will allow the issues under discussion to emerge.

Much of the contemporary discussion owes its origin to Peter Knauer, S.J.[9] In his seminal study of the question, Knauer began with the insistence that moral evil consists in the permission or causing of a physical evil without commensurate reason. In explaining this, he relied heavily on St. Thomas' analysis of self-defense. The defense of one's life against an assailant is not exactly an effect, but rather an aspect of the act. Therefore, the *finis operis* or meaning of an action is not derived simply from its external effect but is really that aspect of the act that is willed. For example, almsgiving is not simply a physical act; it gets its sense and becomes a moral act through the intention of the donor.

Knauer argues that it is with this in mind that we must understand the terms "direct" and "indirect." In the past we have tied these terms too closely to physicial causality. Actually, the "per-

---

[8] I have reviewed some of this in *Ambiguity in Moral Choice* (Milwaukee, Wis.: Marquette University Press, 1973).

[9] P. Knauer, S.J., "The Hermeneutic Function of the Principle of Double Effect," *Natural Law Forum*, 12 (1967), 132–62. Also in *Nouvelle Revue Theologique*, 87 (1965), 356–75.

mission or causing of a physical evil is direct or indirect as there is or is not present a commensurate reason," for when such a reason is present it "occupies the same areas as what is directly willed and alone determines the entire moral content of the act. If the reason of an action is commensurate, it alone determines the *finis operis*, so that the act is morally good."[10]

What then is a commensurate reason? This is crucial to Knauer's presentation. It is not just any reason, meaningful or important as it may be. Rather a reason is commensurate if the value realizable here and now by measures involving physical evil in a premoral sense is not in the long run undermined and contradicted by these measures but supported and maximized by them.

Applying this to control of birth, Knauer argues that a refusal to bear children is only commensurately grounded if it is ultimately in the interests of the otherwise possible child. But this understanding of things is not limited to control of birth. It involves an entire theory. For example, a lie consists in telling what is false without commensurate reason and therefore directly or formally causes the error of another. Theft is the taking of the property of another without commensurate reason. Mutilation is surgery without a commensurate reason. Murder is killing without commensurate reason. Contraception is intervention into the fertility of the conjugal act without commensurate reason. In all these instances, when there is a commensurate reason, the moral content of the act is not the physical evil but the commensurate reason. The physical (or nonmoral) evil is then indirect.

Knauer was convinced that the terms "direct" and "indirect" got too closely bound with physical and psychological realities and in the process lost their original moral sense. So he set out to redress this imbalance. In doing so he shifted the weight of decision-making to the commensurate reason—and in such a way that it is not clear precisely how the terms "direct" and "indirect" really function, though they are retained. Indeed, Grisez says of Knauer that he is "carrying through a revolution in principle while pretending only a clarification of traditional ideas."[11]

Louis Janssens has arrived at similar conclusions from a slightly

[10] Knauer, "The Hermeneutic Function," 141.
[11] Germain Grisez, *Abortion: The Myths, the Realities, and the Arguments* (Washington, D.C.: Corpus Books, 1970), 331.

different point of view.[12] Janssens first analyzes the Thomistic notion of the human act and points out that Thomas never abandoned the position that the inner act of the will must be considered the starting point. With this as the starting point, Thomas stresses that it is the end of the inner act of the will that determines the concrete structure of the action. *Finis dat speciem in moralibus.*

However, the human act is not simply the intent (*intentio*) of an end or a goal. It also includes the choice (*electio*) of means. But the will of the end and the choice of means constitute only one act of the will, but an act that is a composite act. Since the human act is not restricted to the inner act of the will but also involves an exterior event or act, how is the inner act of the will related structurally to the external act? Janssens notes that for Thomas "the end which is the proper object of the inner act of the will is the formal element; the exterior act, as means to this end, is the material element of the very same human act."

After showing that the end is the formal element that specifies the morality of the action, and that the object-event (external act) is the material element, Janssens argues that Thomas insisted that "not any kind of exterior action, however, can become the material element of a morally good end." It must be adequately proportionate to this end. When it is, it participates in the moral goodness of the end. When is it "adequately proportionate" to the good end? His answer: when there is no contradiction between the material (means) and formal (end) elements of the act. He puts it as follows: "Put into terms of the philosophy of values, this means that the means must be consistent with the value of the end."

Janssens illustrates this by several examples of actions involving what he calls "ontic evil." Not every taking of another's property is theft, but only that which undermines the very value of private property. Not every falsehood is a lie, but only that which corrodes the meaning and purpose of human speech. Thus, when the means involving ontic evil is not proportionate, the ontic evil itself becomes the object of the will and is intended. But this may never be, since it vitiates the action.

[12] L. Janssens, "Ontic Evil and Moral Evil," *Louvain Studies,* 4 (1972), 115–56.

In this understanding, the notions of direct and indirect intention have undergone a notable modification. By "intending" Janssens means the following: "Ontic evil should never be the end of the inner act of the will *if by end is meant that which definitively and in the full sense of the word puts an end to the activity of the subject.*"[13] Or again, it can be right to intend an ontic evil, to make it the end of one's inner act of the will "if that end is not willed as a final end, but only as a *finis medius et proximus* to a higher end."[14] Clearly, then, for Janssens it is the *debita proportio* of the evil to the end that determines whether it is intended or not in the moral sense. Practically this means that the notions of direct and indirect have been all but identified with proportionate reason. In this Janssens and Knauer are in agreement.

Bruno Schüller, after noting the areas where the direct-indirect distinction has been used (scandal, killing, contraception), argues that the distinction was used for a different reason where scandal was involved than where killing and contraception are involved.[15] Once this reason is isolated, it will be clear to what extent the distinction can be abandoned.

The sin of another, according to Schüller, is a moral evil and as such is an unconditioned disvalue. It would seem to follow that an action that has such a disvalue as a foreseen effect must be absolutely avoided. But this would lead to impossible consequences. No lawmaker, for example, could attach a punishment to violation of the law because he would know in advance that this would be the occasion of sinful bribery for a certain undetermined number of people. More fundamentally, it is hard to reconcile an absolute duty to avoid foreseen sin with the will of the Creator who created a being capable of sin. The way out of the dilemma has always been sought in distinguishing will, intention, and purpose from permission and toleration—or direct from indirect. The unconditioned disvalue of sin demands only that one not will and intend it under any circumstances. However, for a proportionate reason it may be permitted.[16]

13 Ibid., 141 (emphasis added).
14 Ibid., 141.
15 Schüller, "Direkte Tötung," 341–57.
16 Schüller would argue that "permitting" (not preventing when one could) the sin of another is applicable to God alone and remains mysterious, and hence that "permitting" nonmoral evils is the area of major concern.

Schüller admits that there is something mysterious here but insists on the distinction where active scandal is concerned. But the reason the distinction is necessary is that we are dealing here with moral evil. The unconditioned character of the evil forces some such distinction. However, where we are dealing with nonmoral evils (error, pain, sickness, death, etc.), the reason for the distinction disappears precisely because these disvalues, fundamental as they are, are conditioned (or relative) disvalues. Concretely, sickness must be avoided, but not at any price—not, for example, at the price of plunging one's family into destitution. Schüller argues that when we justifiably cause a relative disvalue in our activity, we should not call it "indirect." Use of this traditional term flies in the face of the meaning of words. For instance, when one administers physical punishment to a refractory child from purely pedagogical motives, should we call the punishment and pain "indirect"? Hardly. Rather it has the character of a means, and we speak of an intending will, a direct choice where means are concerned. We should not abandon this usage. Indeed, it brings out clearly the difference between the attitude to moral evil and that to nonmoral evil. For a proportionate reason we may *permit* a moral evil, but we may directly will and directly cause a nonmoral evil if there is a proportionate reason for doing so.

Traditional theology, he argues, felt it necessary to use "direct" and "indirect" with regard to killing the innocent and contraception because it viewed these actions as "evil in se." It regarded them as evil in se because of certain considerations independent of consequences (lack of right for killing the innocent, unnaturalness for contraception). Once one judges that sterilization is not always "contrary to nature," there is no reason for the designation. Similarly, the intrinsic evil of killing the innocent can be sustained only if the death of a person is an unconditioned evil in the sense of a moral evil. Once it is granted that the killing of an innocent person is the destruction of a fundamental but nonmoral value, there is no need for the distinction direct/indirect. Rather, the assessment is made teleologically.

The thrust of these studies, therefore, is that directness/indirectness of action or intent—at least as traditionally understood

—is not as morally decisive as was thought.[17] The truly key element is proportionate reason. Indeed, the logic of these analyses would suggest that it is the notion of proportionate reason that gives rise to the terms "direct" and "indirect." Thus, it is argued, it is clear to what extent the terms may be abandoned as morally decisive. There is never any reason for intending the sin of another in order to realize a more urgent or "higher" value, because there is no more urgent or "higher" value. No good is greater for man than his moral good. Or negatively, sin is an unconditioned disvalue for man in light of which all other disvalues (for example, sickness, poverty, death) are relative or conditioned. Hence we may never choose and intend it as we may choose and intend other disvalues.

The most formidable opponents of these analytic developments are philosopher Germain Grisez and theologian Paul Ramsey.[18] Grisez's defense of the direct/indirect distinction (and therefore of the so-called double effect) interlocks logically with his over-all moral theory. This moral theory is developed somewhat as follows. The basic human goods (life, knowledge pursued for its own sake, interior integrity, justice, friendship, etc.) present themselves as goods to be realized. They appeal to us for their realization. Thus these goods are the nonhypothetical principles of practical

[17] Others in this school of thought, with modifications of their own, would be J. Fuchs, S.J., "The Absoluteness of Moral Terms," *Gregorianum*, 52 (1971), 415–58, and "Sittliche Normen—Universalien und Generalisierungen," *Münchener Theologische Zeitschrift*, 25 (1974), 18–33; less explicitly but clearly F. Böckle in "Recht auf menschwürdiges Sterben," *Evangelische Kommentare*, 8 (1975), 71–74, and others covered in *Ambiguity in Moral Choice* (C. van der Poel, W. van der Marck, et al.). Others also sharing some of these tendencies would include Helmut Weber, "Der Kompromiss in der Moral," *Trier Theologische Zeitschrift*, 86 (1977), 99–118; Franz Scholz, "Objekt und Umstände, Wesenswirkungen und Nebeneffekte," in Klaus Demmer and Bruno Schüller (eds.), *Christlich Glauben und Handeln* (Düsseldorf: Patmus, 1977), 243–60; Albert R. DiIanni, S.M., "The Direct/Indirect Distinction in Morals," *Thomist*, 41 (1977), 350–80; L. Cornerotte, C.S.C.M., "Loi morals, valeurs humaines et situations de conflit," *Nouvelle Revue Theologique*, 100 (1978), 502–32; Enrico Chiavacci, "La fondazione della norma morale nella riflessione teologica contemporanea," *Revista di teologia morale*, 37 (1978), 9–38.

[18] For Grisez, see footnote 11. Paul Ramsey, W. Frankena, B. Brody, and B. Schüller have written responses to my *Ambiguity in Moral Choice*. They can be found in *Doing Evil to Achieve Good* (Chicago: Loyola University Press, 1978).

reason. "As expressions of what is-to-be, the practical principles present basic human needs as fundamental goods, as ideals." But the appeal of these goods is not the direct determinant of moral obligation. They clarify the possibilities of choice but do not determine why some choices are morally good and others evil.

What determines this? The attitude with which we choose. What, then, is a right attitude? A realistic one. "To choose a particular good with an appreciation of its genuine but limited possibility and its objectively human character is to choose it with an attitude of realism." The right attitude does not seek to belittle the good that is not chosen, but only seeks to realize what is chosen. This open, realistic attitude shapes itself into specific moral obligations. For instance, we must take all the goods into account in our deliberations; we must avoid ways of acting that inhibit the realization of any one of the goods to the extent possible; we must contribute our effort to their realization in others. A final and most important mode of obligation is this: We must never act "in a way directly destructive of a realization of any of the basic goods," for to act *directly* against a good is to subordinate it to whatever leads to that choice. And one may not morally do that, because the basic goods are equally basic.

But clearly not every inhibition of a good that occurs as a result of my action is directly destructive of this good. Some inhibitions are unsought and unavoidable side effects of an effort to pursue another value. Thus one directly goes against a basic good when its inhibition is directly intended.

When is the destruction of a basic good directly intended? Here Grisez modifies the textbook understanding of the double effect. He believes that the modern formulation is too restrictive. It insists too much on the behavioral aspect, the temporal, physical causality, in determining the meaning of the act. In the textbook tradition, if evil is the sole immediate effect of the physical act, then it is directly produced and hence directly intended. For example, one may not "shell out" an ectopic fetus that represents a mortal threat to the mother, though he may excise a pathological tube that contains a fetus. Similarly, one may not abort the fetus to save the mother.

Grisez rejects this understanding. Rather he insists that "from the point of view of human moral activity, the initiation of an indivisible process through one's own causality renders all that is involved in that process equally immediate. . . . For on the hypothesis that no other human act intervenes or could intervene, the moral agent who posits a natural cause *simultaneously* (morally speaking) posits its foreseen effects."[19]

For instance, the saving of the mother is an aspect of the abortifacient act equally immediate, morally speaking, to the death of the child. Thus Grisez writes: "The justification is simply that the very same act, indivisible as to its behavioral process, has both the good effect of protecting human life and the bad effect of destroying it . . . the entire process is indivisible by human choice and hence all aspects of it are equally present to the agent at the moment he makes his choice."[20]

Central in Grisez's analysis is the indivisibility of the action or behavioral process. It is this indivisibility that allows one to conclude to the equal immediacy of the good and the bad effects—and therefore to the direct intent of the good and the indirect intent of the evil. If, however, the process is divisible and the good effect occurs as a result of a subsequent human act, we are dealing with means to end, or with effects not equally immediate. Thus one may not commit adultery to save one's children from a prison camp "because the saving effect would not be present in the adulterous act, but in a subsequent human act—that of the person who releases them." Grisez's defense of the double effect is by far the most subtle, powerful, and consistent in contemporary literature.

Paul Ramsey has much the same notion of "directly turning against a basic good."[21] However, he has a far less systematic understanding of what the basic goods really are and he disagrees sharply with Grisez about the criterion of indivisibility. To make his point about the indivisibility criterion, Ramsey proposes several cases of birthroom conflict. One is the case of a pregnant woman with a misplaced, acute appendicitis who will die from its rupture unless a surgeon goes straight through the uterus (that is, kills the baby first, then saves her life). Another such instance is

[19] Grisez, *Abortion*, 333.
[20] Ibid., 340.
[21] Paul Ramsey, "Abortion: A Review Article," *Thomist*, 37 (1973), 174–226.

that of aneurysm of the aorta in which the wall of the aorta is so weakened that it balloons out behind the pregnant uterus. In order to deal with the aneurysm, the surgeon must first kill the fetus. On Grisez's terms, he could not allow such procedures, for the evil effect is separable, by human action, from the good effect. Ramsey rejects this and sets out to show why in his terms even such a killing is indirect. (It is aimed at *incapacitating* the fetus from doing what it is doing to the mother.) In summary, then, while these authors disagree as to what actions must count as "turning directly against the good of life," they agree that it is never permissible to turn against this basic value directly or against any value that is truly basic. Thus any killing that is permissible must be indirect.

Their oft-repeated argument for saying this, and for resisting analyses such as those of Knauer-Janssens-Schüller, is that the basic goods are incommensurable. Those who shift the major emphasis in cases of conflict to proportionate reason are measuring the incommensurable. If one attempts to do that, he is unavoidably involved in a form of consequentialism that determines the moral rightness and wrongness of an action according to greatest "net good"—not only an incoherent notion, as the long philosophical discussion of utilitarianism has shown, but also one that is at odds with some basic Christian convictions. In other words, one does not suppress one basic good for the sake of another, for that would be to subordinate a basic good to another one *equally* basic. The only way to cut the Gordian knot when basic values are conflicted is only to indirectly allow the defeat of one as the other is pursued. As Ramsey words it: "My own view is that the distinction between direct and indirect voluntariety is pertinent and alerts our attention as moral agents to those moral choices where incommensurable conflicting values are at stake, where there is no measurable resolution of value conflicts on a single scale, where there are gaps in any supposed hierarchy of values, and therefore no way to determine exactly the greater or lesser good or evil. . . . Where there is no single scale or common denominator, or where there is discontinuity in the hierarchy of goods or evils, one ought not turn against any human good."[22]

[22] Paul Ramsey and Richard McCormick, *Doing Evil to Achieve Good* (Chicago: Loyola University Press, 1978), 70–71.

Those who put the major emphasis on proportionality in situations of conflicted goods might respond in any number of ways. For instance, negatively, they might urge that if proportionate reason involves measuring the unmeasurable, then what is the meaning and function of proportionate reason in the standard understandings of the double effect? They might ask why an "indirect killing" does not involve one in turning against a basic good. In other words, they would press the matter of the *moral* (not merely descriptive) relevance of directness as this was understood traditionally.

A concrete vehicle for bringing these questions into clearer focus is the classic even if rare obstetrical case where the physician faces two options: Either he aborts the fetus and thus saves the mother, or he does not abort, and both mother and child die. Both those who defend the moral relevance of the direct/indirect distinction in such instances (for example, Ramsey and Grisez) and those who question it (Schüller, Knauer, and, among others, the present writer) agree on the conclusion. That is not at issue. What is at issue is the reason for the conclusion. The defenders of the traditional distinction would argue that the conclusion is correct insofar as and only insofar as the death of the fetus can be said to be indirect. The revisionists, so to speak, would argue that the real reason for the conclusion is that *in such circumstances* the abortion is proportionately grounded, is the lesser evil. When one is faced with two options, both of which involve unavoidable (nonmoral) evil, one ought to choose the lesser evil. To argue that the intervention is morally right because it is "indirect" is, in this view, to use a notion that is adventitious, unnecessary, and ultimately indecisive.

The common response to such argument is that if this is true, then what is known in philosophical circles as "the Caiphas principle" is valid—that is, one is justified in sacrificing one innocent person to save five. The example often used is that of a sheriff in a southern town in the United States faced with the alternatives in a rape case of framing a black suspect (whom he knows to be innocent) or carrying on a prolonged search for the real culprit. The immediate indictment and conviction of the suspect would save many lives and prevent other harmful consequences. If an action's moral rightness is determined solely by consequences (one innocent killed v. many innocent killed), then it seems that the sheriff ought to frame the one innocent man—a conclusion that shocks our moral sensitivities, but one that a revisionist on the double effect would seem to be forced to draw.

At this point, the revisionist would return to the insistence on the words *in such circumstances* in the abortion dilemma given above. In the abortion dilemma, the situation is not *simply* a save-one-v.-lose-two dilemma. It is not simply quantitative. It must be added that the deadly deed is intrinsically and inescapably connected with the saving of the mother's life, whether that deadly deed be a craniotomy or the removal of the fetus to get at a life-threatening aneurysm[23]—that is to say, there is in the very nature of the case no other way of saving the mother. There is an essential link between the means and the end. By contrast, however, such a link does not exist in the instance of the sheriff. There is no inherent connection between the killing of an innocent person and the change of mind of a lynch mob. For those who hold to the notion of free will in the doing of evil (and good), there is never an inherent connection between killing an innocent person and changing the murderous mind of a lynch mob. In other words, in the abortion case, one chooses to save the life that can be saved because in such circumstances that is the lesser evil, is proportionately grounded. In other circumstances, it would not be the lesser evil, would not be proportionate.

That might bring the revisionist to a further and more positive contention: Seeing proportionate reason as the crucial element in situations of conflict need not at all involve one in measuring the immeasurable.[24] There are times, of course, when genuine measuring in the strict sense is appropriate—for instance, when merely instrumental goods conflict with basic goods. One sacrifices the instrumental for the basic, because instrumental goods are lesser in the order of goods. Thus one prefers life to property. This is a strict *Güterabwägung*.[25]

But such is clearly not possible where basic goods are con-

---

[23] I owe these reflections to Jerome Wiseman, O.S.B.
[24] I say "might" because I do not know what form individual responses would take.
[25] See B. Schüller, S.J., "Neuere Beiträge zum Thema 'Begründung Sittlicher Normen,'" *Theologische Berichte*, 4 (Einsiedeln: Benziger, 1974), 109–81.

cerned. But neither is it necessary. While the basic goods are not commensurable (one *against* the other), they are clearly associated goods. Thus one who unjustifiably takes human life also undermines other human goods, and these human goods, once weakened or undermined, will affect the very good of life itself. Let marriage and birth control be another example. Two distinct but closely associated goods are involved: the procreative good, the communicative good. The manner of protecting the procreative good may undermine it in the long run by harm to an associated good, the communicative good. Practically, this could mean that the possible ineffectiveness, and forced and perhaps prolonged periods of abstention can easily harm the communicative good and *thereby* the procreative good itself. The Second Vatican Council said something very similar when it stated that "where the intimacy of married life is broken off, it is not rare for its faithfulness to be imperiled and its quality of fruitfulness ruined."[26] That seems to be a reasonable account of things. It is precisely concern for the procreative good, but as related to and supported by the communicative good that could lead to the conclusion that interference with fertility is morally right when necessary. In summary, one does not commensurate the incommensurable in using proportionate reason; one associates the associable.

Something very similar could be said of the case of the southern sheriff noted above, and by extension, I believe, of the immorality of obliteration (counterpeople v. counterforce) bombing. The manner of protecting the good (human life—by framing one innocent person) will undermine it in the long run by serious injury to an associated good (human liberty), for by killing an innocent person to prevent others from unjustly killing five innocent persons, one equivalently denies the freedom of these others. That is the very moral meaning of extortion. One supposes by his action that the cessation of others from wrongdoing is necessarily dependent on my doing harm or nonmoral evil. Such a supposition denies and therefore undermines human freedom. And because such free-

[26] Vatican Council II, "Pastoral Constitution on the Church in the Modern World (*Gaudium et spes*)," translated from the Latin and reprinted in Walter M. Abbot, S.J. (ed.), *The Documents of Vatican II* (New York: Herder and Herder/Association Press, 1966), 199–308.

dom is an associated good upon which the very good of life itself depends, undermining it in the manner of my defense of life is undermining life itself—is disproportionate. Here, again, one does not exactly weigh life *against* freedom; one merely associates the associable and reads proportion within such an interrelationship. That is why Schüller seems absolutely correct in insisting that in this and similar cases it is not simply a matter of the life of one v. the life of many others; the entire institution of criminal law is at stake. And that is how proportion must be read.

Ultimately, then, revisionists admit a descriptive difference between actions involving nonmoral evil directly and those involving nonmoral evil indirectly—that is, directness or indirectness of an effect tells us what is being sought and by what means and in what circumstances. These in combination reveal the significance of the action. Whether the action is, as a whole, morally right or morally wrong depends on this significance, for significance reveals what other values are at stake, and therefore whether the manner of the pursuit of the good here and now is destructive of it or not. In other words, it reveals whether in the action as a whole the good outweighs the evil, whether there is a truly proportionate reason or not. And it is the presence or the absence of such a reason that determines whether the attitude of the agent is adequate or not, whether he is choosing rightly or wrongly, whether he remains open to the basic goods or closes off one of them in pursuit of another—whether or not he chooses against a basic good.

This has led some recent commentators to conclude that where nonmoral evils are concerned, the essential line of demarcation to be drawn (as distinguishing right and wrong attitudes of mind and will, and therefore right action as expressive of these attitudes) is not between intending and permitting, as tradition understood these terms, but between intending as an end on the one hand, and intending as a means and permitting on the other.

This chapter represents a brief—and therefore almost necessarily misleading—summary of the way the discussion is being conducted. Because the discussion is ongoing, it is difficult and even inappropriate to draw hard-and-fast conclusions. Furthermore, because the present writer is associated with one tendency (the revisionist) rather than the other, it is even onerous to be fair. But the discussion will continue—as it should—and these inequalities will be balanced out. It is sufficient to note here that in the rather technical doctrine of the double effect—to some curious, to others insignificant—much is at stake: the understanding of moral norms, the solution of some anguishing and delicate moral dilemmas, the interpretation and/or reformulation of magisterial statements, and, finally, the very will of God as man must attempt to discover it in a world of suffering, error, and conflict. For those interested in pursuing this very difficult discussion, further considerations may be found in *Doing Evil to Achieve Good: Morality in Conflict Situations*.[27]

[27] See footnote 18.

INDEX

Index

352–61 (see also Morality; specific aspects, problems); moral right to privacy and, 362–71; physician's automony and, 28 ff.; and preservation of life, 340–51, 352–61, 362–71, 372–80, 381–89, 393–411, 423–30; teaching of medical ethics and, 20

Heenan, John Cardinal, 213 n, 215 n

Hellegers, André E., 33, 120, 149 n, 282 n, 339, 379 n, 384 n

Helsinki, Declaration of (1964), 53–54, 55, 65, 76

Heylen, Victor L., 211 n

Hirschhorn, Kurt, 308 n, 310

Hirschmann, Johannes B., 210–11

Holistic, moral responsibility for health care as, 46–47

Hospitals (health facilities, hospitalization), 36–37 (see also Doctors; Medicine; specific aspects, issues, problems); bioethics and (see Bioethics); living-will legislation and, 412–22; moral responsibility for health care and, 36, 37, 352–61 (see also Health care); moral right to privacy and, 362–71; preservation of life and, 339–51, 362–71, 372–80, 412–22, 423–30; sterilization and, 260–68, 269–78

Houle, Mr. and Mrs. Robert H. T., 339

Howieson, John, 57

Humanae vitae, 209–37, 238–59, 261, 271; tenth anniversary of, 238–39

Human Guinea Pigs, 20, 292

Humani generis, 253

Human relationships. See Relationships, human

Hydrocephalus, 22, 23, 45

Hypothetical test, rights of the voiceless in medical experimentation and, 99–113

"Ideological structures," moral responsibility for health care and, 35–36

Inclinations (tendencies), basic, values and development of moral codes and, 5–8

Individualization (humanization), abortion and issue of, 139–49 passim, 165–68. See also Personhood; Sociality

Individual rights (see also Autonomy; Freedom; Liberty; Self-determination; specific issues, problems): and abortion, 131–32, 133–34, 136, 138–39, 142 ff., 157–59, 166–67, 171; genetic medicine and, 298, 299, 300; living-will legislation and, 412–22, 423–30; medical experimentation and, 93–95 (see also Consent; Decision-making); moral right to privacy and, 362–71

Infants. See Babies

"Informed Consent" (O'Donnell), 58 n, 75 n

Ingelfinger, Franz J., 53 n, 56–57, 65, 76, 342

Insemination, artificial. See Artificial insemination

International Theological Commission, 254

Interventionist mentality, abortion and, 203–4

"Invincible ignorance" notion, 152

In vitro fertilization, 21, 24, 25–26, 40, 195, 281, 283–305, 321–33; ethics of, 321–33

Irish bishops, 242 n

Issue areas concept, teaching of medical ethics and, 18–31

Jakobovits, Immanuel, 314, 317

Janssens, Louis, 242, 246, 248 n, 265, 435–37, 442

Jefferson, Mildred, 363

Jehovah's Witnesses, 369, 373

Jesus Christ, 9–10, 12, 15, 138, 387

John, St., 346; Prologue of gospel of, 289, 290

Johns Hopkins case, 340–44, 351, 408

John XXIII, Pope, 183, 229 n

Jones, William E., 428

Jonsen, Albert R., 402–3, 405, 411

Journal of the American Medical Association, 71, 91, 354 n, 418 n

Jousten, A., 126–27

Judaeo-Christian teaching and tradition, 3–17, 18–31 (see also specific aspects, concepts, individuals, issues, problems); and abortion (see Abortion); and bioethical codes, 3–17 (see also Bioethics); moral responsibility for health care and, 38, 40, 42; living wills and, 416–22; and preservation of life, 345–47, 351, 416–22; and sexuality and the family, 25; and teaching of medical ethics, 18–31

Kant, Immanuel, 94, 263

Kass, Leon R., 11 n, 281 n, 286, 293–98, 302, 303, 304, 311, 323 n, 325 n, 329, 331

Kautzky, R., 401, 405

Keene, Barry, 412

Kelly, Gerald, 347

Kidney transplants, 96

Knauer, Peter, 163, 434–35, 437, 442, 443

Knox, Richard A., 375–76

Komonchak, Joseph A., 248–49

Krol, John Cardinal, 118

Kurland, Philip B., 173 n

Lader, Lawrence, 117

Lancet (journal), 357

Lappé, Marc, 324 n

Laughlin, Dr. James, 352

LaVerdiere, Eugene A., 251–52

Law (legislation), 362–71 (see also Courts; Government; Public policy; specific aspects, cases, courts, issues, legislation); living wills and, 412–22, 423–30; moral right to privacy and, 362–71; and preservation of life, 362–71, 372–80, 381–89, 412–22, 423–30

Lederberg, Joshua, 282 n, 311

Lercher, L., 250

Liberals (liberalism, permissiveness), 124 (see also specific groups, individuals, issues); abortion and, 124, 135 ff., 139, 142 ff., 174–75, 181, 205; and birth control, 258 n

Index

Index

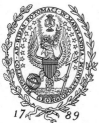

GEORGETOWN UNIVERSITY PRESS
STUDIES IN ETHICS Series

HUMAN RIGHTS IN THE AMERICAS:
THE STRUGGLE FOR CONSENSUS
Alfred T. Hennelly, S.J., and John Langan, S.J., editors
Hardcover and paperback

HUMAN RIGHTS AND BASIC NEEDS IN THE AMERICAS
Margaret E. Crahan, editor
Hardcover and paperback

PERSONAL RESPONSIBILITY AND CHRISTIAN MORALITY
Josef Fuchs, S.J.
Paperback

PERSPECTIVES ON POLITICAL ETHICS: AN ECUMENICAL INQUIRY
Koson Srisang, editor
Paperback

THE MORAL DIMENSIONS OF INTERNATIONAL CONDUCT
The Jesuit Community Lectures: 1982
James A. Devereux, S.J., editor
Paperback

FUNDAMENTALS OF ETHICS
John Finnis
Hardcover and paperback

CHRISTIAN ETHICS IN A SECULAR ARENA
Josef Fuchs, S.J.
Paperback

THE CATHOLIC BISHOPS AND NUCLEAR WAR
Judith A. Dwyer, S.S.J., editor
Paperback

AUTHORITY IN MORALS:
AN ESSAY IN CHRISTIAN ETHICS
Gerard J. Hughes, S.J.
Paperback